I respectfully dedicate this book to the spirit of the late Professor SHŌMA MORITA. *At the same time, I wish to express my deepest appreciation to my own mentor, Professor Emeritus* TAKEHISA KŌRA *of the Jikei University School of Medicine, and to the many other people who have helped me along the way.*

Contents

Introduction

What Is Morita Therapy?

This book is intended to offer a detailed explanation of the therapeutic concepts and system of treatment originated by Shōma (Masatake) Morita (1874–1938).

The author will first examine Morita's therapeutic principles, based on Morita's writings, chiefly *Shinkeishitsu no Hontai oyobi Ryōhō* (The Substance of *Shinkeishitsu* and Its Therapy), formally published in 1928.

To place Morita's work in historical perspective, it is essential that the author first discuss the prevailing cultural, and specifically the psychiatric, milieu in which Morita worked out his theory of psychopathology and his therapeutic principles for the management of *shinkeishitsu* (a type of chronic neurasthenia or constitutional nervosity) at a time when concepts of that kind were still vague.

The author will then attempt to explain the problems that Morita's therapeutic principles and techniques have posed during the period of great transformation in Japanese psychiatry, from his lifetime to the present.

The author sincerely hopes that a large number of therapists will take an interest in Morita therapy, which was developed in the distinctive cultural climate of Japan. To stimulate such interest, the author needs to negotiate his way through a number of obstacles posed by the linguistic and cultural peculiarities of Japan.

If the common goal of all psychotherapies is to expose a patient's erroneous mental set, instill awareness of his or her authentic self and direct the patient toward the life-style that he or she truly desires, Morita therapy, in principle and practice, is no exception.

Most psychotherapies are derived from Occidental concepts, centered around psychoanalysis. Morita therapy also incorporates Oriental concepts. The author believes there is a universal need to utilize Occidental as well as Oriental concepts to achieve the most effective therapeutic results.

Contemporary social patterns, in particular the incessant pursuit of new industrial technologies, have produced a modern age of alienation of the individual in combination with a rational materialization of human values. The contemporary conflict of isolation of the individual in opposition to material prosperity may continue to intensify. No small number of people, in Japan and elsewhere, suffer from a sense of being powerless, out of control, lacking a firm, clear-cut sense of self-identity.

In the author's opinion, Morita therapy is effective not only for resolution of conflicts within a person but also for resolution of conflicts between that person and society. The objective of Morita therapy is to stimulate self-awareness, self-discovery and an authentic perception of the substance of human nature.

Wellsprings of Morita Therapy

Our concern with nature, or the state of being natural, has reached a new peak of awareness in contemporary culture. We must ask why.

To seek the answer, we must examine our current cultural conditions. The material benefits that we have reaped from scientific and technological innovation have given us—at least those of us living in the developed nations—a rationalistic and relatively prosperous life-style. However, once we become accustomed to material comforts, we begin to experience a new sensitivity to a number of internal and external contradictions and conflicts. The contradictions and conflicts arise from the estrangement of modern man from nature, which is symptomatic of an irredeemable alienation that occurred long before we became aware of it. The contradictions and conflicts, moreover, have brought about a situation in which we live in opposition to nature, a condition that is detrimental to ourselves as well as our natural environment.

In Japan, it was traditionally assumed that man lives in essential harmony with his fellow men and their natural matrix. With the swift Occidentalization of Japan, however, nature has become an isolated object rather than the basic matrix of human existence.

At the cost of acquiring the many benefits of a high-technology society, the Japanese have had to abandon that original spirit of harmonious integration with nature.

This dislocation has produced conflicts and brought about a so-called age of anxiety characterized by nervousness, distrust or even indifference toward the social system and the selves of the Japanese. Japan is a battleground of clashes between traditional values and the demands of new technological values.

The modern process of prying men loose from their natural moorings and setting them against nature is similar to the tragic fate of the Emperor Konton in the fable related by Sōshi (Chuang-tzu).[1]

The people of Japan were not aware, for a long time, that technological progress is not a spontaneous (i.e., natural) cultural phenomenon, believing, instead, that it is the result of a foreign (Occidental) mechanization brought into the country from overseas. Only recently has the realization of what the Japanese had to abandon begun to emerge. The traditional creative spirit has receded into the backwaters of the social order. Other conventional values, such as intense respect for human life and labor, or the spirit of mutual service to one another, have been substantially eroded.

The Japanese may be able to see and acknowledge the objective advantages and disadvantages of a modern technological society. However, the people of Japan must also be attuned to the subjective impact, both positive and negative, of this new culture as it is expressed in contemporary Japanese behavior.

Self-awareness and self-scrutiny may be said to arise from an awareness of conflict, either external or internal, or a combination of the two types of conflict. In particular, the contemporary urge to "return to nature" may be attributed to the acute awareness of having been, in some meaningful way, set in opposition to nature, including the authentic human nature of the Japanese.

To live in accordance with authentic human nature is, perhaps, the central psychological concern of the people of Japan. The Japanese have created a sense of self-estrangement by choosing to isolate and evaluate certain aspects of their selves as being abnormal (i.e., unnatural). The Japanese need to see themselves as "whole units" to discover their authentic human nature. However, to do so, the Japanese need to have a process, a series of steps leading to self-awareness and self-acceptance.

This process is intended to restore, to open up, the natural appetite for self-actualization of the Japanese. Not only rational thought, but intuition, imagination and spontaneity need to be exercised.

This was the vision that created Shōma Morita's view of human nature and authentic mental health. Work therapy–coming into direct contact with nature by working with one's hands–became a major element of Morita therapy. In his perception, too much dependence on rationality and too little use of the therapeutic benefits of manual labor contributed to the persistence of mental illness.

[1] Konton can be defined as the condition in which "all" is apprehended as being "one," with no awareness of distinctions or differences. In his fable, the Chinese philosopher Sōshi, who predates the third century, relates that the Emperor Konton once invited the emperors of the North and South Seas to a feast. In return, the two imperial guests decided to confer on Konton the gift of the seven sensory orifices (eyes, ears, nostrils, mouth) that human beings have but Konton lacked. This gift would give him a sensory perception of the world as being distinct from himself. For seven days, they poked holes in Konton's body to create those orifices. However, by the time they had finished, Konton had died.

Morita's lifework was focused on the need to discover and define a therapeutic system that would bring the embattled modern mentality back into a condition of authentic mental health.

Beginnings of Morita Therapy

The rise of science in Europe produced a conflict between the new scientific mode of thought and the strict, religion-based mode of thought of the Middle Ages. The latter was eventually superseded by an epistemology that emphasized the rational application of the intellect. This scientific epistemology has continued to amplify its influence to the present.

The new psychological world of the "scientific intellect" rested on the supports of a dichotomy, namely, the Descartian principle of cognition in which there is a strict division between subject and object, between internal experience and the external world. As a result, men were led into conflict with nature and, further, began to view the human mind as an isolated object. This principle of dualism, which dominates modern civilization, has had a profound effect on human thought, particularly in the form of psychoanalysis, with its subject-object techniques for clarification of mental illness.

The concealed dimension of the human mind was gradually revealed to the intellect in the form of abnormalities. Psychoanalysis came into existence as a technique for revealing deeply concealed mental mechanisms, the underlying causes of mental distress and suffering, and for using that knowledge to induce a condition of mental health.

The Western (scientific) intellect perceived the topographical dissection of nonconscious human mentality as a powerful means for achieving an understanding of authentic human nature and for solidifying one's self in a condition of normality.

Psychoanalysis does have indubitable utility. However, it is still doubtful whether psychoanalysis alone, with its insistence on treating human mentality in dry, abstract terms of "let it be this or that" or "it must be this or that," can lead to a full, comprehensive understanding of authentic human nature.

There is another therapeutic approach, based on stimulation of intuition, in which patients are naturally awakened to a recognition of their authentic human nature. The principle of this approach is having patients discard all discretionary mental artifices and learn to behave in harmony with their authentic human nature. The principles of this approach form the "root" of Morita therapy, one that is grounded in the Oriental perspective of a monistic, nondichotomizing mode of thought.

Role of Morita Therapy and Its Contemporary Relevance

After numerous clinical experiences with the mental condition called chronic neurasthenia, or constitutional nervosity (the concept of which was vague), Shōma Morita defined and developed a new theory of psychopathology (theory of the hypochondriacal basic tone and pathogenesis of *shinkeishitsu*). He also consolidated the factors that are common to this mental condition under the new term *shinkeishitsu.* Under this general term, he classified *shinkeishitsu* into three types: ordinary *shinkeishitsu*, paroxysmal neurosis and obsession.

Morita worked out a therapeutic system based on this theory. This system was called his special, or natural, therapy for *shinkeishitsu.* This treatment modality was so completely his original creation that the system became popularly known as Morita therapy and was already fully developed when it was described in published form. Morita, at the time, was 46 years-old. Morita therapy, as a rule, requires absolute, isolated bed rest, work therapy and social life training on admission.

In simplified form, a number of modifications, such as outpatient treatment techniques, correspondence by means of a diary submitted to a therapist for his or her comments and group discussion formats, were later incorporated into the system.

Psychotherapy, to Morita, was a general term for a variety of techniques whose objective is psychosomatic efficacy, in other words, psychological approaches that are capable of producing therapeutic results. In his thinking, a therapist functions in accordance with his or her therapeutic philosophy and psychiatric principles. Morita therapy was firmly rooted in Morita's philosophical venue. In other words, his therapeutic principles and techniques were derived from his view of human nature, his system of therapy being a scientific product of his philosophy of life.

Morita's mode of thought is clearly and deeply rooted in Japan's distinctive environment and traditional culture (see Part I).

By his own admission, Morita went through a long trial and error period lasting about 20 years to perfect his system of therapy. For that reason, no heavy revision of the principles that form the foundations of his system was deemed necessary during or after his lifetime. Moreover, his system is gaining increased credence and acceptance among contemporary psychiatrists. As Takehisa Kōra, a leading Morita therapist, points out, Morita's therapeutic principles are easy to understand, his therapy is easy to put into practice and the therapeutic effect is considerable.[2] The author agrees with Kōra's evaluation, adding only that Morita's therapeutic principles are solidly based on fact.[3]

Morita therapy was developed on the basis of long-term clinical experience; this subject is discussed in detail in Part III. The author would like to note here, however, that Morita's concept of the hypochondriacal basic tone, his emphasis on *sei no yokubō* ("the desire to live") and his therapeutic objective of inducing an acceptance of *arugamama* ("things as they are") in his patients all stem from his keen clinical observation of human nature and his accurate descriptions of human behavior as a direct result.

Morita therapy, as has been mentioned, was Morita's original creation, and it is unlike other theories of neurosis and psychotherapy in the sense of how the system was developed.

In general, Morita therapy is directed to the management of *shinkeishitsu.* For this reason, it can be considered to be narrow in scope because *shinkeishitsu* is only one type of neurosis. Morita's system, however, has much wider application, being based on an accurate perception of human nature. It is effective, for example, in the management of errors of consciousness that make it difficult to adapt effectively to the environment. Patients who experience such a lack of adaptation frequently resort to ignoring or negating their authentic human nature. This psychological inclination takes precedence over any effort to resolve the problem. Such a patient is captured or enmeshed in his or her network of errors. For example, a patient suffering from a chronic physical disorder, such as diabetes or hypertension, may become so obsessed by the concept of self-preservation that the result is hypochondria. If interpersonal relationships are the major problem, the patient may try to evade reality and thus intensify feelings of inferiority. Because the patient cannot flee from his or her conviction of inferiority, he or she may lose the spontaneous will to be involved in meaningful social activities.

In addition, weighted down by the burden of the activities required in daily living, the pat-

[2] Kōra, T.: Morita ryōhō no konnichiteki igi (A today's significance of Morita therapy) (in Japanese). *Modern Medicine* 6:79–83 (1974).

[3] Human nature, as understood by Morita, consists not only of feelings and drives, including as well a desire for self-improvement or self-actualization rooted in an inherent love for moral and social order (see Part I).

ient can suffer from a fixation on "the meaning of human life," "is life worth living?" or "how to behave" and end up enmeshed in a mental condition of self-estrangement.

There are numerous instances in which Morita therapy is effective in resolving such problems. Morita therapy is effective in such instances because its objective is not to have the patient think in intellectual terms to clarify or deal with the problem but, rather, to have the patient understand that suffering is, in fact, suffering and that suffering is an integral component of human nature. A therapist also guides a patient toward authentic self-discovery by having the patient acquire the attitude of making efforts that are consonant with reality in terms of the patient's inherent *sei no yokubō* (for a discussion of this subject, see Part III).

There was no essential change in that therapeutic goal during Morita's lifetime or afterward. Changing times do not change the desire for self-fulfillment through one's efforts. Suffering must be accepted as an occasional component of human life. In fact, the incidence of suffering will increase in proportion to the effort expended to achieve self-fulfillment, in the same way that the resistance of the wind increases the faster one runs.

Morita thus perceives suffering as being a natural phenomenon. His therapeutic goal is to have a patient acquire tolerance for suffering, not vainly attempt to avoid it, to proceed along the path of self-actualization. In other words, the process of self-fulfillment is inherently painful, and the patient must come to accept that fact.

The basic principle of accepting, rather than evading, suffering has wide application to human problems beyond the limited scope of the management of *shinkeishitsu*. It is a solid psychological support for anyone apt to lose sight of his or her authentic human nature when enmeshed in the complications of contemporary living.

The condition that Morita calls *shinkeishitsu* is, in brief, caused by the pursuit of self-actualization, which gives rise to conflict. *Sei no yokubō* may be best defined as "the desire to live." The "hypochondriacal basic tone" is a condition produced by an inversion; in other words, it is the negative face of *sei no yokubō*. This interfacial relationship of *sei no yokubō* and the hypochondriacal basic tone, which will be examined in detail later, is a major pillar of Morita's theory.

It is natural for human beings to experience *kizukai* (fear, anxiety, uneasiness); this subject will be discussed in more detail in Chapter 2. For the moment, the author wishes to note that, in Morita's view, the struggle for self-actualization inevitably produces contradiction and conflict. The experience of contradiction and conflict is a natural manifestation of human life. Nevertheless, the effective action of a healthy mentality is rendered inoperative if the mind shifts to a fixation on the suffering that has been generated by contradiction and conflict.

Morita therapy seeks to engender the effective action of a healthy mentality and to use that experience of effective action to induce authentic self-discovery through the therapeutic experience.

One concrete illustration of the effective operation of a healthy mentality can be observed in the incident of the canoeload of Pacific islanders who arrived at the World Oceanic Exposition held in Okinawa, Japan. The canoe arrived at the site toward the end of 1975, when the exposition was about to close. The six persons on board the canoe had come from the Micronesian island of Sawataru, approximately 3,000 kilometers away from Okinawa. The islanders had wished to see the exposition because its oceanic theme was closely related to their lives. They had come by canoe because they could not afford the expensive plane fare, and the canoe was a simple craft, paddled by manpower.

The islanders were able to avoid typhoons by accurately observing and interpreting such natural phenomena as slight changes in the strength of the sunlight, the twinkling of the stars, the direction and strength of the wind and the swell of the waves.

The news of this gallant voyage had an exhilarating effect on people who heard about it.

Their reaction was, in part, admiration for this small group of islanders who had exerted their utmost strength and determination to fulfill an objective and who had succeeded by means of a keen observation of nature, without the use of sophisticated instruments. The response to the achievement of the islanders was focused on their demonstration of courage, self-confidence and composure, which are considered to be positive human attributes in any society.

A different viewpoint, however, may also be worthy of consideration. Although the islanders personified the qualities of courage and confidence, they must have experienced anxiety to some degree. They had a certain mutual security reinforced by traveling together as one group in one canoe. However, if one considers the numerous dangers and difficulties of this long voyage to a distant land, it is apparent that the major guarantee of their safety was nothing other than their strength and intelligence. On the whole, human beings experience hardship and anxiety in direct proportion to the scale of their ambitions and efforts. It may be assumed that these adventurous islanders were no exception. However, they accepted anxiety as inevitable, achieving their objective with the experience of anxiety taken into account.

In other words, the islanders knew that they would have to travel with anxiety as a constant, natural companion, and they were thus prepared to keep it under control, to take action calmly as dictated by the conditions that they encountered. If, by contrast, they had become fixated on anxiety as such, they could not have acted as they did and reached their goal.

Although the true feelings of the islanders will never be known, the author believes that this incident contains several elements that can serve as reference points for an understanding of Morita therapy. The psychological aspects of the voyage are worthy of further consideration from that perspective.

Healthful Anxiety and the Desire for Self-development

The Sawataru islanders were motivated by interest and anticipation to undertake their voyage to the World Oceanic Exposition in Okinawa. In other words, they were motivated by what Morita calls *sei no yokubō* (also see Part III). This desire for self-actualization is basic to human life and is one of the two most important concepts of the *shinkeishitsu* theory, the other being the hypochondriacal basic tone, which is discussed in detail in Part III. Morita considered the latter concept to be the central concept of his theory of psychopathology.

The importance of *sei no yokubō* is so heavily emphasized by Morita that the author should summarize Morita's explanation of this concept in his own words. Morita states that "one should examine one's self by returning to one's true human nature. There is a life-force, and a desire for self-development and self-actualization, in any human being who lives with vigor."

This desire is, he continues, a pure (fundamental) desire that is naturally self-motivated but not clearly apparent within the daily complications of modern life. It can, however, be comprehended if one is placed in isolation, when it will come into awareness as the expression of the fundamental life force. The desire arises from the life force, which is inherent to human nature (*shizen no honsei*). The desire is primarily instinctive. (It can be inferred that Morita's trust of human nature stems from his conviction that self-development and self-actualization are psychological priorities.)

The mental transformations that occur in human beings as they interact with specific living conditions are all expressions of *sei no yokubō*.

If, for example, the islanders had become so obsessed by the dangers of their voyage that their minds were overwhelmed by fear and anxiety, the natural manifestation of *sei no yokubō* would have been suppressed and the outcome of the voyage different. Let us suppose that they had been keenly aware that fear and anxiety arise in situations in which the desire for self-actualization is manifested. If they had this awareness, they would have recognized the intimate relationship between fear and anxiety and *sei no yokubō*.

This close-knit relationship somewhat resembles the phenomenon of sensory relativity; the desire will recede into one's sensory background if anxiety is so intense that it dominates the foreground. The anxiety may be so intense that the desire cannot be perceived and acknowledged.

Courage and self-confidence are developed from various kinds of experience motivated by *sei no yokubō*. A person overwhelmed by fear and anxiety is enmeshed so deeply in timidity that he or she craves courage and self-confidence. However, the person retreats more deeply into fear and anxiety, which continue to intensify, holding him or her tightly captive.

The reactions of "the captive" can be observed in the person's daily life. If the person is urged to "take heart," to "be bold, have self-confidence" or to "act with efficacy," he or she may suffer a further loss of those qualities that his or her advisors wish to evoke. The person's sense of suffering will thus intensify.

In the person's awareness, fear and anxiety hold the foreground position, with *sei no yokubō* in the distant background. Nevertheless, *sei no yokubō* will persist and continue to provoke fear and anxiety. If the sufferer makes a conscious effort to override fear and anxiety, the direct result will be an increased awareness of both conditions. Morita disparaged such mental efforts, stating that "any attempt to control the mind with the mind is similar to attempts to lift one's self by one's own bootstraps."

If a person wishes to become "something"–a businessman, politician, scholar, artist–that desire is naturally accompanied by whatever level of exertion is required for reaching the goal. If, however, the person then reacts against his or her ambition, owing to the exertion and suffering caused by fear and anxiety that is experienced in working toward the goal, the original desire will tend to fade into the background of his or her perception. The person will come to think that achieving that goal is not worth the pain and anxiety. Thus, the suffering, not the desire, will come to dominate the foreground of the person's thought.

If, however, the person acts from strength directed by desire, with suffering accepted as inevitable, he or she will find that *sei no yokubō* remains in the foreground. The suffering will recede into the background of the person's awareness.

Living a Natural Life

To live in a state of nature, here and now, accepting "things as they are" (*arugamama*) is to manifest the natural life force in the form of *sei no yokubō*, with pain and anxiety accepted as natural components of life (see Part I).

The life force cannot function efficaciously if it is misdirected, fixated and dissipated on efforts to escape pain and anxiety. The end result of any such misdirected mental focus is a mind that is captivated by pain and anxiety. Morita calls this condition of captivity *toraware* (see Part III). The mind is distracted–wrapped up–in fear, pain and anxiety instead of being absorbed in purposeful activity.

If one is engrossed, for example, in work to the point of forgetting to eat or sleep, there is little, if any, awareness of feelings, only an awareness of the work. A person who is thoroughly absorbed in purposeful activity will probably not feel fearful even if what he or she is doing places him or her in great danger or even the gravest risk of death. The person does not experience fear because his or her mind is fully concentrated on action rather than on emotion.

The islanders appear, in objective terms, to have acted with courage and self-confidence. One may also suppose that they faced a number of frightening situations. It can be assumed, however, that they were not wrapped up in subjective considerations. Their mental focus was one of doing their utmost from moment to moment. This mental focus is a state devoid of "advance mental projection" or "consideration in retrospect." It is a state of total absorption in the present moment, in the immediate action, of being fully in one's "mental present" self. This state includes full reliance on one's natural mentality.

When Morita states that the need to "obey nature and submit to circumstances" is mandatory, his comment can be construed to mean that "the mind shifts fluidly with changes in situations." This process of mental transformation is delicate. Human nature can be readily comprehended if one complies with situational changes. Such changes include emotional reactions to specific events. We experience joy as joy, grief as grief. The self transcends verbalizing and is not controlled by emotions if one has the simple acceptance of "things as they are" (*arugamama*). One trusts one's human nature, including one's mind. Learning to trust the self (i.e., the mind) is similar to progressing along a hill and valley configuration, one that rises and falls and eventually flattens out, vanishes, when we learn to "let go," discarding all sense of discretion, accepting fear and anxiety as such, obeying the actions of nature as such. One's only natural choice is to obey one's mind in that manner. This mental state is one that Morita defines as recognizing that "the fact in itself is the only truth."

The islanders in the canoe were able to act freely because they entrusted their lives to their minds (natural selves) and were thus able to achieve their objective.

We are now confronted by the question of *how* Morita therapy induces a patient to discard "discretion" and, instead, rely on "natural mentality."

The first stages in the therapeutic process are absolute, isolated bed rest, followed by work therapy (treated in detail in Part IV). The initial objective of the bed rest condition is to eliminate interfering stimuli, induce a state of ennui and bring a patient into direct awareness of his or her fundamental desire for self-actualization. Work therapy is intended to invoke spontaneity and engender persistence.

A patient will, of course, continue to exercise discretion by, for example, pondering the question of whether or not pain and anxiety will disappear if discretion is discarded in favor of simple endurance. Silence will not, in other words, be silence at the moment a patient claims to be silent.

However, to take an action that needs to be taken, while enduring anxiety as such, is, in fact, the act of accepting "things as they are." It is the act of striking out in a new direction after one is driven into the corner called "anguish." It is a move in the direction of self-deliverance. On the whole, the process of self-realization in a healthy person begins with the acceptance of "things as they are"–with respect to whatever shifts of the mind arise from situations–and without a keen awareness of what is happening in one's mentality.

Human Health and Human Nature in Morita Therapy

Human health, in Morita therapy, is defined on the basis of Morita's fundamental conviction of the monistic unity of mind and body (for details, see Part I).

In Morita's words, "living is activity, and there is life only when there is activity. The body can be imagined as static and inactive, with the phenomena of 'physical activity' caused by what we call 'the mind'."

Both mind and body can be viewed as either static or dynamic, but these distinctions are simply two different ways of looking at the same object. Morita views human health as a condition in which "activity is appropriate to the goal of existence and improvement, characterized by growth of strength, speed and endurance."

This definition, as such, is not modified by specific reference to either mind or body. It is based on the premise that a full integration of organs and functions is indispensable to human health.

Morita summarizes his position by stating that "human health must be evaluated by examining the entire persona." Needless to say, the entire persona includes the "social persona."

The functioning of human nature, when directed toward self-development, is always self-supportive. Effective functioning takes place by harmonizing the natural activities of the mind, that is, by resolving and harmonizing mental conflicts. Simple impulses and desires may be countered by ethical values to produce a conflict that is then resolved by intentional thought processes to make a choice, to reach a decision.

Morita emphasizes that the mind is capable of delicate transformations for the purpose of adapting to situations. "A free (liberated) mind," he writes, "will function effectively in every situation" if the self "accepts the natural laws of human mentality." There is a natural order in Morita's view of human health. This natural order, or process, is active and creative. Morita indicates this natural order in his remarks that "all phenomena are vicissitudes of life" and that the "phenomena of mind and body also have relativistic shifts and currents."

Morita frequently explains the delicate motions of a healthy mind by referring to the straightforward Zen Buddhist dictum: "Go day by day, that is sufficient (*hibi kore kōjitsu*)." He does not imply that we can be content because every day will be an occasion for feeling cheerful. He points out that the human mentality is involved in continual shiftings of major and minor tensions. Morning and evening, happiness and sadness, life and death–these shiftings are all actualities.

A mentality that includes the evaluation "I did not get enough done today" can exemplify an eager person full of vigor, straining at the bit to accomplish something worthwhile. This kind of mental tension is healthy. It is precisely this kind of mental experience that makes any day a "good day." Morita asserts that this continuous feeling that "today is a good day" can be experienced by anyone, not just people who are "spiritually enlightened."

Another important aspect of Morita's position is that he does *not* define a normal (healthy) mentality as being one that never becomes disturbed or distressed. The natural mentality does acknowledge that summer is hot, winter cold. Nervous stress is experienced in the face of danger, or the fear of dying when confronted by the death of a friend. However, if such phenomena are simply experienced as "things as they are," the mentality is healthy.

The human mind can act with complete freedom only when it accepts "things as they are" and does not attempt to rebel against the facts. This is Morita's sense of the essence of genuine mental health. It is this "natural mentality" that can perceive and appreciate fine details, possessing the spontaneous delicacy to identify with a cluster of tiny wildflowers at the edge of a field, or direct the feet to sidestep and not scatter the pebbles in one's path.

In brief, the author may summarize Morita's position by stating that human health is characterized by a natural integration and harmonization of the mental and physical functions of the human being. This condition rests on a process of rhythmical interaction between mind and body, a sort of pole-to-pole rocking back and forth between a life-forceful desire for self-development, on the one hand, and a cautionary "health-concerned anxiety," on the other. The incessant shiftings toward one or the other of the two poles is, to Morita, indicative of the state of being natural, of accepting "things as they are."

As one of those two poles, the substance of "anxiety," or the hypochondriacal basic tone, is one that Morita considers to be essential to the maintenance of a healthful human temperament. A person with that temperament acts to preserve and improve his or her life because the hypochondriacal basic tone functions for that purpose when observed from the basic focal point of the desire for self-actualization.

The author has dealt with Morita's essential perspective on human nature in this introduction, rather than with his therapeutic system, to lay down the groundwork for a detailed exposition of Morita therapy.

If the author examines Morita's therapeutic system only in terms of techniques, Morita therapy will seem limited to bed rest and work assignments. It is far more important that we see how Morita's thinking transformed the meaningfulness and objectives of those techniques. Morita's therapeutic system is, indeed, his original creation. We can see that originality clearly in the nomenclature he employs for the management of *shinkeishitsu*, which he defines as a "special" or "natural" method of treatment.

The deep foundations of Morita therapy are embedded in his philosophy of human nature. The unique theory that Morita created derived from his recognition that the desire for self-actualization and the disposition toward hypochondria share the same roots in human nature. They vie with each other in a continuous, intimate relationship intended to maintain mental health.

Morita based his treatment procedures on acceptance of both *sei no yokubō* and the hypochondriacal basic tone, at "face value." He did not attempt to invent any detour for a patient to bypass or evade the symptoms of *shinkeishitsu*. His system of treatment is directed to instill, in a patient, a foreground concentration on *sei no yokubō* in a worthwhile context. In that respect, his therapeutic principles have a certain similarity to those of Alfred Adler, who was one of Morita's contemporaries.

In commenting on Morita's therapeutic principles, Uchimura[4] has pointed out that, in Morita's time, the "principal type of neurosis had changed from hysteria to another type of abnormality; namely, *shinkeishitsu*. Morita considered *shinkeishitsu* to be an expression of the fundamental feeling we call hypochondria, or the fear of death. He induced, in the patient, an Oriental discipline which included a 'religion which is not religion' to open up a process not only for treatment of symptoms but also for aggressive development of a goal in life. And this was his own original contribution to psychotherapy."

To conclude this introduction, the author would like to outline the content of this book.

Part I examines the trends in psychiatry and the cultural milieu in Japan during the time that Morita was professionally active. His development of a new form of psychotherapy, his view of human nature and human health with its Oriental, or at least Japanese, mode of thought is discussed in detail. Also explained in Part I is the general approach of Morita therapy in placing greatest emphasis on the entire lives of patients, rather than on limited treatment of immediate symptoms. Part I concludes with an evaluation of the meaningfulness and influence of Morita's contribution to psychiatry in Japan.

Part II discusses the concept of *shinkeishitsu* as an illness and explores the typology of this neurotic condition. Anthropophobia, the most common form of neurosis in Japan, is discussed with an emphasis on its intimate linkages with Japanese culture.

The pathogenesis of *shinkeishitsu* is discussed in Part III. The hypochondriacal basic tone, in being the major concept of Morita's theory of *shinkeishitsu*, is examined in the context of the Japanese family's child care and training and the parent-child relationship.

Isolated bed rest and work therapy, the standard techniques used for treatment in Morita

---

[4] Uchimura, Y.: Seishin igaku no kihon mondai (Basic problems of psychiatry: a view of the structural theory of psychopathology and neurosis), Chapter 15: Theory of neurosis (in Japanese). *Seishin Igaku* 13(11) (1971).

therapy, are discussed in Part IV, along with special features of the therapeutic environment and the therapist-patient relationship.

Part V discusses outpatient therapy, group therapy and concurrent use of drug therapy as modifications of the original Morita therapy. The therapeutic goal, the definition of cure and the prognosis for patients receiving Morita therapy are examined in Part VI.

Comparisons of Morita therapy with other therapies (logotherapy, behavior therapy) are discussed in detail in Part VII. Finally, in Part VIII, consideration is given to the content of Morita's therapeutic techniques, goals and validity in the context of the development and role of Morita therapy in the future.

Part I

Development of Morita Therapy and Its Cultural Roots

The origins of concepts can be an important key to the correct understanding of a theory of neurosis and its management.

Human characteristics cannot be properly viewed only in terms of an academic, objective, scientific perspective. These characteristics spring from the shifting soils of cultural change, in which a number of subjective factors must also be examined.

Shōma Morita's therapeutic approach was derived from a combination of academic scientific factors in relation to his cultural milieu. Because his theory and treatment techniques were structured and applied to relieve the unease and suffering of his contemporaries, we consider it essential to examine the cultural characteristics of his era. However, we will first take a look at the academic origins of Morita therapy.

1

Academic Origins of Morita Therapy

The expression *Morita therapy* was introduced by Morita's professional descendants after his death. Morita called this therapy his "special or natural treatment technique for *shinkeishitsu*."

We need to consider the reasons he used the term *shinkeishitsu* to define his psychopathological basis of neurosis and the reasons his treatment techniques were called "special or natural" to comprehend the wellsprings of his system of therapy.

Psychiatric medicine in Japan, at the time (1902) that Morita began to specialize in the subject, was based on German psychiatric models. Morita believed himself to be a distant student of Kraepelin (1856–1926).

At an even earlier period (the latter half of the nineteenth century), the Japanese practice of psychiatric medicine had been heavily influenced by British studies, notably the study of insanity by Henry Maudsley in *A System of Medicine* (Volume II) first published in 1872 (edited by J. Russel Reynolds) and later translated into the Japanese language (1876).

By the end of the nineteenth century, German medicine had been incorporated into Japanese medical practice, and a great number of Japanese professionals had studied in the German-speaking countries.

Among those pioneers was Shūzō Kure (1865–1932), Morita's teacher, who studied in Austria, Germany and France from 1897. After his return to Japan in 1901, he introduced Western medicine and practices in his teaching. His major goal was to introduce Kraepelin's descriptive psychiatry, Nissl's technique for cerebral histopathology staining and Pinel's movement for liberation of psychotic patients.

Kure first devoted his research efforts to the clarification of the histopathological characteristics of cerebral diseases, following Nissl's footsteps. His attention, however, was eventually directed to the medical treatment of psychotic patients and to the structuring of professional treatment at mental hospitals. He placed emphasis on description of facts rather than on interpretation and explanation of psychological phenomena. In addition to academic research, he was a practical innovator who worked to improve the social position of psychotic persons.

Kure opened the door to mental hygiene activities in Japan and opposed the excessive confinement of mental patients in treatment institutions. His efforts were directed toward producing, in the Japanese people, an awareness of their erroneous social conventions, their ignorance and their indifference toward psychotic persons. He emphasized the need for knowledge and proper treatment of psychotic patients. The influence he achieved was effective in bringing about reforms in Japanese medical treatment and psychiatric research.

Morita was one of the medical professionals who was heavily influenced by Kure into forming the conviction that the principal objectives of clinical psychiatry are an accurate clinical comprehension of psychosis, effective clinical treatment and reintegration of psychotic patients into the social system in a condition of mental health.

Morita took his first step into the field of psychiatry in 1902. His first lesson consisted of experiencing clinical treatment based on observation and description of facts, with a minimum of interpretation. His clinical studies were centered on direct observation of human beings rather than on academic histopathology (in accordance with Kure's instruction).

The reasons he chose psychotherapy as a career will be discussed later in this chapter, but it is probable that his study of work therapy for hospitalized schizophrenic patients, under Kure's supervision, had an important role in that decision.

His humanistic viewpoint as a practicing physician had attracted his attention not only to the special environment of a mental hospital but also to the overall social environment and the neurotic phenomena springing out of ordinary people's efforts to live effectively within that environment.

Morita had suffered from palpitation, insomnia, gastroenteric disturbances and symptoms of beriberi during his student years, frequently experiencing frustrations that made him question the meaning of human life. He had faced a major crisis when his father, because of financial difficulties, had to cut off payment of his tuition and living expenses.

The experience of needing to exert immense effort, in a desperate situation, eventually relieved his suffering and was, no doubt, another major reason for his later interest in the management of neurosis.

The academic trends in psychotherapy at the time Morita received his medical education may be identified with reference to the medical literature of the period.

Of special interest was the wide clinical usage of the term *neurasthenia*. This word was coined by Beard in 1869 to define fatigue of nerve cells as a result of overconsumption of nutrients (based on the theory advanced by J. Brown).

The symptoms of neurasthenia were described as extreme sensitivity and irritable weakness of the nerves, headache, muscle weakness, lack of energy, indigestion, vertigo, insomnia, dysfunction of the vasomotor nerves (with increased reflex function), sensation of mental and physical fatigue, difficulty in concentration, lowering of work capacity and a number of other physical and psychological manifestations.

Neurasthenia was a word generally used, at the time, to describe "culture-related disease."[1] Morita took the view that if fatigue or enervation of physical or mechanical causation actually precipitated a condition of exhaustion in the central nervous system, this condition could be diagnosed as temporary and effectively cured with a proper amount of nutrition.

Nevertheless, he observed many clinical cases in which such treatment actually aggravated the symptoms of neurosis. He was led to believe that two distinct diseases were involved. In his subsequent studies, he divided neurasthenia into two types, which he termed *a priori* (constitutional) and *a posteriori*.[2] He first identified these two types in 1921 and, at the same time, described their differences. The a priori type was identified as *shinkeishitsu*. (He had already used the term *shinkeishitsu* two years earlier in a paper titled "On the Subject of *Shinkeishitsu*.")

It is important to consider the reason that Morita discontinued use of the wider term *neurasthenia* and, instead, chose to use the stricter expression *shinkeishitsu* in diagnosis.

He did not intend to imply that the condition called neurasthenia does not exist. This con-

[1] Sigmund Freud had employed the term *neurasthenia* for a long time. He called it an actual neurosis, together with anxiety neurosis and hypochondria. Between 1890 and 1910, a great many psychiatrists limited the classification of nonpsychotic emotional disturbances to the four groupings of hysteria, hypochondriasis, neurasthenia and psychasthenia in the clinical nomenclature. The hysteria grouping chiefly included conversion reactions or dissociative reactions or, in some cases, psychotic reactions. Hypochondriasis was the term used to identify a neurotic condition that is characterized by excessive worry about physical health and the general condition of the body. Psychasthenia was defined as a condition of tension, obsessive-compulsive states and phobias. The remainder are included in neurasthenia.

[2] A priori constitutional neurasthenia (*shinkeishitsu*): (1) physical hypersensitivity and (2) psychological hypersensitivity (hypochondriasis, obsession); a posteriori neurasthenia: (1) mental and physical exhaustion, (2) hypochondriacal misconceptions and (3) combinations of (1) and (2).

dition is, in fact, a temporary characteristic of early stages of various mental illnesses, physical diseases (e.g., tuberculosis) and psychosomatic fatigue. Even if a specific cause cannot be identified, it is possible to observe changes in symptoms of neurasthenia over time.

What Morita wished to achieve was a specific focus on a priori neurasthenia, and he accordingly gave it the specific name of *shinkeishitsu.* He identified it as a condition that occurs in persons who are hypersensitive to mental and physical irritants and also described it as a condition of "pseudo-irritable weakness."

Although certain symptoms of *shinkeishitsu* were similar to those of neurasthenia, effective clinical treatment could not be undertaken unless the origins of the two respective conditions were clearly differentiated.

Morita referred to Cramer's *Die Nervosität*[3] in his use of the term *shinkeishitsu*, but his thinking was also allied to that of Kraepelin.[4] Nevertheless, his definition of *shinkeishitsu* is different from their definitions of Nervosität, in that Morita does not consider neurosis to be a degenerative disease caused by some sort of hereditary constitutional abnormality. *Shinkeishitsu*, in particular, was not a congenital disorder to Morita but, rather, a condition acquired and exhibited by mentally hypersensitive and excessively introspective persons.

In Japan, Saburo Matsubara had proposed a constitutional theory of hypersensitivity as the cause of neurasthenia. This theory had, at one time, interested Morita. However, Morita's clinical experience seemed to indicate that many cases of *shinkeishitsu* did not spring from a constitutional predisposition.

He concluded that Matsubara's theory placed too much emphasis on constitutional factors. He began to give serious consideration to character, in terms of acquired characteristics, as the cause of neurosis.

We will examine his position in more detail in Part III, but in brief we may comment that Morita perceived certain psychological traits to produce the symptoms characteristic of *shinkeishitsu*, and those traits were attributes of acquired character.

Although the German researchers of the time[5] considered constitutional neurasthenia to be a biological condition, Morita held that *shinkeishitsu* was none other than the same disorder and that it was generated from an acquired hypersensitivity character, not from a constitutionally fixed condition.

He touches on that point in his substitution of the term *shinkeishitsu* as preferable to *neurasthenia.* "The reason," he states, "that I have ventured to use the new term *shinkeishitsu* instead of neurasthenia is that the meaning of Nervosität (nervosity) as a sort of degenerate abnormality lacks clarity; consequently it is not possible to differentiate it from other, similar disorders. In view of this, I felt it useful to substitute the new term. In fact, it is necessary to remove the pernicious influence of a vague term that does not correspond with clinical realities and treatment procedures. When studying the nature of this specific disorder (*shinkeishitsu*), we must restrict its definition."

Morita further defines *shinkeishitsu* as not qualitatively different from a normal mentality but as qualitatively different from psychosis. To him, *shinkeishitsu* was not a true mental disor-

---

[3] Cramer classified Nervosität into three types: Neurasthenie, endogene Nervosität and Hysterie. Morita apparently refers to the second type.

[4] Kraepelin discussed hypochondriasis in terms of the relationship between constitutional nervosity and neurasthenia (nervous exhaustion) in 1896 and afterward.

[5] Krafft-Ebing: Nervosität u. neurasthenische Zustände (Vienna, 1891); Möbius: Zur Lehre von der Nervosität: *Neurol. Beiträge*, Haft 2 (Leipzig, 1894); Jaspers: *Allgemeine Psychopathologie* (Springer, Berlin, 1913). Nervous syndrome is a general term for neurasthenia and a grouping of neurasthenic symptom complexes. In both instances, the word refers to symptoms that occur as a disposition abnormality or that appear during the early stages of various types of illness (Jaspers).

der but, rather, a characteristic mental attitude or mode of living. The author will consider this issue in more detail in the following chapter, but the author can, here indicate Morita's thinking.

This *shinkeishitsu* disposition was included in Morita's classification of various types of functional degeneration.[6] He considered it a functional rather than a biological disorder. If the disposition was mild in degree, he described it as a "psychological trend."

Even if some abnormality is detected in the autonomic nervous system, the trend in itself is a matter of a functional excess or deficiency. A person with a *shinkeishitsu* disposition is in a position between health and illness.

His opinion was an innovative attempt to understand neurosis as a psychological rather than as a biological phenomenon.[7]

The notion of classifying the neurotic disposition as between the poles of illness and health resembled the views advanced by Koch (J. L. A. Koch, *Die psychopathischen Minderwertigkeiten*, Ravensburg, 1891–93) at the time. According to Koch, however, it was possible to have either a priori or a posteriori psychotic states, and even advanced states could not be classified as absolutely psychotic. On the other hand, mild cases could not be classified as mentally "normal."

Koch also believed that an inherent psychopathic inferiority appears as a singular component of various disorders and is, for that reason, an important factor in neurosis. He classified psychopathic inferiority into three categories. It appears from his explanation, however, that the differences among the three types[8] are due to qualitative, not quantitative, differences in the degree of the disorder.

On this issue, there seems to be a basic divergence between the Koch and the Morita points of view.

Near the end of the nineteenth century, such pioneers as Westphal, Krafft-Ebing and other investigators in the German-speaking nations, as well as Janet in France, took an interest in the problem of neurosis. Numerous attempts were made to develop new classifications of mental disorders to sort out the chaos existing during that era.

Morita developed the idea of splitting neurosis into the two types of *shinkeishitsu* and hysteria. Influenced by a paper written by Jolly in 1877, he followed Jolly's notion of discarding the term *neurasthenia* in favor of the two categories of hypochondriasis and hysteria.

Jolly thought hypochondriasis to be a type of disease and wrote that "hypochondriasis is that state of dysphoria (due to a pathological change in self-experience) in which the patient's attention is continually or principally directed towards his own physical or mental state."

---

[6] *Shinkeishitsu*, hysteric, weak-willed, hyperthymic, hypothymic, paranoiac and schizothymic dispositions.

[7] It is believed that the major trend in German psychiatry at that time consisted of the position that degeneration is not affected by cultural conditions and that it is transmitted to descendants without environmental influence. Morita was influenced by that trend. His proposal concerning the disposition concept of *shinkeishitsu* includes references to Cramer and Kraepelin. Although he considers the *shinkeishitsu* disposition and hypochondriacal tendency as a priori trends, he differs from Cramer and Kraepelin in his view that "hereditary" or "a priori" cannot be properly defined in a narrow, specific biological sense but that they can be acquired a posteriori. This is understandable if we consider the implications of the neurotic manifestation of a disposition in terms of the effects of environment on a person. Morita later published a paper on the subject of Kraepelin's definition of *degenerate*, including his own opinion that human character is formed by correlations of disposition, environment and opportunity. Accordingly, human character is not entirely a matter of a priori disposition, fixed and immutable; rather, it can be developed and matured in interaction with the environment. For that reason, Morita stresses character training as "making use of *shinkeishitsu*" and strongly encourages the inclusion of educational treatment in his system of therapy.

[8] 1) Psychopathic disposition is chiefly a neurasthenic condition characterized by increasingly irritable sensitivity and hypersensitivity. 2) Psychopathic hereditary taint is characterized by abnormal mental excitation; violent agony, fear and anguish; unstable emotion; increasing hypersensitivity; obsessive thought patterns; and periodic shifts of emotional emphasis. 3) Psychopathic degeneration is a mental abnormality that coexists with a feeble-minded tendency that precipitates intellectual and moral disorders.

Morita, however, differed from Jolly in not using the term *hypochondriasis* as a noun for a disease. He used it as an adjective associated with the disposition that gives rise to *shinkeishitsu*, the so-called hypochondriacal disposition.

Morita classified neurosis into the two types of hysteria and *shinkeishitsu.* He used the latter term to classify, in one type, various neurotic phenomena exhibited by patients to indicate that the so-called hypochondriacal basic tone arises from a "*shinkeishitsu* disposition" or "*shinkeishitsu* personality."

Another matter that warrants our attention is the development of Morita's treatment techniques in relation to the then-contemporary trends in psychotherapy.

As far as we can ascertain, Morita developed his psychotherapy soon after he began to specialize in psychiatry. In a paper titled "An Example of Curable Obsession" (1905), he reported the case of a patient who had suffered from urophobia[9] and who was cured by hypnosis.

It should be noted that hypnosis was introduced into Japan around the end of the nineteenth century. Morita, as did Freud, took a considerable interest in hypnosis and used it in treatment for at least ten years. He noticed that the effects of hypnotic suggestion were distinctly different in a case of hysteria and a case of *shinkeishitsu.* This comparison helped him differentiate the two conditions and clarify his psychopathological basis of *shinkeishitsu.*

Freud had first used hypnosis for the management of hysteria and later proposed his technique of free association analysis. Morita moved from hypnosis to an isolated bed rest technique.

The major difference between the two men is that Freud wished to elucidate the relationship between the conscious mentality and the unconscious mentality (the ego and the id). Morita, although recognizing the importance of the conscious and unconscious faculties, chose to emphasize purely descriptive phenomena. His notion of the unconscious would probably correspond to what Freudians call the preconscious.

Morita's theory and his treatment concepts were developed over a trial and error period of about 20 years and were first published in 1919. His theory of neurosis was fully developed in 1922 and has stood firm without essential revision ever since.

Freud developed his psychoanalytic theory from his experience with a case of hysteria. Morita drew his inspiration from a case of obsession. These disparate centers of attention probably contributed to the separate development of the two theories. Nevertheless, it can be suggested that Morita was excessively critical of Freud's pan-sexualism and lacked a clear comprehension of unconscious dynamisms. It is interesting to speculate whether Morita, had he lived longer and read more of Freud's output, would have been more positively or more negatively influenced by Freud. Morita died in 1938, the year that Freud began to write his *Abriss der Psychoanalyse* (Abstract of Psychoanalysis). Freud died the following year.

Although Morita had started working with hypnosis, as has been mentioned, we must also note that he had begun to use work therapy for psychotic patients as early as 1904. Emphasis was initially placed on indoor work. Within a year, however, Morita was given charge of occupational therapy and then concentrated his efforts on outdoor work therapy.

Morita allowed his patients as much freedom as was possible but also assigned them a great number of practical tasks[10] to increase their skills and abilities and to enrich their sense of life. His work in this field formed the foundation of work therapy in Japan.

---

[9] Fear of passing the urine.

[10] In 1901, Prof. Kure built a workshop for patients in Sugamo Hospital (the present-day Tokyo Metropolitan Matsuzawa Hospital). He set up rules and regulations for the work program. In his own words, "Work has a close relationship with treatment of psychosis; doctors and nurses should encourage patients to work." He mentions occupational therapy in his book *Psychotherapy*, published in 1915. His therapy program was used first for the management of neurosis. Griesinger was the first investigator to apply it to the management of psychosis.

One of Morita's important discoveries was that *shinkeishitsu* neurotic persons differ from schizophrenic persons in having a keen "desire for self-development" (see Part III). This was a result of his experience in work therapy with schizophrenic patients.

In a similar manner, Morita's experience in treating juvenile delinquents taught him that "weak-willed" persons lack that "desire for self-development." Both delinquents and schizophrenic patients differed from *shinkeishitsu* patients–and from each other–in that respect, even if they had other clinical symptoms in common.

Morita accordingly defines the "desire to live" as an important characteristic of *shinkeishitsu* and as a key concept in his theory of and therapy for the condition.[11] The few books on modern psychotherapeutic treatment available in Japan at that time had little influence on his thinking.

In 1906 he translated Otto Binswanger's *Grundzüge für die Behandlung der Geisteskrank heiten* (Fundamentals of Treatment for Mental Illness).[12] One passage in that book, which we quote in full, held a special interest for him.

"Young people," Binswanger had written, "who are seen to have psychotic disorders of a genetic type (predisposition) will suffer from such mental afflictions as night terrors, enuresis, sleep disturbances and other types of fear. They also exhibit physical symptoms; e.g., vasomotor and endocrine disorders.

"Treatment of these patients is limited, since medical examination and treatment is confined to the physical symptoms only. But we need to expand treatment procedures in the interest of assisting them to live normal lives. We need to use psychotherapy in recognition of their basic character, which is ultrasensitive and tends toward emotional over-reaction.

"The psychotherapeutic program should include preparation of a clearcut timetable that includes work, play and rest in a combination suited to the mental abilities of the patient. Mechanical work associated with farming, gardening and handicrafts is useful. But the basic objective is to lead the patient toward a normal daily life.

"It is very difficult to have this treatment program carried out at home; in particular, mother love, characterized by excessive worry and a strong tendency toward excessive protection of the patient, may pose a major problem, with only a low degree of resultant effect in spite of the therapist's efforts.

"A patient who has a weak mental and physical resistance tends to strenuously evade or escape effortful labor. That tendency can be aggravated by excessive family protection, particularly from the mother. When that type of family environment is recognized, the therapist must stress the necessity of placing the patient in a hospital for treatment."

Morita had gained similar perceptions from his observation of juvenile delinquents and other patients with psychoneurotic complaints. Binswanger's remarks reinforced his commitment to work therapy for treatment during a patient's hospitalization. We need to consider, in that context, his mode of thought on the subject of human labor. (The fundamental meaning of "work" as Morita defines it will be examined in detail in Part IV.)

Binswanger's method of guidance toward normal life was carried out by imposition of intellectual or mechanical work assignments, such as gardening and handicrafts, in accordance with a strict timetable. However, Morita was doubtful about this approach. He did not consider it undesirable to lead a life in an ordered manner, but he realized that a patient's interest in

---

[11] Morita defines *sei no yokubō* as a pure desire in the human heart that is put into action naturally. However, in complex conditions full of contradictions and errors, it is not easily recognized. The natural motion of *sei no yokubō* arises within the self only in a lonely environment isolated from society. This motion is the strength to live. It does not arise from normative criticism, or sense of duty or sense of purpose. It is, rather, the strength to live exhibited by children, who are engaged in activity all the time. (Also see the next chapter.)

[12] Binswanger, O.: Grundzüge für die Behandlung der Geisteskrankheiten. *Vorträge für praktische Therapie*, Haft 3.

work and in persistence would not develop spontaneously if the patient was instructed to perform the work mechanically as a daily task.

Morita took the position that work in actual life must be felt to have life and warmth in itself. To have natural feeling appear during work activity, the type and timing of work selected by the therapist, although not introduced to a patient in a nonspontaneous manner, should be introduced in such a way that the patient will carry out the work assignment on his or her own initiative, without the imposition of fixed rules.

Patients will suffer more, when they try to find work but cannot find any, because they will become absorbed in the issue of what sort of work would be most efficacious for them and how it can serve to defeat their suffering.

In other words, if a patient begins to think about self-generating interest in work, and tries to acquire this interest by mental concentration, the work he or she may have been instructed to perform may become ineffective. The patient will be seized by a compulsion to take action on everything immediately.

Morita is in favor of not imposing work on a patient in a nonspontaneous manner. However, the therapist must seek a means of manipulation or guidance that will generate spontaneous activity in the patient—a self-generated desire for work—as distinct from activities that are essentially recreational or that provide mental diversion.[13]

In actual life, according to Morita, there is natural activity. There is, further, a natural desire or appetite for activity, and that desire should be given opportunity for expression in the form of work therapy. The imposition and regulation of work activity, as in Binswanger's scheme, is not the point. The point is to lead a patient to a state of experiencing a natural, heartfelt need for activity.

To Morita, no matter what sort of work a patient is assigned, the patient's condition will improve. To recover from *shinkeishitsu*, the patient will seek work for the purpose of overcoming *shinkeishitsu*. However, this effort will be to find no avail, and the patient will experience anxiety. The therapist must guide the patient to work for the sake of work, not as a means of defeating *shinkeishitsu*.

However, work that requires a concentration of attention based primarily on feelings should be avoided. A patient's sense of success or completion in working is acquired by eliminating the issue of work selectivity by exercise of value judgments. The therapeutic plan is designed to cultivate an essential patience and persistence, to foster a fundamental self-confidence and courage toward work in an unconscious manner.

Morita instituted bed rest to precede work therapy as an effective means for accelerating the initial step toward spontaneous activity. By placing a patient in absolute, isolated bed rest, mental ennui as well as physical ennui are experienced. The complete deprivation of external stimuli and activity has the effect of arousing an appetite for "something to do."

Morita first instructed a patient to "sleep as long as possible, with the notion that 'nothing is more pleasant than sleep.' This," he continues, "is a remark that follows hard labor. At other times, nothing is more 'distressing' than too much sleep. This sense of distress leads, within several days, to a rising desire for activity. The condition of ennui becomes unbearable. It is the same as experiencing starvation once the appetite is roused. We can describe this sensation, following prolonged bed rest, as a 'desire for action' or a 'desire for work' but it is fundamentally a 'desire to experience life.' A person cannot relish the taste of food if obliged to eat three times

---

[13] W. R. Dunton of the United States published a report on occupational therapy in which he states that ordinary laborers are fortunate: their illnesses are readily cured because they engage in work. He also insists that working is better than recreational activities or attention-diverting activities for therapeutic usage (*Occupational Therapy*, Saunders, Philadelphia, 1915).

daily regardless of lack of appetite. Overeating can result in a pursuit of ever richer delicacies to stimulate a sated palate. The true desire for food can only be experienced in a situation of starvation."

"The next step is to release the patient from bed rest and let him stand outdoors all day exposed to fresh air and sunlight. He will, without conscious direction, extend his arms and try to touch something. Or he will begin to clean the entire yard, take care of plants, observe growing things, or track down an ant hole. This is spontaneous activity driven by mind and body. When we accept our situation and concentrate our attention as we are naturally directed to do, there is no sense of anticipation, or value criticism, or sense of duty in the experience. There is no anxiety in the mind. We function without question, just as we swallow food smoothly when we are hungry. This is a natural phenomenon of the human mind and body. This desire–this appetite for activity–cannot be comprehended theoretically or by imagination. It will be aroused and experienced only when we are actually placed in such conditions."

At the time Morita wrote this, Otto Binswanger was a professor in the psychiatry department of Jena University. His nephew was Ludwig Binswanger. When the elder Binswanger wrote his paper on the need for work to restore a patient to normal life, psychoanalysis was not accepted by orthodox German psychiatry.

Otto Binswanger was critical of psychoanalysis. In his book on hysteria, however, he included an academic evaluation of Freud's *Studien über Hysterie* (Study on Hysteria). At the same time, his nephew Ludwig, then an assistant in the psychiatry department of Jena University (1909), contributed a paper titled "Versuch einer Hysterieanalyse" (Attempt at analysis of hysteria) for a yearbook (Jahrbuch für psychoanalytische u. psychopathologische Forschungen), edited by Bleuler and Freud. Ludwig's professor (and uncle), Otto Binswanger, had directed Ludwig's attention to a psychoanalytic study of a case of hysteria.[14] It was extraordinary for an orthodox German-speaking university to accord such recognition to psychoanalysis.

Morita's interest in work therapy was, as has been mentioned, influenced by his translation of a paper by Otto Binswanger. Although Binswanger was strongly critical of psychoanalysis, he showed an interest in psychoanalytic techniques. Morita's major interest in this paper, however, concerned Binswanger's explanation of the role of work therapy.

During the same period, Morita had also translated a paper titled "Grundsätze für die psychische Behandlung der Psychoneurosen" (Principles of Psychiatric Treatment for Neurosis), written by Dieckhoff.[15]

Among the points that interested Morita was Dieckhoff's assertion that the basic attitude that a psychotherapist must adopt is to win the trust and respect of a patient by treatment with thorough sympathy and understanding. The mental state of a patient must be accepted as such, but with the therapist inducing a mood of hope, so that the patient will cooperate and continue to remain in treatment.

The patient must, further, be led to an awareness of his or her essential mental competence in terms of health and work. The therapist should not express overgeneralizations about the illness that would have a negative effect on the patient's psychological condition. Rather, the therapist should have the patient understand that anxiety over health, or concern to overcome such anxiety, is a common form of human weakness that can be reduced or eliminated by strengthening the mind with work and gradual development of self-control.

Dieckhoff strongly opposed, as an error, the notion that bed rest is essential if a neurotic

---

14 *Erinnerungen an Sigmund Freud*, Bern, 1956. *Mein Weg zu Freud in der Mensch in der Psychiatrie*, Pfullingen, 1957, by Ludwig Binswanger. Translated into Japanese by N. Takeuchi and M. Takeuchi. Iwasaki Gakujutsu Shuppansha, Tokyo (1969).

15 Grundsätze für die psychische Behandlung der Psychoneurosen von Chr. Dieckhoff, Streitberg, *Medizinische Klinik*, No. 11, 1906.

patient is exhausted from too much work and must be forbidden to work at all. He took the opposite position that work is the basis of mental and physical health. In this contention, Dieckhoff basically agrees with Binswanger.

Morita, on the contrary, was totally opposed to the format of furnishing a hospital environment where work is conducted in a communal life-style characterized by strict order, hardship and obedience. It is better, he says, to have a daily work schedule appropriate for each patient.

Immediately after Morita translated the two papers discussed in the preceding text, he published his thesis "Psychotherapy," in 1908.[16] There are a number of points in that paper that deserve special mention. The author will consider a few of them at this time.

First, Morita discusses the relationship between mind and body and the relationship between consciousness and unconsciousness. Concerning the mind-body relationship, he says that we need to know the nature of this relationship to have an understanding of psychotherapy.

Mind and body are not abstractions and are closely related. Mental concepts have physical effects. The intimate relationship between mind and body must always be considered. We cannot, in the final analysis, treat either one in isolation from the other.[17] We must discover the exact nature of the mind-body cause and effect relationship in each specific instance for proper treatment.

Mind and body are essentially the same. When we view mind-body in a static and material manner, we call it body, and when we view it, on the other hand, as a process of dynamic change, we call it mind (see Chapter 4).

Mind, according to Morita, is a process of action but an action that is intangible, like the rings around a source of light. The mind is generally supposed to be something *concrete* but something that is constantly changing. It must be understood that feeling and consciousness are attributes of the mind. The notion of curing mental disease by "spiritual power" or the "influence of concepts" is a form of suggestion therapy that does not include the whole of the mind and can thus constitute only a small part of psychotherapy.

Morita explains the relationship between the conscious mentality and the subconscious mentality as basically characteristic of human mental activity. Conscious activity consists not only of immediate sensory perceptions. It also includes a full recognition of what one is thinking and doing. On the other hand, one is "unconscious" when there is no recognition of activity, with the psychological effect of acting without knowing, without being aware of one's activity.

"The unconscious aspect of activity," he says, "is of utmost importance in psychology. Our lives are governed largely by unconscious factors.

"The relationship between the conscious and unconscious aspects of activity may be compared to the whole of one's personal property and that small portion of it carried around in one's pocket. In other words, unconsciousness is a warehouse full of merchandise, and consciousness a small display stand showing a 'surface' sample of what the warehouse contains.

"Unconscious activity deals with a great number of functions essential to living. But when its functioning is impaired or misdirected, it can generate illness and disorder in our lives."

Morita extends his comments on the subject with a few more examples and then con-

---

[16] Morita, S., in an article titled "Seishin ryōhō" (Psychotherapy). *Igaku Chūō Zasshi* 5(19):39–55 (1908).

[17] Morita discusses in detail the relationship between body and mind in his book (*Lectures on Psychotherapy*), published in 1921. There were quite a number of long-standing theories on the subject, but the theory of materialistic monism was particularly influential during Morita's era and was accepted by most investigators. However, this relationship was, from the perspective of action, interpreted in terms of the interacting mind-body theory, also known as psycho-physical parallelism, which dominated the field of medicine. Morita holds that body and mind are different aspects of the same entity and differ only in terms of how we choose to view the matter. He divides his perspective into four points of view: (1) the physical organs and physical growth in relation to the mind, (2) the relationship between the functions and activities of the body and the mind, (3) the relationship between the mind and internal physical fluctuations and (4) the relationship between the mind and physical disease.

cludes: "Unconscious activity exerts so much power in respect to psychological effects that we must formulate a clear procedure in order to obtain effective results from psychotherapy."

He then refers to Freud's discussion of the symptoms of hysteria and indicates his interest in Freud's point of view.

In this thesis, Morita recognizes the motivational force of unconscious activity. In his opinion, the "concealed" motivational aspect of the human mind, as expressed in human action, must be understood so that we can correctly interpret psychological phenomena–including symptoms of neurosis–and make use of psychotherapy.

We do not know whether Morita acquired this perspective as a result of his experience with hypnosis as a treatment modality or whether he acquired it by studying Freud's theory. It is interesting to note, however, that Morita does not include any discussion of unconscious activity in his thesis "On Aspects of Psychotherapy,"[18] written about ten years later, in 1920.

His emphasis in that paper is centered chiefly on the utility of absolute, isolated bed rest as a therapeutic device. So we can only conjecture why he switched off the light focused earlier on the unconscious mentality.

One reasonable supposition is that he shifted more toward a position of thinking in terms of totalistic, unified and intuitive understanding–rather than adhering to a narrowly focused analytical, systematic and theoretical view of human nature–and included his human experience as an important factor.

Another feasible reason is that he had read Freud's literature a few years before 1912, when psychoanalysis was first brought into Japan, and thereafter moved toward a strongly critical position, evaluating psychoanalysis as an academic theory generated from a mechanistic point of view (that the libido, for example, is a universal determinant of human behavior).

Morita had moved decisively in the direction of interpreting psychological phenomena from a descriptive, phenomenological standpoint. Accordingly, from about 1910, Morita combined criticism of Freud's earlier ideas while in the process of consolidating his own ideas.

Nevertheless, the actual turning point was probably Morita's decision that humanity has a cultural history that is quite separate from the academic scientific recognition of human psychology but that scientific analysis can coexist with cultural awareness without contradiction. (For a detailed explanation of this point, see the next chapter.)

Morita also emphasizes in his later thesis, the applications and limitations of psychotherapy, which he saw as consisting of more than a mere description of conscious and unconscious activities. One must also take into account the professional qualifications of the psychotherapist, his individual character and the need to perceive the individual characteristics of each patient as well as the generalized evaluation of the patient's behavior.

This thesis had a major impact when it was first published, and it remains equally meaningful in present-day psychotherapy.

It is also worth noting that as early as 1902, Morita began to take an interest in hypnosis and the efficacy of suggestion for psychotherapeutic studies of neurosis.

He eventually settled on the position that suggestion therapy is not altogether useless but that it is of limited utility in the management of neurosis. He believed that there must be techniques more effective than hypnosis for rational management of neurosis if the psychopathological factors that operate in a patient's behavior are quite clear.

It still took Morita 15 years to develop fully his system of psychotherapy. During that formative period, he frequently referred to the psychotherapeutic literature written by Ziehen, Löwenfeld and Veraguth.[19]

---

[18] Morita, S.: Seishin ryōhō ni taisuru chakuganten ni tsuite (On aspects of psychotherapy) (in Japanese). *Igaku Chūō Zasshi* Nos. 7 and 8 (1920).

He did not confront Dubois's persuasive psychotherapy in the earliest phase of this formative period. He does not refer to it in his paper "Outline of Psychotherapy," published in 1908. His only reference to Dubois is to cite "Die Psychoneurosen und ihre Seelische Behandlung" (Psychoneurosis and Its Mental Treatment).[20]

Morita must have, nonetheless, been aware of the predominant trend in Japan to define and publicize psychotherapy as meaning *persuasive psychotherapy*. Between the end of the nineteenth century and the beginning of the twentieth century, most books on psychotherapy published in Japan were written by literary figures and stressed the need to *rescue* a disordered mind by means of confessional or persuasive techniques that had distinct religious or philosophical tinctures. Within this main current, Dubois's brand of persuasive psychotherapy gained rapid, widespread acceptance.

The premise laid down by Dubois is that a patient's process of thinking is illogical. The role of a therapist is to furnish interpretation and explanation, followed by instruction and persuasion.

To Morita, however, this procedure was too theoretical, too abstract, for effective use with patients who exhibit symptoms of obsession. There are numerous instances in which a patient's anxiety will increase because of the influence of abstractions. For that reason, Morita did not use this psychotherapeutic approach.

Dubois, however, did use with difficult cases not only persuasive techniques but also simultaneous bed rest or a weight-increasing dietary regimen. Another therapist, Dejerine,[21] also reported the use of isolation treatment.

Morita recognized the usefulness of bed rest and isolation, combining these procedures with other techniques recommended by Weir Mitchel and Binswanger. He began to work out a correlation between absolute, isolated bed rest treatment and work therapy.

In his consolidation of the definition of his absolute, isolated bed rest method, Morita emphasizes its importance for both mental and physical relief, which was based on the premise that a patient needs to be withdrawn, isolated from the general environment and the family matrix, hospitalized and shielded from as much external stimulation as is possible.

Morita stipulates three types of bed rest: absolute bed rest, ordinary bed rest and voluntary bed rest. One of these three types is selected for treatment in response to a patient's mental condition.

This division of bed rest into three types does not have as much importance as the basic concept of bed rest. However, of the three types, absolute, isolated bed rest does have a special effect according to Morita's clinical experience.

One case that contributed most to Morita's strong emphasis on bed rest was that of a female patient who had long been hospitalized in a mental institution for management of obsession (mysophobia) but who had been discharged without appreciable improvement.

The patient then came to Morita, who tried hypnosis, persuasive techniques and regulation of her daily activities, without success.

Since Morita had exhausted his therapeutic resources, he left the patient alone for awhile. Believing that he had abandoned her case as hopeless, the patient initially experienced severe distress and despair. However, this reaction was followed by an experience of courage wrung out of sheer desperation. The symptoms of mysophobia abruptly disappeared.

---

[19] Ziehen, T.: *Psychotherapie, Lehrbuch der allgemeine Therapie und der therapeutischen Methodik*, Herausgegeben von Eulenberg und Samuel, Berlin and Vienna, 1898. Löwenfeld, L.: *Lehrbuch der gesammter Psychotherapie*, Wiesbaden, 1897. Veraguth, O.: *Psychotherapie, Lehrbuch der Therapie innerer Kranheiten*, Herausgegeben von Krause und Garre, Bd. 1, Jena, (1911).

[20] The publication date of this paper is not clear because the source and year are not indicated. However, Dubois had published papers in 1909 and 1911. It is probable that Morita used them as references.

[21] Dejerne, J.J., and Gankler, E.: *Psychoneurosis and Psychotherapy*. Lippincott, Philadelphia (1913).

With an objective examination of the process by which the patient had effected her own resolution of the problem, Morita discovered the therapeutic benefit of bed rest.

The treatment procedures previously used for this patient had consisted of approaches to control and remove the obsession. When the patient, feeling abandoned, relinquished that position of dependence and was reduced to relying on her own resources, she effected a cure on her own. Her previous efforts to struggle free of the obsession had amounted to trying to ignore it to overcome it. Such efforts had simply strengthened the obsession.

This case might have seemed to be one in which the intention of defeating the obsession was more and more intensified by previous treatment techniques, such as rational self-persuasion, imposition of work, regulation of daily activities, hypnotic suggestion or similar techniques for management of mysophobia. In this way, these techniques alone did not, in fact, produce improvement.

Placing the patient in a situation that could be interpreted by a patient as being abandoned by the therapist had served to provoke this patient into a new level of self-awareness. All the subterfuges used to evade self-confrontation were now unavailing. The resultant reaction was one of being left without protection, stripped naked.

After Morita had observed this patient's mental shift, he adopted it as a treatment procedure, identifying the defeat of evasive mental "arrangements" as an effective treatment technique.

Morita afterward built up more experience with this technique, which brought him to a direct recognition of the "desire to live," that is, the desire for self-development through growth and progress. All patients possess that desire, but the psychopathological nature of *shinkeishitsu* has a smoke-screen effect that prevents patients from being conscious of the desire.

Morita sought to identify the mainspring mechanisms of *shinkeishitsu* through studies of patients' dispositions and by chance insights into the condition. His cumulative experience in dealing with *shinkeishitsu* led to his formulation of the concept that he calls the "hypochondriacal basic tone," a fundamental psychological state that underlies and causes the onset of *shinkeishitsu*.

The psychological mechanisms that trigger *shinkeishitsu* will be examined in detail in Part III. It is more important, at this juncture, to focus attention on Morita's use of the absolute, isolated bed rest technique for the purpose of disrupting and defeating the *shinkeishitsu* mechanisms. Once this is done, the therapist seeks to induce, in a patient, a self-awareness of *sei no yokubō* (the desire to live), for which Morita devised a series of progressive treatment techniques. These techniques were directed toward strengthening the character of the neurotic patient by increasing spontaneity and endurance by means of work therapy; in other words, by putting the patient to work.

Morita explains the essential need for absolute, isolated bed rest in the management of *shinkeishitsu* in a number of papers.[22] Condensed to its essence, his position is as described in the paragraphs that follow.

It is first necessary, in Morita's view, to understand the physical and psychological effects of absolute, isolated bed rest. Almost all patients who have severe symptoms experience pain and physical fatigue. A patient's mentality is focused on that pain and fatigue. In some cases, physical motion is no longer possible, and the patient will lie down to achieve direct relief of the suffering.

For treatment of patients with mild symptoms, it may seem that bed rest could be contrain-

[22] Morita, S.: Shinkeishitsu no ryōhō (The therapy for *shinkeishitsu*). *Seiikai Zasshi* No. 452 (1919); Morita, S.: Seishin ryōhō ni taisuru chakuganten ni tsuite (On aspects of psychotherapy) (in Japanese). *Igaku Chūō Zasshi* Nos. 7 and 8 (1920). In *Morita Shōma Zenshū*, Vol. I, edited by T. Kōra, et al. Hakuyōsha, Tokyo (1974).

dicated. This may also be the assumption if the condition includes various types of worry or if it occurs in conjunction with severe distress due to disease. Bed rest, in those instances, could be considered harmful because it will give the patient more time and opportunity to produce even more worry about the future or to arouse unpleasant associations. Reading or light work would seem preferable as a form of management. This is, however, a somewhat superficial point of view.

Confinement to bed is clearly the most restful position for body and mind. In general, it is true that body and mind become stronger and more vigorous as an effect of activity. In absolute, isolated bed rest, however, there is no external stimulus to provoke worry, uneasiness or severe distress, and there is no opportunity to express any such thoughts or feelings. The patient is fully at rest, with all else left to take its course, and time passes more quickly than anticipated.

There is a similarity to neuralgia. Pain in neuralgia intensifies if tampered with in various ways. However, if a patient is left alone and bears the pain with fortitude in a condition of rest, the pain will become less intense and fade away in a shorter time.

Mental and physical pain are much the same. It may seem better to admonish or console a mental sufferer, to massage or rub or manipulate parts of the body, in response to the patient's feeling, or in terms of how someone else may perceive the patient's condition.

In the instance of acute restlessness, a patient may be so confused or so overwhelmed by disappointment and despair that it may seem, to the patient or to other persons, that bed rest is not possible. This is not the case. It is possible to relieve and eliminate the restless condition within several days if the therapist insists on bed rest. The patient will then find bed rest rather easy to experience.

If a patient is assailed by various types of external stimulus, confusion and suffering may intensify. When external stimuli are not present, the patient can genuinely rest. For this reason, proper management of nervous ailments must begin with a period of absolute, isolated bed rest, as the best method to arrest the condition.

On occasion, during the management of *shinkeishitsu*, the therapist discovers that a patient has complained of symptoms of neurosis and has been in voluntary bed rest, sometimes for several weeks. The bed rest technique will, however, have a marked effect only if precaution is exercised by the therapist in putting the patient into bed rest for a few days to a week.

Ordinary bed rest is quite different from clinic-enforced bed rest. Patients in voluntary bed rest at home, for example, sleep or get up when they wish, perform light tasks, read, play chess or cards. This type of activity is not absolute bed rest. It is, rather, a self-indulgent idleness, with neglect of recuperation and health.

Relaxation, taking walks, playing games, conversing and visiting people are pastimes that we would ordinarily consider comforts for the mind and the body. However, most of these activities contribute to fatigue. Greeting and chatting with visitors, for example, causes more mental fatigue than does light work, in most cases.

In the absolute, isolated bed rest prescribed for the management of *shinkeishitsu* , all visitors and conversation are prohibited, as is reading or any other attempt to divert a patient's attention away from the condition of *shinkeishitsu.* As a result, most patients experience qualms, uneasiness and keen suffering by the second or third day in absolute, isolated bed rest. However, they must accept the condition as it is, not seeking mental diversion but enduring the condition patiently.

By doing so, the patient will settle down more quickly than anticipated and will acquire courage by finding the suffering less intense than was expected, with the result that the initial qualms will disappear.

Remarkable results have been obtained with absolute, isolated bed rest for a fixed period, followed by work therapy of a fixed type.

The bed rest technique is only the kernel of the therapeutic system devised for the management of *shinkeishitsu.* There are many elements of the bed rest technique that need to be singled out and developed from a psychological point of view.

Morita, when writing at this time, already had a well-defined perspective of the psychopathological basis of *shinkeishitsu.* In his view, the symptoms of *shinkeishitsu* are expressions of a *true selfhood* that has become covered by a mask while a patient has been involved in the struggle for growth and self-development. The mask is a psychological overlay that consists of viewing that process chiefly in terms of an "inherent disposition" or a "psychological trend" that seems to be an a posteriori type of acquisition. It is, accordingly, the acquisition of authentic self-expression–in which the pure mind or self that desires to live to the full is able to take command–that generates the cure for *shinkeishitsu.*

Morita thus takes the position that psychotherapy should be applied after the therapist has formulated a full understanding of the psychopathological basis, characteristics and conditions of the problem, that is, after the therapist has clarified the diagnosis.

Morita was chiefly interested in devising psychotherapeutic procedures and activities suited to the actual nature of the problem. Because of that, he did not begin to use his knowledge of absolute, isolated bed rest treatment, work therapy, normalization of life-style, adjustment and persuasion techniques or any means of diverting attention until he had assimilated all these elements in his thinking and until he had produced his therapeutic program, as a whole, to deal with the psychopathological nature of *shinkeishitsu.*

The historical process that gave rise to Morita therapy, as discussed in this chapter, was presented mostly in terms of Morita's academic stance and his achievements in relation to the psychiatric literature and influences of his era. The content of this chapter, and the one that follows, will hopefully contribute to a better understanding of Morita therapy.

2

Morita's Thought and Its Cultural Matrix

In Chapter 1, the author examined the academic background in which Shōma Morita proposed his theory for the psychopathological clarification of *shinkeishitsu.* Further, the author described the process by which Morita therapy was systematized.

In this chapter, the author will extend his examination of Morita's thought to the sociocultural matrix of his age and try to point out how that matrix supported the psychological framework of Morita therapy.

Morita first thought of *shinkeishitsu* as a single concept of disease called hypochondria: a pathological fear earmarked by excessive concern for one's health and well-being, as explained in the preceding chapter. He gradually moved beyond that initial position, however, and identified the root cause of *shinkeishitsu* as what he calls the hypochondriacal basic tone.

Shinkeishitsu, in concept, is a condition in which a patient is concerned not only about the pathological condition but also about (worried about) all aspects of human life. The condition is characterized by a wide-ranging concern to sustain psychological and social well-being, along with a strong desire for self-improvement and self-development to guarantee that well-being.

According to Morita, that anxious concern to secure the guarantee of a good life is, indeed, the basic attitude of human nature: the hypochondriacal basic tone. This basic tone is the concept that forms the theoretical core of Morita's theory of *shinkeishitsu.* (Stemming from this core concept, as the guideline of Morita's psychotherapeutic system, is the concept of self-realization of *arugamama* (things as they are), which the author will explain in detail in Chapter 3).

The attitude of anxious concern is an emotional disposition identified, in the Japanese language, by the word *kizukai,* meaning the experience of incessant solicitude, fear, anxiety, uneasiness or apprehension. In this chapter, the author will first explore the relationship of *kizukai* to the hypochondriacal basic tone as the keystone of Morita's *shinkeishitsu* theory.

Kizukai and *Shinkeishitsu*

The Japanese word *shinkeishitsu* has long been used to identify a certain type of nervous temperament. It is believed that, around the beginning of the twentieth century, the word was pressed into service in the field of psychiatry to signify a "degenerate" condition. At the time, "nervousness" did not identify a type of psychological illness in terms of cause, symptoms, course and prognosis, as at present, but was, instead, used to denote a certain type of temperament, or various disorders, such as nervous exhaustion, constitutional neurasthenia and hypochondriasis. This usage caused a lot of confusion, however, because most of those terms had vague meanings.

Morita consolidated the generally vague concept of *shinkeishitsu*, on the basis of clinical observation, defining it as a disorder with a precise psychopathological character.

Because the word is still used in its alternative general sense to indicate a type of temperament, Morita's definition is expressed as "Morita *shinkeishitsu*" or "*shinkeishitsu-shō* (shō = disorder; according to Kōra[1]).

There can be no doubt that Morita was aware of that confusion, although he still insisted on using the word *shinkeishitsu* for his theory. His explanation of the matter has been examined. The author can appreciate the confident manner of Morita's explanation. However, it is apparent that other considerations, not included in that explanation, led to his use of the word to identify a specific type of disorder as well as to his use of the word, in its original sense, as a general term for degenerative nervousness. This contention is conjectural, of course, but as evidence the author points to Morita's attempt to assign a nosological (classification of disease) niche to *shinkeishitsu* in his therapeutic method. It is safe to assume that Morita tried to view *shinkeishitsu* as an attitude or mode of human mentality rather than as a type of illness.

There is no disputing the fact that *shinkeishitsu* is a form of mental disorder because it lies squarely within the scope of neurosis. In spite of this situation, Morita did not consider a *shinkeishitsu* patient to differ from a healthy person merely because of the disorder. His theory of the superiority of *shinkeishitsu* proposes that *shinkeishitsu* is a superior composition of the temperamental tendency called nervousness.

He affirmed the *shinkeishitsu* temperament. Further, he did not consider character immutable, a view that was unusual for his time. Because of that, his treatment technique was later criticized as being too optimistic.

The temperamental tendency characterized by *shinkeishitsu* is introspective and delicately hypersensitive, with the emotional attitude of *kizukai*. This tendency is not, however, a *kizukai* limited only to self-concern, or concern for one's self and environment. It also includes an intense resistance to one's self in reaction to one's shyness and timidity. Kōra remarks[2] that this tendency is characterized by competition between sthenic and asthenic factors, with a double structure of characteristics.

The temperamental quality of *kizukai* is present in most human beings, which is why most people tend toward introversion. The Japanese, in particular, seem to have an affinity for the *shinkeishitsu* temperament and manifest it in the *kizukau* attitude. Accordingly, they have a general personality characteristic of thoughtful consideration.

Overall, the temperamental tendency of nervousness is characterized by an inclination toward introversion, reserve and hypersensitivity. Nonetheless, this type of personality is methodical and fastidious, has a strong sense of self-respect and is constantly introspective. Not unrelated is the fact that the Japanese make much use of such words as individuality, self and self-consciousness. It can be said that the Japanese are excessively self-conscious and much too inclined to show that attitude.

It is not possible to discuss excessive self-consciousness and the *kizuki-kizukau* (become aware of—be self-concerned) attitude on the same level, but both concepts seem to be related in having the same origin from a psychological point of view. Worth noting is the large number of words in the Japanese vocabulary that incorporate the *ki* prefix; for example, *kizukau* (self-concerned), *kizuku* (become aware of), *kigane suru* (feel constraint), *ki ga haru* (become tense), *ki wo momu* (worry about), *kizumaru* (feel ill at ease), *ki ga seku* (be restless), *ki ni suru* (feel anxious), *ki ga hikeru* (feel inferior) and *ki ga chiru* (be distracted).

---

[1] Kōra, T.: Shinkeishitsu no mondai (The problem of so-called neurasthenia) (in Japanese). *Psychiatria et Neurologia Japanica* 42:755–796 (1938).

[2] Kōra, T.: ibid.

Of special interest in this regard is the treatise by Nakai[3] on the changing usages of *ki* (and *ke*) in the Japanese language and the relationship of *ki* to the verbal expression of self-consciousness.

Ki is commonly used as a term for soul, spirit, mind or consciousness. According to Nakai, *ki* is used in the *Kojiki* (the oldest record of Japanese history, completed in 715 A.D.) with two meanings. This is also true of its usage in the *Nihon Shoki* (another historical volume, completed in 720 A.D.) and in the *Man'yōshū* (the first and greatest anthology of classical Japanese verse written between the third and eighth centuries).

One of those two meanings is that of the original Chinese ideograph applied to the Japanese word having the same definition. The other meaning is derived from applying the consonant of the Japanese word to the sound of the Chinese ideograph. In later Japanese literature, *ki* goes through gradual transitions of new meanings under the influence of Japanese historical and social transitions. For example, the first appearance of the word *keshiki*, as a Japanese adopted Chinese ideograph, has the meaning of human attitude, human expression or natural description. This word is used to describe psychological expression in the *Taketori Monogatari* (The Tale of Taketori, written in the early eighth century) and in the *Ise Monogatari* (Tales of Ise, dating from the tenth century).

Within another 50 years, *keshiki* took on a widening range of meanings, to include actions, aspects and motions. In the *Genji Monogatari* (The Tale of Genji, representative of Japanese classical literature, written in the eleventh century), it is used mostly to express internal psychological phenomena, such as joy and anger, expression and motion. Interestingly enough, the same word is in simultaneous usage to describe the phenomena of nature: weather, wind and rain, mountains and rivers, fields and plains, grass and trees. Nakai explains this double usage as follows: "It appears that the people of this era lived in a simplistic harmony with nature. They experienced their own existence as flowing in the loneliness of eternity, with a sympathetic understanding of man and nature that is not yet self-conscious, having no awareness of themselves as set apart from and observing their natural environment. They show a simple, innocent astonishment with the phenomena of life which is sensitive and emotional. The self is mere substance. The fine sensibility of that substance does not come from self-scrutiny, but simply overflows from a non-introspective sense of being 'here and now'."

In the latter part of the twelfth century, the word *ki* began to evolve from the original *keshiki* into a new word, *keshikishite*, expressing the sense of one's self being seen by other people and of feeling to appear dignified. With the rise of the *samurai* warrior class, the word was used to express a sense of people in opposition who scrutinize each other or the appearance of a superior who issues orders to a subordinate. These usages appear in the militaristic literature dating from the latter part of the twelfth century to the fourteenth century, when Japanese culture was undergoing an important transition, including a shake-up of feudal control by excessive expansion of foreign commerce in Japan, along with an increased volume of currency circulation. The feudal authorities were confronted by the danger of crumbling power. This danger signified the beginnings of self-consciousness as an effect of germinating foreign commerce. A second influence during this period was the emerging cultural exchange with China. Japanese visitors to China were heavily influenced by Chinese art and science. Chinese culture flowed into Japan, leading to the rise of neo-Confucianism[4] and a cultural revolution. Devotion to learning had a massive impact on Japan.

The word *ki* now took on metaphysical and Buddhist meanings. It began to have an important linguistic role of not expressing matters of purely personal psychology but, rather, of

---

[3] Nakai, S.: Ki, ke no nihongo to shite no hensen (Transformations of the Japanese words *ki* or *ke*) (in Japanese). *Teikoku Gakushiin Kiji* 5:18–36 (1947).

the psychology of groupings of people who were split into friends and enemies. The Japanized *ki* was fused with the Buddhist word *ki* to mean "a chance, an opportunity," which involves an awareness of time. In this new meaning, *ki* has the sense of a collective straining against the bit to fling one's group into action while, at the same time, engaged in a constant struggle for self-suppression, which results in feeling high-strung. *Ki* further takes on the meaning of one's anticipation of a moment of decision that one must eventually confront.

In this new usage, *ki* precedes, and is linked to, terms that express a sense of actual glimpses of specific moments of time, with the resultant meaning of a delimiting condition, such as an end to the existence of one's self, or of a restrictive condition, such as the dangers posed by a style of existence that tries to exempt the self from the reality of time (a type of personalized psychological expression).

In the sense of restrictive condition, we find *ki* in the terms *ki wo ushinau* (to lose one's consciousness), *ki wo nomareru* (to be overawed) and *ki wo ushinau* (to miss an opportunity). Thus, *ki* now has a meaning of its own in relation to delimiting conditions of human life and in relation to the self discovering its linguistic existence (logos).

Watsuji[5] says that the Muromachi Period (1336–1573) in Japan corresponded to the Renaissance in Europe. It was, in Japan, a time when the feudal system began to break down under the impact of widening currency circulation and advances of commoners into the fields of creative art and science, combined with a new interest in foreign travel. Individual consciousness began to take form. Appropriate words were coined to express this new self-consciousness, among them *ki-tsukai*, meaning solicitude for self. According to Nakai, this word already carries a distinct sense of individual consciousness and clearly indicates that it is the self that controls the process of self-reflection and self-examination. This linguistic means of indicating that the self is the major source of self-evaluation has appeared in various verbal expressions ever since.

Under a feudal system that endured throughout the Edo Period, which lasted more than 300 years–a sort of culture freeze unheard of in the rest of the world–much of Japanese culture was in the hands of the common people. New words came into use to express their distinctive living conditions. The cultural effects of neo-Confucianism, as well as the Jōdo and Zen Buddhist sects–the bases of Edo Period art and science–were transmitted from the *samurai* class to the common people, with consequent new usages of *ki* to express new living conditions.

These new usages are exemplified in the *Yōjōkun* (Regimen Rules of Ekken Kaibara), a book of the period that has a dash of neo-Confucianism but that is largely devoted to a discussion of psychological and physiological matters: circulation of the blood, the relationship between the blood and respiration and hypersensitivity. There is much use of *ki*-linked words: *kekki* (youthful vigor), *seiki* (vitality), *genki* (vigor, energy), *kishitsu* (temperament), *kishō* (weather), *kizukai* (solicitude), *kifusagari* (depression), *kizuyoku* (daring) and *kizumari* (constraint).

Changes in the use of *ki* also occur in the ordinary conversational vocabulary of the common people. Such changes are obvious in the drama scripts written by Monzaemon Chikamatsu (1653–1724), in which approximately 2,550 *ki*- (or *ke*-) linked words appear. In order of usage frequency, these words are *kizukai* (solicitude), *kigen* (humor), *kishoku* (feeling), *ki* (spi-

[4] Confucianism is the doctrinal philosophy first advocated by the Chinese scholar Confucius and is a system of education in which religion and politics are brought into accord. It was transmitted to Japan during the fourth and fifth centuries as a system of practical ethics as well as a political and philosophical system of education and was adopted as a means to unite the government. It was subsequently developed in Japan in terms of neo-Confucianism as a practical ethical system. Together with Zen Buddhism, it attained great popularity during the thirteenth century but was gradually assimilated thereafter into a distinctively Japanese doctrinal system, in both practical and philosophical terms.

[5] Watsuji, T.: *Sakoku* (National Isolation). Chikuma Shobō, Tokyo (1950). (Printed in Japanese)

rit), *rinki* (stinginess), *kyōki* (insanity), *byōki* (ailment), *kiniiru* (to be pleased), *kiniirazu* (to be displeased), *kiotsuke* (caution), *kimi* (sign), *kanki* (censure), *tanki* (short temper), *kenage* (courage), *kinikakaru* (to be anxious about) and *kizuku* (to take notice of).

Nakai explains that *kizukai* (solicitude), the most frequently used *ki* word in the Chikamatsu dramas, also appears several times in the *Akizuki Monogatari* (The Tale of Akizuki), a drama penned by a *samurai* playwright of the same period.

The *ki* of popular usage during this time represents the complete consciousness of the individual. Its chief substance is the self, and it suggests that human beings experience uneasiness. Nakai goes on to remark that *kizukai* has great meaning. It is a high-water mark in Japanese linguistic history, representing the point in time at which the common people have become self-conscious in the modern sense.

This is a record of word creation by conscious concentration of attention in an aggressive manner and with reflection on the motions of consciousness. By contrast (although not aggressive), the conscious attitude in which the self must concentrate consciousness is expressed by *ki ni kakaru* (to be anxious about). In the instance of *ki wo momu* (to worry about), we have an expression for a consciousness of profound unease mixed with bitter struggle.

Ekken used *ki* in a medical diagram based on a metaphysical system. With Chikamatsu, however, *ki* has been detached from physiology and is used to express an attempt to move in a direction that one is obliged to take. *Ki wo kubaru* (to be watchful), *ki wo kakeru* (to bring one's self to do) and *ki ga susumu* (to be willing to do) are unquestionably expressions of individual consciousness and of a self-conscious life structure. These words categorize a life system established by self, a system in which one has learned, by a process of self-awareness, that the existence of the self is "here and now."

By authenticating, chiefly through an examination of the literature, the changes in the meanings and uses of this one word *ki*, Nakai indicates the process by which words are changed in accordance with transitions in living conditions, and this is actually a process of self-recognition.

The author has devoted several pages to the subject of word creation to make clear it that the attitude of self-solicitous consciousness (*kizukai*) in both individual and group awareness is closely related to a distinctive philosophy of life. Morita's conception of the hypochondriacal basic tone has clear associations with *kizukai*. It is probable that the historical evolution of this word was inherent in Morita's consciousness, in his philosophy of life.

Shinkeishitsu and Cultural Change

The Japanese, particularly the common people, swiftly increased their self-awareness of individual consciousness, beginning from the middle of the Edo Period. Mental states of *ki wo tsukau* (anxiousness) and *ki ni sezu ni wa irarenai* (compulsion to worry) were prominent, as shown by the manner in which these expressions were used.

The mental state of *kizukai* conveys the unease of the individual mentality. This uneasiness is not neurotic, however. Living conditions contributed to the formation of a mental state that was "solicitous," regardless of whether or not the social matrix conveyed any indication of unease.

The author may surmise the so-called neuroses of the period by examining its literature. In 1757 (the midpoint of the Edo Period), the Zen priest and writer Hakuin published a modest book called the *Yasenkanna.* Its content consists of subjects of conversation discussed by a number of people on a boat trip. Hakuin took great care to write in a style that anyone could understand, as requested by a certain book publisher of Kyōto. What the publisher wanted was a book that would teach any and all readers the proper means of training mind and body to live a long life in good health. A large number of people were looking for a book of that kind.

Hakuin offers a number of recommendations that are basically introspective. To cure mental and physical fatigue, with the internal organs in poor condition, he recommends rejection of medicines and mental activity. First sleep well, he says, and when you wake up, stretch out both legs parallel, concentrate all attention on the body, from navel to lower legs, and experience this as the entire sum of one's self. Seek to know exactly what is the self, what the self is supposed to do in this life. What is mind? Is the self a Buddha? Repeat these injunctions and inquiries. Then tell yourself to engage in extended introspection. By means of prolonged introspection, the strength of the entire body will shift to, and fill up, the lower half of the body. When this introspective regimen is continued for at least five days or as long as two or three weeks, mental and physical fatigue–and whatever intimation of illness was present–will fade away and disappear. However, one must not stop yet. After the initial recovery, one must devote more time to religious meditation.

Hakuin goes on to say that he had suffered from mental and physical illness and sometimes thought of putting an end to it all by committing suicide. However, he recovered fully, after learning this introspective process from an instructor named Hakuyu. The people of this era, he says, suffer in the same way. He has continued this process for three years and, as a result, has become healthier and more energetic.

This is the gist of the book, which concretely conveys Hakuin's experience.

The mental and physical ailments dealt with in Hakuin's book can be identified as psychosomatic or neurotic in present-day psychopathological terms. The introspection process is a form of psychotherapy.

The book was a popular treatise written by someone who was not a physician. What attracts the author's interest, however, is the fact that a publisher of the period wanted to put out a book on the subject of therapeutic introspection because of popular demand. By reading it, the author can draw a number of conclusions concerning the nature of neurosis and forms of management during the middle of the Edo Period.

The author's understanding is increased by considering the book in relation to the previous discussion of the uses of *ki*. When *ki* first appeared in the Japanese language, sometime during the seventh or eighth century, it was used only to express a natural depiction of human attitude, or complexion, or natural scenery. After about 800 years, it has become invested with the meaning of *kizukai*. The gradual changes in the consciousness of the common people infused *ki* with a variety of new meanings needed to express various new facets of individual self-consciousness. These variegated usages of *ki*, in combination with the content of Hakuin's volume, offer numerous insights into the typology of neurosis common to the Edo Period.

About 150 years after the publication of the *Yasenkanna*, the author has Shōma Morita formulating a theory of neurosis and a treatment technique rooted in Hakuin's therapeutic approach. Nevertheless, in Morita's time, social formations, developments and changes have become more complicated, compared to the society of Hakuin's time, and movements of social ideas are far more diverse. The individual consciousness is also considerably more complex.

The author will now attempt to correlate these historical developments with the development of Morita's treatment technique.

Awareness of pathology and a method of treatment spring up in response to the importance of the disorder and the number of patients seeking treatment. This was true in Hakuin's time and has been in our own. The same considerations prompted Morita. His specific interest, in studying psychiatry, was the field of psychotherapy. Morita was a case in point: he had suffered from neurosis.

And he suspected that Japan probably had a large number of neurotics. Further, a number of popular books on the management of neurosis had been published for the general reader.

The concept of neurosis was still vague. Statistical data were not available. All commentary on the subject of neurosis was little more than conjecture.

It is frequently pointed out that neurosis is sociocultural in origin. The relationship between social factors and the onset of neurosis is well-known. Among those factors, the author can specify urbanization, culture shock, political and economic instability, poverty, war and natural disasters. From ecological and epidemiological perspectives, there are differences in the contributing factors and in the typology of neurosis. The specific forms and incidences of neurosis are also related to race and geographical area. Taking into account those conditions, what was the situation in Morita's time?

The author first notes the immense transitions in politics, economics and other cultural conditions beginning with the Meiji Restoration of 1868, with Japan moving out of the long island-nation isolationism of the Edo Period into active communication and impact with the Western world. Japan was set firmly on the road to modernization, with intense effort directed toward public education. The entire country was swept into an all-out effort to construct a modern social system in all respects, from the late nineteenth through the early twentieth century.

As a result, the author can find indicators of European-style modernization throughout the Japanese culture of the period; for example, the establishment of democratic government, the use of capitalism in economics, the development of productive power by progress in technology and mechanization and a modern view of man and racial consciousness.

In Europe, modernization was built on the historical foundations of the ancient Mediterranean civilizations and of the Middle Ages, the Renaissance and the Reformation. In Japan, the process of modernization, drawn largely from Western Europe, occurred chiefly by political reformation in confrontation with a distinctly Japanese cultural history. The transition included two wars within the short span of ten years (1896–7 and 1904–5). National policy took swift strides in the direction of territorial expansionism and colonial imperialism. In spite of the promotion of democratic freedoms and institutions, the formation of an absolutist, bureaucratic character tinged with racist overtones was prominent.

Nevertheless, opportunities for the common people to improve their social position were not lacking, with rapid progress evident. Individual self-consciousness, in a fully modern sense, was clearly emerging. However, individual freedom was still restricted. This restriction was due chiefly to a culture lag for which the common people were responsible, as pointed out by Ogburn.[6]

Notwithstanding the time period, the timing of this cultural revolution has an important implication in relation to the consciousness of the common people. Various conflicts broke out in their lives at sensitive contact flash points of the old and new cultures. The frictions provoked between the traditional cultural values and the new, modern values gave rise to neurotic behavior. In Morita's time, tradition still had a dominant grip on the individual, with a strength that has since vanished between his time and ours.

The people of Morita's era showed a more candid, confrontal reaction to foreign cultural inroads in their lives, with a simplistic consciousness distant from the complicated structure of human consciousness in our era. The comparative lack of complication probably made it possible for Morita to perceive the underlying rivalry, in the mentality of his contemporaries, between the hypochondriacal basic tone and the desire for self-actualization, when he encountered people exhibiting neurotic symptoms.

---

[6] Ogburn, W.F.: *Social Change; with Respect to Culture and Original Nature* (1922).

It is unquestionable that solicitude for self and other persons was still a predominant cultural force in Japanese consciousness during Morita's lifetime. This mentality was mentioned by Lafcadio Hearn in one book he wrote late in life, *Japan, an Attempt at Interpretation* (1940). Hearn's opinion may be summarized as stating that the Japanese people have not, in their tradition, had the freedom to do as they wished (within the range of individual self-expression permissible in Western society). The Japanese are still in that condition. When the Western concept of individual freedom is explained to them, they evaluate it as animal-like. In Japan, what the individual "must do" is far more important than anything one "must not do"; in Europe, the mentality is quite the reverse.

Although this older Japanese mentality has changed substantially since Hearn's time and the end of the Second World War, his opinions are still worth consideration. He believed that the restraints placed on individual freedom were rooted in traditional ancestor worship. Not only were these restraints exercised within family units, but they were moral forces inherent to Japan's provincial society and, by extension, the welfare of the nation.

It is true that policies of isolationism and collective concern tended to immure the individual within a particular group (which we will discuss later). Any attempt to escape from the intense pressures of collective behavioral criteria could threaten the existence of the individual. In this traditional context, group consciousness was powerful, individual character rather weak. The individual was proscribed to consider the group welfare in advance of any individual action and to attach great importance to human interaction. Keen consideration was paid to group concerns and obligations. The resultant mental tensions were considered normal. The group-think mentality was prone to introspection and to sensitivity in self-expression, whether or not the individual was aware of such mental phenomena.

Self-consciousness of one's social position is a frequent concern in Japanese life, a mental condition that characteristically leads to formation of a personality type in which fine gradings of discernment in social relationships must be cultivated. It also creates an obsessive concern for self-protection based on the social character that the self imposes in behavior.

Morita thus differs from Freud in posing obsession rather than hysteria as the origin of his theory of neurosis and his treatment technique. This is not unreasonable, when we take into account the foregoing factors of the Japanese mentality.

Morita's Interest in *Shinkeishitsu* and His View of the Human Persona

Given the considerations noted in the preceding section, what was the actual motivation for Morita's intense interest in nervousness? The author can, at this time, find no immediate answer to that question. It is plausible to suppose, however, that the Japanese people of Morita's era had given voice to complaints of neurosis. Further, with the concepts of neurasthenia and hypochondriasis still vague, neurotic patients were diagnosed as being congenital degenerates. Effective treatment affording relief was not available. These considerations were, we believe, instrumental in motivating Morita's spirit of inquiry. That motivation was fueled by the the humanism he espoused as a practitioner of modern medicine.

When we specify what we define as "modern times," one of the characteristics we may single out as "modern" is the phenomenon of *disintegration*, in other words, the split identity that human beings experience in having lost a sense of integration with nature.

The scientific spirit that drove men forward into modernization was itself a product of the opposition of humanity set against nature. It has created a world that is universal and objective.

This universal scientific culture, with its own nomological structures, has been instrumental in creating a self-awareness of the value of subjectivity and humanistic perception. Nevertheless, "modern" in the Western world's definition of the word does contain the bipolar opposition of self and nature.

Japan adopted Western-world modernization with the inclusion of that bipolar dichotomy but, nonetheless, with certain idiosyncrasies that have been noted and reported by a number of social commentators.

What it all means is that, in terms of Morita therapy, we must be aware of the cultural context and the social structure in which it was thought out and put into practice.

The major factors included a relationship between foreign ideas and traditional notions that was both agglutinative and counterreactive, both positive and negative. This situation was complicated by the prevailing thought of the ruling class, the trends affecting the common people, the relationship of the individual to society and the exact manner in which Western modernization had an impact on the distinctive sociocultural conditions in Japan. By focusing attention on the consciousness of the people of Morita's era, we may be able to clarify the underpinnings of Morita's view of man and nature.

First of all, let us examine the hypochondriacal temperament in terms of what it means to Morita. He discovered the phenomenon that he defines as the hypochondriacal basic tone by digging into a long-standing, vague sort of mental condition–which could not be precisely defined as temperament, or disease or syndrome–covered by the blanket term of neurasthenia or nervosity.

Concepts of hypochondria differed from the standpoints of individual investigators, but in its original sense the word was considered synonymous with "spleen" and had, as its root cause, physical ailments associated with pain of the spleen, solar plexis and hypochondrium. The original meaning of spleen, however, was blended with a French expression during the late eighteenth century and took on the connotations of a melancholic gloom or sadness.[7]

In the Japanese language, the expression *kokoro wo itameru* (to hurt the heart, that is, to feel the distress of worry) is used when someone is profoundly worried and thus experiences a keen uneasiness. However, it appears that Morita defines this expression, in his terminology, as the hypochondriacal basic tone, which includes certain physiological sensations, such as *shimetsukeru yōna itami* (a pain akin to that of choking), combined with psychological factors, such as *ki ni suru* (to become concerned about something). One's psychosomatic condition is subjected to incessant self-surveillance governed by an attitude of *ki ni sezu ni wa irarenai* (something that cannot be ignored or disregarded). Morita studied, in detail, the psychological process that develops out of this emotional wellspring, a process that combines with and consolidates casuistic material. He then devised a fixed-symptom theory and clarified, as much as was possible, the psychopathologic basis of nervosity.

A number of questions spring up at this juncture. Why was his attention drawn to what he calls the hypochondriacal basic tone? Why does he interpret this concept from the standpoint of correlating it with disposition? Why does he fixate on that "basic tone" as the keystone of his symptomatological structure? And why does he disregard the importance of symptom dynamics in the unconscious? Further, what were his thoughts on the relationship between the hypochondriacal basic tone and the desire for self-actualization? The unique ingredients of his symptomatological theory must be kept constantly in mind throughout our discussion of his work in this chapter.

The author has considered the process by which the word *ki* was adopted and transformed in the lives and social conditions of the common people. The author has recognized it as a

[7] Ladee, G.A.: *Hypochondriacal Syndromes.* Elsevier, Amsterdam (1966).

key component in the self-consciousness of the individual that came into prominence in the seventeenth century.

The author has learned that it includes the meanings of *kizuki* and *kizukau* (*kinisuru*) as these two expressions are now used. In particular, we can see that the attitude of *kizukai* forms a special pattern in correlation with the Japanese social structure.

According to Nakamura,[8] for example, this attitude is one of attaching importance to humanity in and of itself. It is a placement of emphasis on interpersonal relationships, of one individual in relation to any other individual, and on the form of their concern for each other.

By extension, it is an attitude of stressing the fixed structure of social classes (based in the feudalistic social order) and a consciousness of class distinctions so intense that it gives rise to hypersensitivity. The manner in which one's self is perceived by society becomes a major problem. Because of the innumerable situations that give rise to the interplay of *kizukai* between one person and another, we witness many types of neurosis rooted in the stereotyped phenomenon of anthropophobia, with a characteristic symptom structure. (The author will discuss this topic in more detail later.)

This attitude of *kizukai* can be said, however, to be universally human, not restricted only to the Japanese people. It is a manifestation of self common to all human beings. Morita postulates *kizukai* as being an expression of ordinary human attributes and gives it the clinical identity of the hypochondriacal basic tone. In its position as the key concept of his psychopathological basis of *shinkeishitsu*, it is in itself neither a disorder nor a symptom of a disorder.

Morita's Thought and Its Cultural Context

Morita's attention was drawn to the attitude of *kizukai* most likely by intuition, but just as likely due to his philosophy of human life. To understand this point, we need to examine Morita as a private individual and as a clinical professional.

His system of treatment is often compared to Frankl's logotherapy. However, Frankl's logotherapy is more theoretical and systematic than Morita's system of treatment. Morita, by contrast, is intuitive and emotional in his approach. His thinking is expressed in a certain perspective of man and nature embodied in his treatment technique. The most characteristic element of that perspective is an attitude of attempting to affirm the importance of the environmental matrix, of factual data or objective conditions, an admission of reality as it is. In other words, what is real, or true, is the world as we experience it. Along with the inclination to recognize and accept the objective world of the environment as it is, Morita affirms an attitude of accepting and approving of authentic human feeling and desire as it is, with no intention of suppressing or opposing the natural manifestations of human behavior. This inclination toward "naturalism" is a characteristic feature of his treatment technique.

To avoid any misunderstanding of what is involved in the acceptance of natural feeling and desire, the author should note that this is not an acceptance of unbridled egotism or amoral self-indulgence but, rather, an acceptance of self and the environment based on moral sensibility, on an ordered sense of humanitarianism that the author can term "virtue" or "the good."

Nakamura[9] refers to certain ascetic paractices that incorporate many religious precepts, such as Buddhist teachings, and points out that these practices are not readily accepted by the Japanese. As a result, the content of Buddhism was gradually modified in Japan to include

---

[8] Nakamura, H.: *Tōyōjin no Shii Hōhō* (Ways of Thinking of Eastern Peoples) (3). Shunjūsha, Tokyo (1962). (Printed in Japanese)

[9] Nakamura, H.: ibid.

greater affirmation of human feeling. In the nineteenth century, the various Buddhist sects in Japan began to discard their religious precepts. Responsible for this movement was the conviction that it is difficult to adopt an attitude of egotism and amoral self-indulgence, notwithstanding an outright affirmation of human feeling and desire, because the essential moral and humanitarian order will be naturally respected and maintained, with no need for formalistic religious precepts to support it.

Morita shares that conviction with the great majority of the Japanese people. What he discovered is that the distortion of the attitude of natural acceptance is the root cause of *shinkeishitsu.* His treatment technique is directed toward the removal of that mental distortion. The aim of his treatment is to have a *shinkeishitsu* patient acknowledge and accept the pain of the condition as his or her own pain, to assimilate it and to learn to live with it.

Morita uses such expressions as *shizen-ni* (in a natural manner) or *arugamama* (in this instance, to leave the symptoms as they are and to lead life as it is). His frequent stress on these expressions comes from his conviction that it is important to engage in direct self-examination of changes in feeling and desire, as expressed in human behavior, and to accept these natural manifestations of self without distortion.

Morita was a deeply emotional, highly intuitive human being. However, at the same time, he took an objective view of psychological phenomena through his training in medical science and placed emphasis on objective analysis rather than on subjective value judgment. His overriding view of human life was empirical, with a recognition of the "facts of human nature" (mentality) acquired by cumulative clinical experience rather than abstract academic cogitation. Ideas had no meaning to him if he did not see them concretely revealed in human behavior. He respected observable facts and lashed out at ideas that are divorced from concrete facts and bandied about in an academic game of abstractions.

He had little interest in the Dubois school of persuasion treatment because it did not attach importance to the reality of human emotion. His criticism of Freud came from his conclusion that Freud was engaged in a game of inference and interpretation of human behavior based far too much on juggling around with all sorts of abstractions.

There is no doubt that Morita studied the psychiatric literature of the German-speaking countries. However, his commitment to go into psychotherapy as his lifework drew him away from the mainstream trends of German psychiatry. With a risk of overgeneralization, it may be said that nosological studies were advanced in the German literature, but practical education in psychotherapy did not get into the limelight. It is true that Freud created psychoanalysis. However, its practical development for psychotherapy occurred outside the German-speaking academic milieu. The German psychiatrists were devoted to a profound pursuit of theory but did not produce much in the sphere of practical application. Morita, by contrast, was a clinical physician who respected practical matters far more than ideological involvement.

It is worth noting, in that context, that the Japanese educational system was shifted from a British to a German model, in terms of academic policy, during the period of modernization in the late nineteenth century. Japan was chiefly interested in the Anglo-Saxon models of civilization. In many respects, that interest was an inevitable phenomenon, as a matter of practical survival in the modern world. An Anglo-Saxon model was adopted in politics. Interest was shown in the progressive educational system rapidly advancing in France. The Anglo-Saxon impact not only was political or educational but affected the arts as well.

The full changeover to the German educational model took place at the end of the nineteenth century. This changeover was accomplished without full understanding of that model as a purely German system created to keep pace with the other advanced nations of Europe. What Japan adopted was a formal copy of the German model–and nothing more. We will not attempt to explore all the consequences of that decision in subsequent Japanese history.

However, its effect in the field of psychiatry was to shift it away from the pursuit of concrete studies for practical application–contrary to Kure's original intention. An ideological priority of "pure ideas" came to the fore, enforced by authoritative guidance centered on the government-administered academic institutions, under the banner of "natural scientific understanding." The true facts of the German educational system were not taken into consideration; only the form was copied.

In that context, we can see the importance of Morita striking out on his own to establish an original system of practical pychotherapy, in confrontation with the general academic trend (also see Chapter 7).

That individual commitment illustrates and underlines his essential character of respect for fact and action, placing emphasis on ideas drawn from the realities of human experience. "An idea," he states, "must essentially be a reflection of actual human behavior and cannot be divorced from the facts of human life."

His medical knowledge and writings were based on the premise: "Arrive at ideas by starting with actions." It was most important to Morita that we observe our mental operations in exactly the same manner to achieve a clear understanding of ourselves. His thinking, in this context, has the attitude of positivism. (His view of human learning is similar to those of actuality theory, empiricism and pragmatism.)

It was from this standpoint that he produced the form, the operation and the idea of "action" and "actual gain," as exemplified in Morita therapy. For the same reason, he was attracted to Weir Mitchell's "treatment regimen" by recognizing its importance as a treatment technique derived from clinical experience.

The practical slanting of Morita therapy was, by inference, due to the effect of neo-Confucianist thought, which held sway in Japan prior to the shift toward Western-world modernization. In brief, this neo-Confucianist position can be summarized as follows: Knowledge becomes genuine knowledge by means of action; knowledge alienated from action has no actual existence; disintegration of reason and knowledge is a result of splitting knowledge away from mind, of making reason a matter of knowledge and action a matter of mind. However, reason is inherent in mind. Mind and reason are essentially conjoined. We become aware of reason through its manifestation in the mind by means of action.

Accordingly, the basic principle of neo-Confucianist philosophy is that native (inherent) intelligence is present in the mentality of all human beings. Native intelligence comes into operation from the desire to have the mind produce an ethical standard. Because this native intelligence is based in the mind, there is no need to suppress any human feeling or desire as being intrinsically evil. The presence of feeling and desire is an affirmation of the human way of life. There is, in fact, both good and evil in all human beings. This duality is based on *kishitsu no sei* (the nature of temperament), which is formed by the *ki* allotted to humanity. There are differences of clarity and turbidity in this "nature of temperament." When we have clarity, the intuitive faculty of authentic human nature is clearly manifested, and we have essential goodness. If turbid, intuition is clouded over and our authentic human nature is obscured. For that reason, we lack goodness. Nevertheless, anyone can achieve goodness if clarity is attained. For that purpose, there is a system of learning to cultivate our minds and our introspective abilities.

This practice-oriented system of learning dominated the intellectual life of the Japanese until they turned toward European culture. It was reinforced by amalgamation with Zen Buddhism and formed the style and structure of their consciousness.

It was studied in Japan initially as an abstract metaphysical system incorporated into formal education. It gained in importance during the early seventeenth century and was given profound attention not only in Oriental studies but also in the coupling of Oriental with Occidental studies, in a practical manner, during the latter half of the eighteenth century. The "enlightenment thought" of the Meiji Period in the latter part of the nineteenth century combined with it to produce an emphasis on blending formal education with the practical needs of daily living.

Morita's thought was presumably formed by the natural scientific recognition evident in modern medicine and by the practical outlook that underlies that recognition. His attitude of monistic empiricism brought him to attach importance to the whole modality of the *shinkeishitsu* patient living in *toraware* (self-captivity) rather than to sift through each of the various symptoms. The monistic overview of *shinkeishitsu* was more important to him than analysis of individual details.

His straightforward appraisal of human beings as they actually behave supported his intuitive insight into the attitude of *kizukai*. However, this attitude was not evaluated as essentially normal or abnormal. Morita considers it a universal human attribute and simply indicates the psychological reactive process by which the attitude can be empirically examined as the hypochondriacal basic tone.

The first question that may surface in that area is: What is the factor that makes the *shinkeishitsu* persona seem to be neurotic, or the factor that amplifies *kizukai*? A second question is: What is the relationship of self-solicitude to the desire for self-actualization?

Morita's reply to the first question would stem from his perception of "disposition" as the determinant factor. His response to the second question would come from his understanding of authentic human nature as possessing the inherent desire for self-improvement, for growth and progress. The fulfillment of that desire is essential to human life.

As the author sees it, however, self-concern over this natural desire is the point of origination of the hypochondriacal basic tone. The self-concern aroused by the desire for self-actualization is apt to give rise to the hypochondriacal basic tone and to lead to inner conflict. This is the disposition of the *shinkeishitsu* persona (also see Chapters 1 and 8).

Morita's straightforward, empirical perspective of human nature was constantly present as a supportive cornerstone for his edifice of academic knowledge. His treatment technique was an outcome of his cumulative clinical experience. However, his incisive insight was a powerful contributing factor.

In bringing this chapter to a close, the author wishes to summarize a number of the points that have been covered.

First of all, with the rapid advance of Japan toward modernization after 1868 (the year of the Meiji Restoration), social opportunities for the individual also showed a rapid advance. The Japanese who lived in that period struggled to raise their social status to the greatest possible degree. It seemed to them that everyone had an equal chance to get ahead and that they had complete freedom of social mobility. However, mixed with this individual striving, and exercising restraint on it, was the traditional self-imposed attitude of *kizukai*, with its sense of self-delimiting solicitude coloring interpersonal and group relationships.

In their social life, the common people were conscious of an aggressive desire for individual initiative and action. At the same time, they had an ever-present sense of self-inhibiting social solicitude. The conflict between these two mental polarities is, in itself, the original signpost of the relationship between the desire for self-actualization and the hypochondriacal temperament.

Morita was probably capable of recognizing that conflict–in light of its historical background in Japan–as the trigger of the *shinkeishitsu* disposition. He accordingly exposes it to open view from his straightforward standpoint.

3

Phenomenology of *Arugamama* and Orientalism

The sociocultural situation in Japan that underlay the origins of Morita's *shinkeishitsu* theory and therapy has been examined in the previous chapter, along with Morita's thoughts. In particular, the author discussed the hypochondriacal basic tone as the core concept of the *shinkeishitsu* theory from the phenomenological standpoint of the culture of *kizukai*. The author took a historical look at how the *kizukai* mentality was formed and how it gave rise to the Japanese predisposition toward *shinkeishitsu*.

In this chapter, the author will examine the importance of *arugamama* condition–awareness and acceptance of things as they are–as the guiding principle of Morita therapy and, as the underlying basis of its importance, its historical position in Oriental thought.[1]

Origins of Morita's Thought Process Concerning Human Nature

The author readily notices, in reading Morita's writings, that Morita has an academic orientation that is inclined chiefly toward the "live mentality" of human beings. The motivation that is responsible for that perspective and the process by which it was concretized and developed are of great interest. An examination of Morita's view of human nature can be meaningful in relation to the essential postulates of Morita therapy. Morita's studies of human nature can be construed as a lifelong academic effort to create his therapeutic system. Much of what the author covered in Chapter 1 was a summation of that effort.

Any such lifelong study is closely related to personal experience. Morita is no exception. In Chapter 7, this author will explain his own views on this point in detail. Here, the author will concentrate on how Morita's immersion in Oriental thought and experience was incorporated into Morita's theory and practice of psychotherapy.

As the author has noted, Morita's professional interest was centered exclusively on the actual mental activities of human beings. Through this focus, Morita first wished to comprehend the essence of human nature. From his perspective, human life is characterized by a mentality that continually asks: "How should human beings live?" This question contains a basic contradiction: that of imposing limitations on human life in a world that, in essence, poses no such limitations. Morita wished to clarify this dilemma through the application of a natura-

[1] "Oriental thought" refers to the Indo-Chinese culture of East Asia, which became the foundation for the formation of Japanese thought. Indian thought did not have a direct influence in Japan. It was transmitted through the medium of Buddhist thought translated into the Chinese language. It is probably most accurate to say that the Oriental thought of primary influence in Japan was of a Chinese cultural character.

listic scientific approach that he defines as materialistic. What he consequently apprehended as an intrinsic characteristic of human nature is *sei no yokubō*, the desire to live, which in relation to the hypochondriacal basic tone of human nature forms the character of the *kizuki/kizukau* mentality.

However, the more human beings strive to live a "better life," the more limited their options in living become. The essential contradictoriness between the reality of "what is" and the human desire for "what it should be" is a constant presence in human consciousness. This is what Morita means by "contradiction in thinking" (see Chapter 5). To have the individual become aware of that contradiction is Morita's ultimate objective.

He takes the position that if the characteristic attitude of the *kizukau* mentality accelerates the process of development of contradictory thinking, without the application of practical measures to handle problems, the autonomous, integrative function of the mind, which works to resolve conflicts and adjust actions,[2] becomes too weakened to maintain overall mental harmony. The individual is then trapped in disharmony. When the conflict of contradiction becomes uppermost, the *kizukau* mentality is inclined toward hypochondria, and the essential desire for self-actualization fades away in awareness. By contrast, when the inclination toward contradiction-conflict is reduced, *sei no yokubō* becomes foremost in awareness and functions as the prime mover to start the process of conflict-adjustment consolidations.

For Morita, *sei no yokubō* is ambivalent. It can be the prime mover of healthful, harmonious mental activity, or it can function as the prime mover furnishing power to conflict-contradiction "captivity" if the *kizukau* mentality shifts primarily toward hypochondria.

Morita based his observations of human nature on a naturalistic scientific type of cognition that posited the external world as an objective reality, without an overlay of preconceived value judgments. His insistence that we must "attempt to perceive the phenomena of the world as they are" or that "the fact in itself is truth" pertains to both natural and social phenomena. The efforts of the Japanese to search for and recognize absolute meaning in the phenomenological world can be construed as a search for the "roots of truth."[3]

Morita's naturalistic and, let us say, secularistic[4] view of nature and human nature did not seem refutable to him. As we have pointed out in Chapter 1, he experimented with a number of different therapeutic techniques and pursued them further only when they had objective, observable effects. Perhaps the most original facet of his therapy lies in his rediscovery of the therapeutic values inherent in the traditional, native psychology of the Japanese people during his experimentation with various therapeutic techniques.[5]

Although it is true that Morita's cognitive view of human nature sprang from a naturalistic scientific perspective, which included psychiatry, it is arguable that the Oriental wellsprings of his thinking served to support and reinforce his cognitive processes.

---

[2] Activities of conflict and adjustment in human mentality are discussed in detail in Chapter 5.

[3] Nakamura, H.: *Tōyōjin no Shii Hōhō* (Ways of Thinking of Eastern Peoples) (3). Shunjūsha, Tokyo (1962). (Printed in Japanese)

[4] According to Morita, there is no form of existence after death; to believe in human life after death is to labor under a misconception.

[5] Kondō, K.: Morita ryōhō ni kanren shite (In correlation with Morita therapy) (in Japanese). *Seishin Igaku* 17:1348–1354 (1975).

Phenomenological Structure of *Arugamama*

From that standpoint, the author can suggest that the special character of Morita's view of human nature appears most vividly in the actual practice of Morita therapy, which emphasizes strictly therapeutic values, as distinct from psychopathological descriptions of neurosis. The author will thus explore this special character of Morita's thought[6] by focusing on the structural importance of *arugamama* (things as they are) condition as the central guideline for his therapeutic system.

As has been explained in the previous chapter, Morita considers the hypochondriacal basic tone to be the cornerstone of his *shinkeishitsu* theory. Underlying the phenomenon of *kizukai*, which bolsters the hypochondriacal basic tone, is the human capacity for vigorous growth and development.

Morita therapy has, as its guiding principle, the intention to restore the human mentality to its original *arugamama* condition. Exactly what is that condition?

In the practice of Morita therapy, three factors stand out: (1) the patient's specific symptoms are ignored, to bring him or her into essential confrontation with reality; (2) the patient is induced to return to and accept his or her authentic human nature; and (3) the patient begins the process of self-realization within the context of actual living conditions.

The various symptoms are ignored or, in effect, left as they are for the time being. In other words, a Morira therapist does not attempt to resolve them immediately but leaves them in *arugamama* (as they are). A patient is guided to exert effort to perform the activities of living while in confrontation with his or her living conditions. This is a training process of reaching a subjective awareness of "here and now" on his or her own. The premise underlying the initial disregard of specific symptoms is that the symptoms of *shinkeishitsu* stem from the same roots as healthful human nature.

Morita had an intuitive understanding of the rules of internal order that integrate and harmonize mental activities, namely, the interaction of the desire for self-actualization, with its persistent impulse for growth and development, and the factor of self-solicitude as an expression of the struggle to fulfill that desire. These two elements are basic to human nature and cannot be artificially manipulated. This basic view of human nature espoused by Morita also suggests the meaning of "truth" as the recognition of what harmonizes the contradiction of life and death in human existence.

Restoring a patient to the original mental state of recognizing "things as they are" must include, of course, the patient's subjective acceptance of his or her authentic human nature.[7]

The third factor is to grasp that the action, *as it is*, that expresses one's life and moves it in the desired direction is to take place with a full subjective acceptance of whatever mental phenomena happen to crop up and then pass through the natural, ongoing process of sifting and assimilation performed by the mind.

Morita perceives mental activity as a process of ceaseless change and flow, quite similar to natural and social phenomena, which reflect the same unending change and flow.

In his words: "All phenomena of the universe are enmeshed in relative relationships,

---

[6] This peculiar or distinctive characteristic should probably be construed as an integration of the Japanese mental-emotional modality, or the style of life subsumed in Japanese cultural foundations, which underlies Morita's conscious knowledge or thoughts but which contributes, nonetheless, to his thought process.

[7] A. Kondō calls this "creative-passive activity" in Acceptance: Its meaning in psychotherapy (in Japanese). *Shinkeishitsu* 3(1):13–18 (1962).

adjustment activities, and 'balancing acts.' Mental phenomena are no exception. Our mentalities endlessly flow and change, never coming to a halt or becoming stationary for even a moment." Further, he asserts, "the mental phenomena experienced by human beings change in relation to changes in environment."

He points out that consciousness is invariably aware of "something more than what it has attained in any localized area during the flow of mental activity; we may forget something partially or entirely, or retain it vividly in memory" due to the nature of consciousness itself.

"Forgetting," he says, "is a function of human nature to free the mind from a present association, to sever a relationship with something so that it passes out of our awareness; it does not remain as a component of our ongoing mental flow; it goes out of consciousness altogether."

Morita does not accept the notion of mental repression. Whatever we forget or remember is, in his thinking, determined by the incessant changes of mind in the flow of time and space. Forgetting and remembering are one aspect of the constant flow of mind and represent consciousness engaged in retaining or terminating certain relations as it continually forms and reforms its own content in interaction with the environment. (This interpretation corresponds to the Buddhist conception of history as a process of chance formations of relationships. See Footnote 28.)

Morita's thought can be summarized as stating that mental phenomena do not constitute an individual, fixed object but, rather, that they represent one phase, or aspect, of the overall time-space conditions in which we live, conditions that constantly change and flow. The actual fact of the "human condition" is that we have a mental makeup that forms, develops and changes without becoming fixed–unmoving–for even one instant. In the same way that natural phenomena function in accordance with a "natural order" (the so-called laws of nature), mental phenomena form and change in accordance with an internal mental order. This is the core truth of human nature.

It is also the standpoint of Morita that characterizes his view of human nature. As Miyoshi[8] points out, Morita takes the position of "putting human beings into connection with a certain 'wholeness' in order to entrust their lives to the strength of something in human nature that is truly fundamental."

When Morita's concept of *arugamama* is viewed from that perspective, it signifies that we live on the basis of an "eternal law"[9] that maintains our basic human nature. If we accept this, we can comprehend that human beings cannot manifest their authentic selves unless they obey their essential nature.

Morita's position on human nature was the outcome of a Japanese type of thought process based on Japanese (and, by extension, Oriental) cultural foundations.

The author has attempted to clarify the meaning of *arugamama* to give this concept its proper weight for an accurate evaluation of Morita's *shinkeishitsu* theory and therapy. However , the term *arugamama* has a diversity of meanings in the Japanese language, which give rise to controversial views on its exact definition with respect to Morita's usage. With this background of controversy taken into account, the author will examine the concept of *arugamama* in more detail.

---

[8] Miyoshi, I.: Seishin bunsekika wa Morita ryōhōka tari uru ka (Kann der Psychoanalytiker gleichzeitig als Morita-Therapeut tätig sein?) (in Japanese). *Practice and Theory of Psychotherapy* 2:37–46 (1971).

[9] The "law" (*dharma* in Sanskrit) has a rather simple and comprehensible meaning. It provides a basis for human beings to become fully human without a need for external change. In universal meaning, living as one's authentic self is living in accordance with whatever one internally possesses for genuine human life. From the Confucianist standpoint, the basis for genuinely human life is completely furnished by Heaven.

Akirame (Resignation) and *Arugamama*

There are indications that Morita therapy, with its guiding principle of recognition and acceptance of "things as they are," is influenced by Zen Buddhism, although Morita denied it.[10] Nonetheless, the traditional philosophy of the Orient did have a definite influence on Morita's thinking, and his therapeutic system contains teaching material that embodies the essence of Oriental religion.[11]

Criticism of the *arugamama* condition in contemporary psychotherapy is common to the thinking of a large number of Japanese psychiatrists today. Most Japanese psychiatrists who subscribe to that criticism have the impression that *arugamama* is to be understood as a submissive, passive or relinquishing state of resignation (*akirame*). Another common trend in Japan is to advocate an acceptance of misery as a normal component of human life, in line with an overall acceptance of "things as they are." To the degree that misery is accepted with passive resignation, Morita therapy is seen to be effective.[12] Nevertheless, Morita therapy is attacked for allegedly advocating "obedience to nature and submission to environment," which can be construed as a reflection of feudalistic ethics taught to the general public to secure unquestioning obedience to both the natural and the social order of things.[13]

This, in turn, has given rise to criticism of Morita therapy for advocating acceptance of "things as they are" as a process aimed at fusing the individual–who is isolated and frightened by the protective matrix of his or her environment–back together with that environment.[14] Viewed in that manner, Morita therapy would have principles and goals quite different from those of Occidental therapy, with its emphasis on individualism and individual responsibility for one's life.

When the Morita's thought of "things as they are" is explained without a refutation of such criticism, it is hardly remarkable that one might choose to draw the conclusion that Morita therapy is, indeed, intended to induce a dependent and regressive psychological character, quite the reverse of the modern psychotherapeutic mainstream methodology of strengthening individual character to contend effectively with modern-day living conditions.

Doubtless, a number of Japanese psychiatrists do interpret Morita therapy in that manner and, accordingly, reject it as unsuited to modern-day psychotherapeutic goals. Much of the criticism of Morita therapy has sprung from Japanese advocates of psychoanalysis.

The confrontation between Morita therapy and the psychoanalytic school is not new. It began to take place while Morita was still alive. The dispute has had a positive, constructive influence in accelerating the subsequent development of Morita therapy and other schools of psychotherapy in Japan, as one result of the continuous, mutually critical dialogue.

Morita therapy and psychoanalysis have contrasting principles and methodologies. This is not simply a difference of logical thought structures but, evidently, stems from the great disparity in thought modalities fostered by important differences in the cultural foundations–Oriental and Occidental–underlying each of these two disparate psychotherapeutic systems.

---

[10] Sakurai, T.: Morita *shinkeishitsu ni tsuite no dansō* (Random thoughts on Morita *shinkeishitsu*) (in Japanese). *Practice and Theory of Psychotherapy* 1(2):3 (1969).

[11] Kasamatsu, A.: *Textbook of Psychiatry*, 602. Chūgai Igakusha, Tokyo (1959). (Printed in Japanese)

[12] Katō, M.: Taijin kyōfu wo megutte–Shinkeishō no nihonteki tokusei (On the problem of anthropophobia (*taijin kyōfu*) in Japan) (in Japanese). *Seishin Igaku* 6(2):107–112 (1962).

[13] Katō, M.: ibid.

[14] Doi, T.: *Seishin Ryōhō to Seishin Bunseki* (Psychotherapy and Psychoanalysis). Kaneko Shobō, Tokyo (1973). (Printed in Japanese)

There has been no meaningful concord between the two schools over the past 75 years or so. The various psychotherapeutic theories developed out of the psychoanalytic school may be fully integrated into Japanese psychiatry in the future. However, if this integration is accomplished, without a concomitant acceptance of the underlying premises of Occidental philosophy, the applications of psychotherapy in Japan will still be subject to criticism as being "Japanized eclectic systems which consist of packaging innumerable fragments collected together in a rather haphazard, irrational manner."[15]

Disputes relating to theory will continue between the two schools, without any constructive concord, as long as criticism of Morita therapy continues to be confined to a theoretical level. To move away from that, the author must examine, in more detail, the modality of thought intrinsic to Morita, with a special focus on the precise interpretation of "resignation" (*akirame*) and "acknowledgment of misfortune" (*fukō no shōnin*) within a system or instruction that posits misfortune or suffering caused by human beings as essentially the same as misfortune of suffering caused by the natural order of "things as they are." The author must further explore the grounds for contention centered on various interpretations of "reconciliation with the environment" or "reversion to totalitarianism," which give rise to criticism of the phenomenon of *arugamama* (conditions as they are).

In general usage, *akirame*[16] is defined as synonymous with *dannen* (resignation). It follows, in critical thinking, that the acceptance of "things as they are" in Morita therapy should be interpreted as inducing a patient to give up all thoughts of curing his or her mental disorder by his or her efforts and, instead, to submit completely, with unquestioning obedience, to the instructions of the Morita therapist.

The acceptance of "things as they are" is not, however, synonymous with "resignation" but, rather, is used in Morita therapy in the sense of "clear discernment" (*akiraka-ni mikiwameru*). It is synonymous with *dōsatsu* (discernment) and pertains to deep insight into the condition in which the mind is shackled by *shinkeishitsu*. In other words, *arugamama* is nothing other than comprehension of one's authentic human nature, a realization of one's authentic self. It is also a process of assimilation,[17] in which a patient attains self-awareness.

This is not a process of obedient dependence on the therapist. Such expressions as "candid compliance with the facts" or "obey nature and comply with the environment" are not intended to induce a patient into unquestioning resignation or blind compliance. Morita perceives that a

---

[15] Nakane, C.: *Seiyō bunka juyō ni okeru shomondai–Indo to nihon no baai–*(Problems in acceptance of Occidental culture–The case of India and Japan); Lecture, Oriental Thought 9, Orient and Occident II, *Bunka to Bungei Shichō*, 3rd Edition. University of Tokyo Press (1974). (Printed in Japanese)

[16] *Akirame* is the noun form of the verb *akirameru*. It can have the meaning of *dannen* (resignation) in the sense of giving up in situations that show no prospect of resolution. It can also have the meaning of *akiraka ni mikiwameru* (clear discernment) or *kuwashiku shiru koto* (knowing in depth). Etymologically, the latter meaning is derived from *satya* (the meaning of truth) in Sanskrit and signifies a practical principle of Buddhism. The condition of *arugamama*, which is the guiding principle of Morita therapy, has a meaning akin to that of clear discernment.

[17] According to Morita's view of human nature, all human beings possess the essential *sei no yokubō* desire for self-improvement and self-development. This desire is exhibited without limit throughout one's life, with a looking forward toward self-realization. Once a *shinkeishitsu* patient becomes aware of his or her symptoms, an attitude of considering the symptoms "foreign matter" appears (intra-self separation) and the patient becomes captivated by the symptoms in a phenomenological manner. As a result, the patient loses sight of his or her authentic human nature and falls into a captivated condition of fear and anxiety. The process for dissolving intra-self separation, that is, restoring *honrai no jiko* (authentic self), is also present in the condition of *toraware no jiko* (the captivated self). This process is manifested as the consciousness of one's mind taking a new turn. Morita considers the relationship of intra-self separation and dissolution of *mujun* (contradiction) as being the essence of mental activity (antagonistic action of the mind). T. Kōra (1958) remarks on this point: "When we strongly desire something, anxiety arises over the possibility that what we desire may not necessarily materialize. This process of conflict is essential from the standpoint of actual life; our actions are harmonized by the presence of this antagonistic action of the mind."

patient is suspicious of, and antagonistic toward, a therapist, owing to suffering from excessive anxiety, and these attitudes are natural phenomena of the human mind. Morita's intention is to bring a patient's mind to a new turning point, when the patient has reached the extreme point of suffering and hopelessness. This "turning point" is akin to a condition of "profound doubt as the beginning of profound enlightenment."

That process of enlightenment begins with a fundamental recognition of the facts of human mental activity. Contradiction and conflict not only give rise to mental suffering but also provide the material that the mind consolidates to create harmony, stability and rhythm in living. Without the presence of contradiction and conflict, there can be no mental growth.

Thus, the meaning of the acceptance of "things as they are" is quite different from the common notion that it signifies "resignation to misfortune" or "acceptance of misfortune caused by human beings as being the same as misfortune caused by natural disasters." Because the Japanese often tend to include a submissive fatalism in their mental makeup, they tend to conclude that what Morita means is consistent with that sense of passive, submissive resignation to misfortune.

Morita means that "facts are facts" and that misfortune is, indeed, misfortune. It is to be confronted and acknowledged as such. One is not to run away, negate and hide from "things as they are." One is to recognize and acknowledge the facts. In the instance of the human mind, the facts of mental operations are to be acknowledged and accepted "as they are" according to one's authentic human nature, in order to resolve problems.[18] A passive, dependent psychology of resignation is of no avail in that regard.

Criticism of *arugamama* thus misses the point if it is based on the notion that the Japanese are taught to resign themselves to human-caused misfortune as being quite the same as any natural disaster.

To see how absurd that is, we need only ask ourselves what sort of historical transitions the Japanese social system would have gone through if the common people, after the feudal era, had simply resigned themselves to accepting social misfortune in the same way that they had suffered the effects of natural calamities. It is far from certain that the great majority of the Japanese population was ever given any such instruction and guidance at any time.

The author cannot, on the other hand, deny that the Japanese do have a habit of *figuratively* equating man-made misfortune with natural dispensation. It is more reasonable, however, to surmise that this attitude arises from their characteristic life-style (the so-called monsoon type life-style in Watsuji's description[19]), rather than from any formal program of education and guidance. However, their characteristic stance of acceptance, or even submissiveness, is not passive, dependent, powerless or unresistingly persevering.

Likewise, Morita therapy does not define "things as they are" in association with unresisting submission to man-made events as equivalent to natural phenomena. Acknowledgment of "things as they are" is a process of discerning the actual facts and of taking practical action in accordance with the facts of one's human nature. Candid recognition and practical action characterize authentic human nature. Nature is what nature is. Acceptance of nature "as it is" gives rise to the sort of endurance described by Watsuji[20] as well as to decisiveness and a tranquil spirit of *akirame* (acceptance of facts as facts).

The author must take note that Morita uses such expressions as *arugamama* (things as they are), *shizen sono mama* (nature as it is), *shizen no kokoro* (natural human mind) and *junna*

---

[18] One of the notions in opposition to this concept is that of "sour grapes." The fox cannot accept the "as it is" anger, vexation and misery of his failure to get the grapes and tries to defend his failure to attain that objective by a process of rationalization.

[19] Watsuji, T.: *Fūdo* (A Climate–Philosophical Study). Iwanami Shoten, Tokyo, 23rd Printing (1958). (Printed in Japanese)

kokoro (authentic or intrinsic mind; pure-mindedness) as, in essence, synonymous. In this, he typifies a common Japanese tendency to make figurative equations between natural and human phenomena. If this is, indeed, characteristic of the Japanese thought process, it is evident that differences in modes of thought do occur between the Japanese and Occidental peoples concerning human relationships with natural phenomena.

It is true that Morita's thought of "things as they are" involves an attempt to understand activities and transitions of natural phenomena. His point of view is clearly nomological.

The author will now move on to examine criticism of the *arugamama* condition by interpreting it as a term that connotes a "fusion" of the human being with the environment, that is, a "coupling" of the human being with the "wholeness" of all things.

Arugamama Condition and Reintegration with the Environment

There is some truth in the remark that "attainment of the condition of *arugamama* brings the individual who suffers from a sense of alienation from environment back into a protective reintegration with environment."[21]

This idea can be understood by supposing that if "the condition of an individual who wishes to presume on someone else's love, but cannot do so, continues–this becomes constraint and prejudice, the reflection of which appears as captivation by *shinkeishitsu.*"[22]

An individual is released from the condition of self-entrapment by fusion, or reintegration, with the environment: the condition of *arugamama.* This line of thought agrees with the idea that the condition of *arugamama* is that of coupling with and reverting to something that is fundamental and holistic.[23]

A number of Japanese psychotherapists criticize the notions of fusion and reversion in Morita therapy because they believe it will engender a dependent and regressive condition that is not in agreement with their concepts of the "modern self."

What is this fusion and reversion, this condition of accepting "things as they are"?

The goal of modern-day psychotherapy is to produce, in effect, an automous human being who accepts responsibility for his or her life and who achieves self-direction in a condition of internal freedom. Nevertheless, the tendency to seek harmonious fusion with the environment and to identify oneself with something all-embracing is a powerful factor in the ethos of the Japanese population.

Yanagida[24] once remarked that the Japanese, during the past thousand years, had a style of life centered on reverence for power. This concept is similar to what Masuda[25] refers to as a "migratory bird disposition." Migratory birds aggregate in flocks; the weak birds obey the

[20] Watsuji calls the life-style of peoples living in the monsoon regions "monsoonic." With that perspective, he remarks that the cultural character of the Japanese has a double structure of receptiveness and submissiveness. He points out, as distinctive characteristics of the monsoon region, the double character of tropical and frigid climatic conditions, with such phenomena as the typhoon, which is seasonal but which also has an unpredictable, outbursting character. The double structure of a tropical zone that receives abundant moisture, and a frigid zone that receives little rain, is distinctive of the monsoon culture. Receptiveness and submissiveness are not patient, strong-willed or powerless *akirame.* Rich emotion persists while changing, the unexpected is contained in each moment of this persistent changing, and a frank and tranquil *akirame* is concealed behind an unexpected upsurge. This sense of *akirame* is not, however, at the core of the cultural character trend of the Japanese.

[21] Doi, T.: ibid.

[22] Doi, T.: Shinkeishitsu no seishin byōri–Tokuni toraware no seishin rikigaku ni tsuite (Psychopathology of *shinkeishitsu*, especially regarding the psychodynamics of its *toraware*) (in Japanese). *Psychiatria et Neurologia Japonica* 60:737–744 (1958).

[23] Miyoshi, I.: ibid.

[24] K. Yanagida (1875–1962) established the field of *Nihon minzokugaku* (studies of Japanese folklore).

strong ones as a matter of self-protection. Social and cultural changes have heavily eroded that disposition, but it is believed that it remains apparent in the tendency of the Japanese to live within tight-knit groups known as *nakama shūdan* (associative groupings)[26] or *seken* (a circumscribed world that serves as a personal sphere of reference and that delimits the range of one's activities).

Doi's definition of environment, in the sense of fusion with the environment, is precisely that of the *nakama shūdan* or *seken* environment. The style of life in this type of environment is governed by the principle of *kizukai* and is a modality for human relationships and activities. A person makes decisions within a system of self-controls that eschew shameful actions and that conform to the expectations of his or her *nakama shūdan* or *seken.* It is important to receive feedback from this environment to carry out one's duties with an enhanced recognition of what the group thinks about oneself.

In Occidental societies, the achievement of being a "modern self" is given priority. The notion of *nakama shūdan* would necessarily be construed as dependent and regressive. The considerable differences between Eastern and Western cultures in their respective definitions of the "normal self" in relation to other selves and groups have been frequently pointed out in the past. The development of self-consciousness in Europe and Western Asia, where life was centered around a pastoral culture attentive to natural features of the surrounding environment, was unquestionably affected and shaped by considerations of time and place. These conditions were determinant factors for human action. It was important to exercise self-assertion and to have an individualistic view of the benefits and penalties of one's behavior.

By contrast, a domicile-type life-style centered around farming was indigenous to Japan. Mutual dependence and cooperative thinking, rather than individualistic self-assertion, had priority. The natural features of the land were conducive to a collective spirit of *wa* (concord).

This collective concord embodies the concept that "everything occurs by *en* relation, *or* by *engi no ri* (the principle of *pratītyasamutpāda*)."[27] Namely, nothing in this world can exist by itself; all things exist in a "whole cloth" of mutual, interdependent relationships.

For example, one can become a parent only if parents and children exist to create that relationship. Likewise, relationships between males and females, and between life and death, cannot be excluded from this principle, which is one of *sōtai* (relativity): whatever exists must be apprehended in terms of mutual relationships.

The relationship between Morita's *sei no yokubō* (desire to live, desire for self-actualization) and *shi no kyōfu* (fear of death) can be discussed and apprehended in terms of that selfsame principle of relativity.

In Japan, the relationships between a person and his or her social grouping are also subject to this principle of *sōtai.* A person who belongs to a *nakama shūdan* does not display a passive dependence but, rather, manifests his or her individuality in the process of acting out the relationship between self and group. In this context, genuine selfhood is not possible if one lives a life of isolation and nonrelationship with the rest of the world. Selfhood is produced and manifested in a natural human life modality of interpersonal and social relationships (see Chapter 9).

In a universal sense, the notion that a human being cannot live properly in total isolation gives rise to the concept and consciousness of *kū* (a void)[28] or *mu* (nothingness).[29]

The concept of *mu* is exemplified in the individual mode of living in Japan. It is embodied

---

[25] Masuda, K.: *Minzoku no Shisō* (Thoughts on Ethnic Customs), edited with commentary. Chikuma Shobō, Tokyo (1964). (Printed in Japanese.)

[26] Yoneyama, T.: Nihonjin to wa nanika (What are the Japanese?). In *Nihonjin no Kokuminsei*, edited by S. Iijima and T. Sabata. Nihon Keizai Shimbunsha, Tokyo (1973). (Printed in Japanese)

[27] A basic Buddhist doctrine: everything occurs by chance relationships (see footnote 28).

in such expressions as *mushin* (nonvoluntary mentality) and *musō* (a mental condition of discarding discretion in psycho-physical movement; similar to *mushin*). These expressions are used in Japanese arts and military science and refer to a psychosomatic condition of impartiality, of an unrestrained mental flexibility that is free, elastic and wholly self-illuminating. It is exactly this condition that Morita calls *junna kokoro* (authentic or intriusic mind; pure-mindedness) and *hakarai no nai kokoro* (mind without design). This condition is the *michi* or *dō* (road),[30] which leads to the state of casting aside everything artificial and living in reliance on one's authentic human nature to handle and resolve whatever occurs in living.

The *mu* condition is strictly autonomous and noncritically active. It leads to the mental state of *engi no ri* or what, in other words, is called the appearance of the state of *nehan* (nirvāna).[31] The human mind becomes aware of *engi no ri* (i.e., the principle of *pratītyasamutpāda*). The opposite state is that of artificial self-assertion and entrapment in self-opinionated designs of the mind. This limits the optimal expression of selfhood; that is why, in Japan, excessive self-assertion and self-expression and considered improper, in that they are self-delimiting.

When Doi et al interpret the state of *arugamama* as an opening of the self to the universe of "things as they are," that is, a fusion with the environment, they can see that it leads to a recovery of the realization that in self-isolating entrapment, what they judged to be fearful and abnormal is, in fact, the self-liberating world of interdependent, mutual relationships of any one thing to everything else. The author believes, however, there will still be some objection, a certain disparity of interpretation of Morita's thoughts on *arugamama* in Morita therapy even if it is understood in this above sense.

By extension, the therapeutic goal that Morita set for a *shinkeishitsu* patient to achieve is a condition for living in which one has full mental flexibility, with the goals of self-actualization and self-development. One is imbued with the conviction that human life has endless potential or, in Morita's words, that "human life is hope."

To reiterate Morita's standpoint on *arugamama* and its importance in Japanese thought: (1) ignore the symptoms and confront the condition of *shinkeishitsu* itself; (2) return to an acceptance of one's authentic human nature; and (3) exert one's efforts to move toward a practical actualization of one's authentic self.

The mental phenomenon common to the *arugamama* condition in all three of these stages is the *attitude* by which one expresses one's self. It is the attitude of progressively discarding *hakarai* (fixed mental set or design). The author might call it, in other words, an attitude of temporary "suspension of judgment"[32] pending the attainment of the *mu* state of mind.

The attitude that Morita considers natural, which is one of discarding egotism and returning to (human) nature, is manifested in the day-to-day behavior of the Japanese. It can be understood as it is, with no need for additional comment or explanation. The concept of nature (*shizen*) is integrated in the Japanese sense of life. It has the same meaning in Morita therapy,

---

[28] The notion that everything on earth occurs and exists by *innen* (cause and effect) and that this in itself is not a fixed reality of existence. Nāgārjuna (circa 150–250, comes from South India) propounded the theory of *kū* (śūnyatā) along with *engi* (pratītyasamutpāda) and *mujishō* (aśvabhāva) and stressed its aggressive aspect. *Kū* is sometimes used as a synonym for *nehan* (nirvāna).

[29] *Mu* is not a relative concept in opposition to *yū* in the sense of being a negation of *yū*. Rather, *yū* is defined in association with *mu* as *mu kara yū wo shōzuru* (something comes out of nothing). That "something" is absolute and unlimited. From that standpoint, it is also called *michi* or *dō*. Chuang-tzu (a philosopher of the Chinese Civil War Period in the latter half of the fourth century) once remarked that *mu* is a negation of the knowledge and decisions made by human beings and that it is indicative of the ultimate goal of individual ethics rather than a metaphysical point of view.

[30] *Michi* is the teaching of reason and the fundamental concept on which human beings should rely.

[31] Suffering is transcended in practical terms by conforming to reality.

[32] The definition of "suspension of judgment" in this sense is the attitude of accepting any phenomenon as it is and setting aside any decision to cope with it.

in the sense of a "return to nature" (*shizen ni kaere*). For Morita, it signifies a condition of acceptance of nature, in the course of events, and expresses the authentic nature, in terms of the principles of the life of the mind and body, that is present in all human beings. It is not an artificial construct but, rather, a nature that is nonconscious and inevitable for normal human life.

Similar to the rhythms of other natural phenomena, human nature has natural rhythms that need to be recognized and delineated in the sciences of mind and body to comprehend the foundations, the essence, of a human being.

The conception of human nature as basically akin to other natural phenomena was already present, as a distinct point of view, in the literature of Japan's Man'yō Period (circa fourth to eighth centuries). The manifestation of authentic human nature is both *onozukara* (naturally spontaneous) and *mizukara* (of one's self).

In other words, it is a state of mental activity embedded in the recognition that nature includes one's self and that one's self is, indeed, nature itself. This conception of human nature as natural in itself, or as being as natural to itself as is anything else in the universe, is characteristic of the *dōka* thought (Taoism)[33] that has probably permeated the Japanese mentality with so much historical forcefulness that it is now simply taken for granted without reference to any specific thought process. It is not uniquely Japanese in origin but, rather, inherent in the ground roots of Oriental thought as a whole.

One particular facet of *dō*ka thought that is often remarked on is the need for assimilation with other natural phenomena, such as the growth of vegetation,[34] which lies at the roots of the Oriental thought process. The notion that human nature has an active participation in the evolution of heaven and earth existed in China ages ago as one manifestation of it, along with a sense of the importance of integrating the human being with nature.[35]

Morita's view of nature is similar in essence. The authentic nature of the human mind is restored when a person heeds the instruction to "let go of the self-opinionated mentality (*gashū*; ātma-grāha in sanskrit)" "and return to the natural self" or to "pure mind," as Morita puts it. The condition of the mind in a state of authentic human nature is one that does not require any superficial overlay of "presence or absence" of self. It is a condition in which self and mind are no longer enmeshed in a subject-object relationship. Self and mind have become an absolute "one." There is no division between subject and object, no opposition of nature and human being in any sense of "seeing" and "being seen."

Morita's standpoint on restoring the individual to this authentic selfhood rests on his absolute trust of essential human nature. In Morita therapy, this means a patient's restoration of trust in his or her human nature. To discard all mental artifice and place absolute trust in one's essential human nature, regardless of the consequences, is the goal of Morita therapy. This, again, is the condition that Morita calls *arugamama*, the condition of casting off the artificial ego and returning to authentic human nature. It is a condition probably equivalent to the *jinen hōni* concept[36] expounded by Shinran.[37]

The author might add that what Morita refers to as the self-opinionated mentality (*gashū*)

---

[33] *Dōka* (Taoist School) is a collective term for those who subscribe to the doctrines of Lao-tzu and Chuang-tzu.

[34] *Taidan* (A conversation) in: *Tōyō no Kokoro* (The Oriental Mind), edited by T. Morohashi and H. Nakamura. Taishūkan Shoten, Tokyo (1976).

[35] This notion appears in the *Chūyō* (or *Chung-Yung;* one of the Chinese classic doctrines) written by Shishi (Tzu-ssu; ca. 5th century B.C., grandson of Confucius). His intent was to explain the oneness of nature and humanity. This notion means that nature creates and fosters all things.

[36] This concept means being based on truth itself and that it is "as it is." Discard the activity of designing by one's strength. Leave all in the hands of *nyorai* (*tathāgata*; Buddhahood). It also means that a human being can discover his or her nature only by discarding and cutting off all self-designing.

[37] Shinran (circa 1172–1262) is a founder of the Jōdo-shinshū Buddhist sect. This sect is one of the most influential in Japanese Buddhist thought.

is the condition of the entrapped and captivated self. Even in a condition of captivation, however, the self cannot discard itself or its desire for self-actualization. What Morita means by discarding or letting go is the cessation of self-designed captivating acts. He recommends that the natural desire of the self for actualization is to be manifested as it is, in essence, without artificial mental set or design. The desire to live (*sei no yokubō*) is the essential motive power for self-actualization. Morita therefore directs a *shinkeishitsu* patient to recover essential trust in and reliance on the self.

When Morita discusses the "desire for what is *as it is*," he identifies the first stage in the recognition and acceptance of "things as they are." This condition leads to the state of *fudan bonno soku nehan* in Shinran's terminology. This expression means living in a constant state of carnal desire. This carnal desire should not be discarded but, rather, affirmed as exactly what it is. When that is done, the factor of *nehan* (the nirvāna mentality) comes into awareness. *Fudan* (daily life) is then lived in the process of confronting it directly, as it is. And this life is, of course, one's life here and now.

In the condition of *arugamama*, as Morita defines it, the mind has set off in a new direction. The pain of *shinkeishitsu* does not change, but it is now accepted with equanimity because the mental design that promoted it and drove it forward has been cast off, after the patient has been taken to the peak of suffering and then beyond it. Living conditions do not change. However, there is now a selfhood that is completely natural. The patient has returned to his or her authentic human nature. And to all of nature.

In Morita therapy, the human condition of *arugamama* is completely reliable. This conviction of reliability is reinforced in traditional Japanese thought. Emotion and will, that is, are considered natural to human nature. Further, the desire for self-improvement and self-development is evident in any attempt to recognize it as being internally present a priori. It is not an artificial construct. The implication of this desire is that it manifests the hope of a *shinkeishitsu* patient to return to the world (his or her *nakama shūdan* or *seken*) by means of an ethical process that the patient recognizes and accepts on his or her own. This ethic is motivated by a compassionate, empathic caring for, and by a sense of service toward, other human beings.

The psychological mechanisms that motivate this conception of human nature cannot be ascertained. However, it is probable that Morita's thought process in this regard was motivated by the trends of thought of the age in which he lived and worked. One of these trends was the influential "natural law" mode of thought[38] prominent in the late nineteenth-century Meiji Period. This trend appeared, in a cultural context, as the so-called Meiji Enlightenment. It consists of cultivating a self-loving, independent mentality and a free-minded independence, present together with an innate sense of ethics as the true nature of human beings.

Nakamura[39] points out that there was a trend toward acknowledgment of natural emotion and will in the thinking of the Japanese far back in their history. This trend can be described as an acceptance of the external, objective, natural world as it is, combined with a tendency to

---

38 The "natural law" mode of thought was not dependent on custom or legislation; rather, it was a regulation or standardization based on society or human nature and a correct reasoning based on harmony with nature. The Japanese natural law mode of thinking is considered as a sense of ethics existing within human beings as true human character. Under the influence of neo-Confucianism, this true character becomes the standard for social order and, at the same time, is related to natural reason as the original order of the universe. In the natural law mode of thinking called the Meiji Enlightenment, however, the characteristic features of human will and emotion, which should be inhibited according to Confucianism, were accepted as authentic human nature, together with a natural moral and social order. Consequently, the self-loving, independent mentality, or the free-minded independence (not shackled but genuinely free), was considered the primary attribute of human nature (self-love in itself is neither good nor bad but a natural feeling for self-preservation).

39 Nakamura, H.: *Tōyōjin no Shii Hōhō* (Ways of Thinking of Eastern Peoples) (3). Shunjūsha, Tokyo (1962).

accept the natural emotions and desires of human beings as they are, without any attempt to suppress or come into conflict with them. In the sense that the Japanese constitute a closed and humane social order, they do not perceive any loss of moral order, even if natural desires are affirmed or if Buddhist ethical precepts are set aside.

Morita makes no comment on the similarity between this view of human nature and the philosophy of humanism or on the affinity between the Meiji Enlightenment and the older, traditional Japanese thinking. However, the author can assume, to some extent, the influence of neo-Confucianist philosophy on Morita's thought process. (Refer to Chapter 2 for a discussion of the development of neo-Confucianist thought in Japan.)

The acceptance of the natural internal character of human beings was, for Morita, based primarily on his psychological and psychiatric methods of recognition. Combined with that, in importance, is the practical, scientific, pragmatic viewpoint that he adopts.[40] His materialistic, even utilitarian, concepts of value, and his emphasis on experimentalism, do not exclude the influence of the foregoing Oriental modes of thought.

The author can see, in Morita's outlook, one concrete manifestation of his constant emphasis on coupling naturalistic scientific recognition with what actually happens in human life, from an experimentalist perspective.

The keynote motivation of his continual insistence on "fact" and "nature" is none other than the entire body of Oriental thought that lies beneath it. Morita brought his patients into a condition of self-discovery through practical, everyday activities. In effect, he used techniques of "practical confrontation" and "practical inrush" of insight, with attainment of the state of *arugamama* as the final therapeutic goal. The therapeutic process rests on an essential trust in human nature. However, the culture in which Morita lived and worked, and carried within himself, was a powerful support for his therapeutic principles and methodology.

[40] Morita frequently refers to this viewpoint.

4

Psychosomatic Theory of Identity; Psychosomatic Activities as Natural Internal Phenomena

Morita views mental phenomena from a monistic standpoint, as was pointed out in Chapter 1. In this chapter, the author will examine that standpoint in greater detail. Morita's fundamental concept is that "mind and body are nothing more than verbal terms for different views of one and the same thing." Thus, at all times, Morita examined the functions of psycho-physical phenomena from a descriptive phenomenological perspective.

"Mind," he declares, "is simply the activity of life itself; there is nothing recognizable about mind except that activity. We have no knowledge of mind except in reference to human behavior: laughter, blushing, vocalizing, volitional thinking, moving the limbs, etc. This so-called 'mentality' is not a hypothetical entity called 'soul.' The fact that wind blows or iron rusts is a phenomenal change; if we wish to know how these changes occur, we take for granted the existence of certain causative forces or energies, but what we know directly is not those forces or energies, but only the phenomenon of the change as it is.

"This is also the case with mind. What we directly recognize and design, in daily life, are those shifting phenomena we display in our physical behavior. By analogy, if we see a fire burning at the tip of a motionless, unchanging stick, we observe a strictly physical entity; if we choose to view it as an active, changing phenomenon, it is analogous to what we call mind. The stationary stick with the fire at its tip–or a ring of fire visually produced by swinging the stick in a circle–are not different entities at all. The only difference lies in the way we choose to view things: as static or dynamic. The ring of fire is something created by choosing to view the stick and fire in circular motion rather than stationary position."[1]

From his fundamentally monistic viewpoint, Morita considers psychosomatic (mental/physical) activity as manifesting the natural character of a human being. This activity is free, however, only when one's life is a manifestation of genuine human nature.

Human beings realize more than the content of whatever comes to the threshold of consciousness, in localized terms, during the incessant process of psychosomatic activity. Some of the material brought into consciousness, for example, may or may not persist; it may be slightly forgotten; it may recede immediately and forcefully from consciousness; or it may remain as a deep imprint.

Morita rejects the notion that forgetting occurs by repression, as Freud maintains. He insists instead that forgetting is a purely natural phenomenon. Consciousness is freed and withdrawn from present thought associations by the process of forgetting. This is not a conscious option–to forget (or remember)–but is inherent in the natural operation of the inces-

---

[1] Morita, S.: *Seishin Ryōhō Kōgi* (Lectures on Psychotherapy), 1922. In *Morita Shōma Zenshū*, Vol. I. Hakuyōsha, Tokyo (1974). (Printed in Japanese)

santly changing mental activity of the self. It is not a process that is subject to the volitional activities of consciousness.

Kondō[2] later explains this: "In other words, forgetting is understood as one phase or aspect of the fluid changes in human mentality as it flows in the timestream. Material is brought into consciousness, as necessary, at whatever point in time the mind happens to intersect with reality."

Morita states that emotion, when "left alone as it is, or when it rises from natural activity as it is, will follow a mountain-type curve, going up and then down, and will finally disappear (into forgetting)." He also points out that "neither desire nor suffering can be clung to indefinitely, due to the fourth dimension: namely, the timestream."

The action of a healthful attentiveness is one in which "the whole mind acts with adequate efficiency, possessing a sense of caution (keeping on guard) which maintains a certain level of mental tension to prevent rampant release of any momentary impulse to let go and overflow."

For Morita, therefore, the changing, developing and flowing phenomenon of mental activity is, in itself, the manifestation of human life. It is a fact of reality. He considers "the activity of daily living as true human education, as truth itself." Life, mind, meaning, emotion, desire and attentiveness all function in relation to time–which essentially flows. He mentions that ideas, that is, the effects of concept formation, lead one to lose awareness of this essential flow of the mind in time. The author will explore this notion in more detail later. Here, the author wishes to examine Morita's psychosomatic theory of identity.

Morita's view of human health and of psychotherapy is, needless to say, embedded in his view of human beings. The roots of that view include his psychosomatic theory of identity. In brief, he advances the idea that "life is activity; there is life only when there is activity. If one views living as a 'still form,' then that 'still form' is what we call 'body.' If we look at the functional phenomena of physical activity, that is what we call 'mind.' Accordingly, 'body' and 'mind' are two aspects of the same entity, either viewed statically or dynamically."[3]

The close correlation between mind and body is, of course, a fundamental fact of human psychology. Changes in mind bring about physical change, and vice versa. This intimate interrelationship has been confirmed in numerous observations. In simple terms, bodily ingestion of drugs can effect mental stimulation or tranquility. Emotions of joy or sorrow, as such, arise as expressions of physical change and activity. Exterior changes correspond to internal processes. Such is the interacting correlation. Any number of theories advanced by philosophers have equated the mind/body phenomenon with the issue of "mind and matter." No end is seen to those debates, but in the final analysis, such theories boil down to some essential postulates of what is mind and what is body and, moreover, what is the cause-effect

---

[2] Kondō, A.: Morita's theory of neurosis compared with the psychoanalytic theories of Freud and Horney (in Japanese). *Tokyo Jikeikai Ika Daigaku Zasshi* 73:2077–2123 (1958).

[3] The prefix *mi* in the Japanese language is useful in grasping the meaning of Morita's psycho-physical theory of identity. The Japanese reading of the original Chinese ideograph is *mi*, but when read phonetically, *shin*. Both readings mean *body*. The prefix does, however, have a number of other meanings. In the *Kōjien* (A dictionary of Japanese Words, edited by I. Shinmura, published by Iwanami Shoten), the Japanese readings of *mi* encompass the following meanings: body, oneself, status, mind (or true heart), flesh, inner part of tree bark, blade in a sheath, placement of substances in covered containers and an actor's gesture. In general usage, *mi* means oneself, one's life, one's welfare, one's heart, one's character or one's lot in life. In combination, the meanings of *mi* range from *mi ni naru* (to put oneself in someone else's position) to *mi ni shimiru* (to feel something profoundly), *mi ni amaru* (to rise above oneself), *minoue* (one's lot in life) and *mi wo tsukusu* (to do all that one can). Implied in this range of meanings is that life itself, including the lives of individual human beings, whose minds and bodies are inseparably integrated, is subject to and circumscribed by fate or circumstance. Thus, although *mi* is essentially body or flesh, that is, substance as object, it also has the meaning of *oneself* as the subject. This meaning suggests the existence of mind and body as one integral entity. Although Morita does not make specific reference to *mi*, it is reasonable to assume that his psycho-physical theory of identity is based on this type of psychocultural concept.

correspondence between the two. We detect, in the controversy, the age-old conflict between spiritualism and materialism, as well as the notion of dualism, which defines the essence of each–mind and body–from two different points of view.

We also have theories of mental/physical parallelism and interactionism. There have been attempts to explain mind-body interaction by dual causation and dual effect, and other theories that postulate some form of psychic energy.

One point of view worth noting is that of Sakuma,[4] who comments that "the various manifestations of mind, or consciousness, as phenomenal facts that emerge in the sphere of intuition, as well as the composition of the body, or of various material substances, must be strictly differentiated from the facts of the non-intuitive sphere of phenomena produced by the dynamics of condition formation: in other words, that sphere of reality, concealed behind surface phenomena, which is not susceptible to explanation in terms of the simple realism of modern physics.

"It is necessary to first differentiate the spheres of phenomenon and function, and to examine the formation of the concepts of so-called mind and body from the perspective of reformulating those concepts and to clarify the conceptual causes of confusion."

From that standpoint, Morita's psychosomatic theory of identity is seen as a strong negation of the dualist interpretation in which objective and subjective, mind and body, are mutually independent–two separate entities causally related to each other in some manner.

Simple monism postulates a certain essence common to both, and in this essential sense both mind and body are nothing more than phenomenological forms.

Morita's monism, though, is of a quite different kind, and it may have been derived from the major advocates of "Identitätslehre" ("theory of identity"), who wielded an apparently immense influence over the science of psychology during the nineteenth century, specifically G. T. Fechner (the mind is an auto-phenomenon of the body) and W. Wundt (the mind is the integrated interior presence that we recognize, from the exterior, as the body). Morita's theory of mind-body identity does bear certain resemblances to these earlier theories of identity.

Nonetheless, the objective of Morita's theory of psychosomatic monism is to define mental/physical functionalism in the process of apprehending the actual facts from a phenomenological point of view. A special feature of Morita's theory is his discussion of the mutually integrative functioning of mental/physical phenomena.

In his view, the human being has a holistic nature composed of a kinetic oneness of external nature (environment) and internal constitution (human nature). It could be called "integrative anthropology" with a penchant for pragmatic development.

A different methodological position is taken on this issue in the actual application of Morita therapy. However, it can be said to resemble the notion of the "integrativeness of mind and body," which is heavily stressed by the mainstream school of contemporary psychology that evolved from Meyer's psychobiology and pragmatism.

The concept of the holistic nature of human functionalism is to be understood as a combination of mental and physical motivations, in which the mental and physiological spheres stem from the selfsame functional source and are directed toward the same objective.

Morita's psychosomatic theory of identity also takes the position of viewing, in an integrated manner, the whole human being as a living physical entity. The basis of his perception of human health is that health is present when "the activity of living exhibits strength, speed and endurance in conformity with existence and improvement" and "a condition in which there is neither excess nor deficiency." This condition is without reference to such adjectives as mental or physical.

---

[4] K. Sakuma (1888–1970) was a major representative of Gestalt psychology research in Japan.

Morita does not attach any special importance to such terms as self or personality in his definition of human health. The expression of what he calls *sei no katsudō* (the activity of living) includes self or personality as the subject. In his definition, adaptation does not mean simply reactive accommodation with the environment; rather, it involves a complex colligation of introspection, emotional and contemplative experience, sense of ethical standards and social responsibility. These are the natural interior phenomena of his psycho-physical theory of identity structure.

In conclusion, the author might say that Morita's perception of human health is based on a sociocultural *ethnos* that defines human health in thoroughly holistic nomenclature. Health can be ascertained only by examining all the aspects of any human being.

Holistic motivation aimed at constant improvement and development within the social systems in which human beings function is the basis, in Morita therapy, for psychotherapeutic goals. The goal of the therapeutic process is to instill, in a patient, a harmonizing of the inevitable need for activities in day-to-day living. This is an autonomous process of choosing, determining and acting, guided by the antagonistic effect of, on the one hand, sensitive impulses and, on the other, intentional control, within the context of never-ending mental contradiction and conflict.

5

Human Nature and the Incidence of Psychological Phenomena

The developmental processes of psychotherapy have contributed to an elucidation of the psychopathological basis of neurosis in relation to our understanding of human beings. This has given psychotherapy a more rational formulation.

How does Morita therapy stand up in that regard? How are human beings perceived according to Morita therapy?

In a previous chapter, the author discussed the processes of the conventional usage of *kizukai*, considering the sociocultural context of linguistic transformations relevant to what Morita calls the hypochondriacal basic tone. The author will once again briefly examine the meaning of the hypochondriacal basic tone in conjunction with the content of this chapter.

In Morita's explanation of the hypochondriacal basic tone in his book *Shinkeishitsu no Hontai oyobi Ryōhō* (The Substance of *Shinkeishitsu* and Its Therapy),[1] this trait is defined as an expression of human nature, specifically of *sei no yokubō*, the desire to live and self-actualization. The term originally meant "to mind or pay heed to." An introvert, for example, is scrupulously aware of his or her mental and physical distress and abnormalities, "minding" them too much. When this tendency is intensified, the hypochondriacal trait emerges.

Kōra reinterprets Morita's concept of the hypochondriacal basic tone in depth and, instead, uses the term "inadaptability anxiety." Kōra defines his concept as the mood in which an introvert feels himself or herself placed at a disadvantage in relation to his or her mental and physical states; in other words, the introvert experiences the anxiety of his or her inadaptability to his or her environment.[2] In both Morita's and Kōra's explanations, this concept is characteristic of a mental attitude by which an introvert takes swift notice of even trifling changes in his or her physical and mental condition and worries about them.

This condition is, however, not objectively abnormal. It is a normal psychosomatic condition of human nature. Nevertheless, an introvert tends to be psychologically uneasy, considering these mental and physical phenomena as disadvantages and handicaps.

Therefore, the psychopathological basis of *shinkeishitsu* casts light chiefly on the processes by which an introvert interprets essentially normal psychosomatic phenomena in that manner, along with the subsequent processes by which he or she begins to focus excessive attention on those phenomena, worries about them and is finally captivated by them.

The principal goals of Morita therapy are to free a patient from that captivation during the activities of day-to-day living and to have the patient discern that his or her captivation is subjective and fictitious.

The author will first consider how Morita came to understand what it is that captivates an

---

[1] Tohōdō, Tokyo (1928). In *Morita Shōma Zenshū*, Vol. II. Hakuyōsha, Tokyo (1974). (Printed in Japanese)

[2] Kōra, T.: Shinkeishitsu no mondai (The problem of so-called neurasthenia) (in Japanese). *Psychiatria et Neurologia Japonica* 42(10):755–796 (1938).

introvert, in other words, what it is that constitutes the therapeutic target: those psychosomatic phenomena based on Morita's descriptive definition of human nature. The author will also clarify Morita's view of human nature in more detail.

When speaking of human nature, we sometimes go beyond strictly human attributes and include such ideological considerations as individual rights, freedom, equality and intellect. In the present context, however, we are concerned solely with the facts of human mental activity.

Morita's views of human mental activity were, of course, derived from his direct clinical observations.

Our mental activities include a phenomenon that we may call antagonistic, relative or modulating action. This mental antagonism or relativism can be meaningfully compared with muscular motion. For example, the extensor and flexor muscles of the upper arm are called antagonistic muscles. When we bend or stretch an arm, these muscles work in opposition to facilitate the desired mode of motion–at a fast or slow speed, or in a strong or weak degree. If we did not have this antagonistic muscle structure, our muscular motions would be similar to those of a marionette. If these antagonistic muscles become too tense, spasms may occur and the arm will not move; if the muscles are overstimulated, tremor or convulsion may occur. If one of the muscles is paralyzed or becomes tonic, the arm will go into a bent or stretched state.

Mental antagonism is similar. When we experience fear, for example, we mentally oppose it. When we are praised, we may have a guilt reaction. When we grow rich, we may feel poverty-minded–fixated on the notion of wasting money when we want to buy something. Our will dictates the degree of strength we exert when we close a door or hammer a nail. These are all examples of natural mental phenomena.

It is impossible for us to regulate these muscular and mental antagonisms voluntarily.

When antagonistic mental action is deficient, behavior becomes impulsive, without restraint, like that of an infant or an idiot driven by simple desires. If the action is too slack, behavior becomes rash and imprudent, like that of a drunkard or psychotic. If restraint is too intense, freedom of speech and action is often completely impeded, as is characteristic of depression.

The confusional excitation or stupor observed in catatonia can be compared to a clonic or tonic muscle convulsion. Thus, it is evident that the various types of suffering and loss of mental freedom characteristic of *shinkeishitsu* will occur through obsessive concern over the antagonism between desire and self-control. In Morita's explanation, this antagonism of desire versus control, or one notion versus its opposite, is precisely what gives us adaptability to living conditions, so that we naturally work out our own adaptive actions. Morita considered this mental antagonism a natural action of the mind, a psychological phenomenon rooted in human nature. However, there is a widespread range and variety of differences in such adaptive mental actions, from the relatively simple antagonistic psycho-phenomena experienced in day-to-day living to situations of acute complexity. Morita studied these mental activities in the context of individual mental development.

The symptoms of *shinkeishitsu* include certain psycho-phenomena closely related to mental antagonism.

For instance, when we look down from a great height, we may experience vertigo and shudder, or we may even feel the sensation of having fallen. When we carry valuables, we may be fixated on our fear of their loss or breakage. We may feel anxious about ourselves when we receive news of the accidental death or illness of an acquaintance. All these examples can be considered manifestations of antagonistic mental activity. Because of this natural antagonism, we are able to devise practical, coordinative ways of living and to live a balanced life. The antagonistic, adaptive action is a sort of safety valve for our daily lives, something that functions in us as bio-positive.

By contrast, antagonistic mental activity functions in a bio-negative manner if we behave in opposition to this natural action of the mind.[3]

A person with a morbid fear of not being able to be perfect is likely to be anxiously fixated on the inadequacy of his or her behavior, even in such routine matters as mailing a letter, putting documents or other articles in a drawer or locking a door. Consequently, the person tends to closely monitor each action, to confirm that it is perfect. The person intends to firmly believe in the perfection of his or her action but soon wants to reassure himself or herself by repeating it again. Repetitive actions for confirmation of perfect conduct continue to occur as a result of the same inevitable psychological effect. Finally, to eliminate the uneasiness caused by nonconfirmation (quite apart from the factual content of any prior confirmation), the person is compelled to reconfirm the action again and again, which leads by gradual degrees to the formation of a compulsion. In other words, antagonistic mental action takes an impulsive operational role, snagged between the fear of imperfection and the opposing desire to prove that past, present and future actions are faultless, thoroughly perfect.

If, in a healthful way, we pay attention to the scope of our practical abilities in accordance with our natural mental activity, we can conduct ourselves in harmony with the facts of life and, as a result, antagonistic mental action becomes bio-positive.

By contrast, a person afflicted with *shinkeishitsu* combats his or her natural mentality and devotes considerable attention to setting himself or herself free of uneasiness, rather than behaving naturally, in consonance with his or her own mind. Consequently, the person's mental antagonism is bio-negative. In that condition, there is no harmony, no natural attitude. The person wishes to win the incessant assurance of the perfection of his or her conduct in opposition to natural mental activity.

Harmony and Antagonistic Mental Activity

Natural antagonistic mental activity leads to mental adaptability. In our life situations, we encounter mutually contradictory conditions. By means of so-called mental ambiguity, we compromise, to find a way out of any such situational impasse. An example is taking a trip by airplane despite reservations about the safety of flying. We compromise by giving priority to our travel objective, without a guarantee of perfect safety. We can also observe this process of compromise, in difficult situations, taking place in the mentality of a person afflicted with *shinkeishitsu*. This antagonistic mental activity is similar to what Frenkel-Brunswik calls mental ambiguity.[4] In her explanation, mental maturity is not defined by the presence or absence of mental ambiguity but, rather, by the method one uses to deal with it.

According to Morita, the difference lies in whether this ambiguous mentality is accepted as it is. The ambiguity is harmonized by accepting it without mutual contradiction. Free action then develops naturally. This becomes the mental motion of a mature human being.

However, if the ambiguity takes the form of a "psychological rigidity," all the problems of a life situation will be judged in absolutist, either-or terms: healthy or unhealthy, clean or dirty, safe or dangerous, good or bad. When relativistic judgment is lacking, what Morita calls *shisō no mujun* (contradictoriness in thinking) will become more intense. Klein points out that this

---

[3] Kōra, T.: Shinkeisuijaku oyobi shinkeishitsu to seikaku (*Shinkeishitsu* and its character) (in Japanese). *Tokyo Iji Shinshi* 2659(60, 61) (1930).

[4] Merleau-Ponty, M.: *Éloge de la Philosophie. L'Oeil et l'Esprit.* In *Me to Seishin*, translated by S. Takizawa and G. Kida. Misuzu Shobō, Tokyo (1966). (Printed in Japanese)

condition in itself is not morbidity[5] but may be termed a condition in which the ability to confront contradiction is missing. The thought process is often stalled and an absolutist confronts a wall because he or she tries to create a simple, clear-cut, either-or solution owing to this condition of psychological rigidity. The absolutist ends up going around in circles, having lost harmonic fluidity, the mental flexibility of adaptation to the facts of situational realities.

Various symptoms of *shinkeishitsu* stem from hypochondriacal feelings of unease (discomfort). Certain theoretical errors made about them arise from observation of secondary symptoms. The principle of psychotherapy for the management of *shinkeishitsu* places emphasis on practical learning through emotional experience rather than relying on intellectual understanding. Morita made extremely scrupulous observations of feelings and emphasizes consideration of the following points.

1. Feeling is one kind of reflection of human life.

Most people are prone to feel nervous on public view or in front of persons of prominent social standing or shy in the presence of young women of great beauty. Such emotional expression is a reflection of one's life and cannot be avoided or suppressed by the exercise of rational ideas. Most persons suffering from *shinkeishitsu* make poor choices in such situations because of their bio-negative mental attitudes.

2. Emotion will gradually fade away in a parabola if it is left alone, as it is, to run its course naturally.

Suffering, pain and anxiety produced by a particular stimulus will tend to fade away with the passing of time as long as a reinforcing stimulus does not arise. In Japan, there is a proverb: "If you wish to quarrel with someone to quench your own resentment, you must take the decisive step within three days." This proverb suggests that anger will fade away as time goes by. However, if we try to stifle and uproot that natural feeling, exactly that mental reaction of opposing and combating the feeling will in itself function as a reinforcing stimulus, giving rise to one powerful surge of emotion after another.

A fit of anxiety is a pertinent clinical example: the more a patient reacts in being upset about it, the more the anxiety will intensify and persist. Morita compares this mental situation to another proverb: "If one tries to smash a wave, then the wave, on the contrary, breaks into a thousand waves one after another."

A person afflicted with *shinkeishitsu* often seeks to resist unpleasant feelings, such as fear and anxiety, in an idealistic manner or tries to struggle free of them in various ways but in most cases ends up ensnared by the same feelings. This self-defeating process is thoroughly dealt with in the proper management of *shinkeishitsu.*

3. Emotion levels off and fades away once it reaches a peak.

If, for example, we eat, on the verge of starvation, the pangs of hunger, no matter how acute, soon disappear. A person suffering from *shinkeishitsu* often chooses ineffective routes to alleviate pain. The person may reveal painful feelings to family members to divert his or her mind. The person may cry to escape inner reality. The person may satisfy his or her resentment by smashing inanimate objects. All these actions are nothing other than temporizing measures and do not provide effective relief. The person, consequently, worries and regrets his or her actions. Therefore, it is essential, in the management of *shinkeishitsu*, to have a patient learn to live as naturally as is possible in accordance with his or her mental reactions–to accept the unpleasant feelings exactly as they are.

We need to learn from our emotional experiences that emotional events are reflections of the external, as well as the internal, world. Morita comments: "Once we discover there is no

[5] Cited by M. Merleau-Ponty; ibid.

way to run away, we have no choice except to accept suffering and to work out a new life-course which leads to a higher level of perception (*satori*)."

He also declares that "in treatment of *shinkeishitsu* the most important concern is to have the patient let go of his attempts to struggle to get free of the condition." He goes on to add: "In other words, the important point is for the patient to learn how to naturally recognize his mental actions for exactly what they are."

These comments may seem to imply a passive posture of accepting unpleasant feelings as they are, but this acceptance is not a merely negativistic *akirame* (resignation). The term *akirame* has the etymological source meaning "to penetrate," that is, to express a positive mental attitude of discerning one's present life situation. Our emotional experience is a reflection of a real-life situation, and we need to have a strong attitude of dealing with real-life situations with a desire to let our mental activity run its course (See Chapter 3).

4. Emotional intensity will be reduced when we become accustomed to any specific sensation.

When we meet extremely important or attractive people, we may be more tense than usual. When we express ourselves in public, we may become so serious that we experience palpitation. We may sweat or feel thirst, blush–and consequently take little notice of what other persons have to say. Or we may feel so absentminded that we cannot remember what we said. We do not feel relaxed in such situations but, rather, ill at ease. However, we do become accustomed to such situations if we experience them repeatedly and become less shy and nervous. In the meantime, we can still act to the best of our abilities. We often experience such situations not only in playing sports or while seeing theatrical performances, but also in our daily lives.

If we attempt to push down or evade the feeling of nervous discomfort, we achieve the opposite effect of feeling it all the more. If we attempt to avoid meeting the persons who provoke, in ourselves, the variety of sensations associated with nervous discomfort, we come to feel more nervous than ever before.

5. We cling to unpleasant feelings.

An emotion will persist as being unpleasant when it is associated with behavior that is incomplete. This is quite the same in content as point 3 but is the reverse phenomenological relationship. In general, we feel burdened down and discomforted when we avoid or do not do whatever it is that needs to be done. Any attempt to avoid work or study because it is difficult can give rise to suffering owing to feelings of incompletion. It is essential to make the effort to complete a laborious task, after due consideration of its difficulties. For example, a student with *shinkeishitsu* will not exert his or her best effort to master his or her studies. The student will attempt to cling to a pleasant ambience because he or she cannot settle down to study, cannot concentrate, cannot feel inclined to get to work. The result is that indispensable learning may be neglected. The effort that accompanies the learning experience becomes entangled with the unpleasant feeling of incompletion caused by evading that effort. This condition tends to cumulate, so that learning is experienced, more and more, as a tortuous burden. This redirects us to Morita's assertions that "we should not live on feelings but on facts" and that "we need to live as we naturally are."

6. We become accustomed to feelings garnered from experience.

We learn to have certain feelings by going through one experience after another. We gradually become accustomed to those feelings. We cultivate courage and develop confidence from repeated experiences of effort and success. We become accustomed to painful effort while we experience the subsequent enjoyment of success. A series of such behavioral exercises can be called operant conditioning.[6] If, however, we experience repeated failures after great effort, we may be unable to forget those unpleasant feelings. We become timid and fainthearted.

---

[6] Grossery, J. M.: Behaviour therapy: A review. *Psychological Bulletin* 62:73–88 (1964).

Emotional experiences, as we have noted, are closely related to our perceptions and our activities in day-to-day living. Such experiences become more cultivated as we elevate the level of our perceptions and activities. The cultivation of positive feeling is based on performance of daily activities and on the elevation of our perceptions. This approach was advocated by P. Janet with a type of mental exercise theory linked to the history of human growth and the development of human feelings. Our cultivated ability to appreciate and love literature and plastic arts, work and study, and other human beings can be traced back and attributed to the perceptions and activities of our everyday lives.

In healthful persons, sound and proper emotional attitudes are formed from repetition of experiences. A person with *shinkeishitsu* may, instead, experience an emotional attitude of withdrawal and escape as a result of repeated experiences of effort followed by failure, leading to the formation of negative feelings that disarm the person for the functions of living. The person comes to accept his or her mood as more important than effort and action. The person's attitude of "seeking" self-completion, dominated by idealism or self-centrism,[7] is intensified. He or she tends to evade ordinary day-to-day activities, to flee from discomfort or pain that accompanies those activities, and remains enmeshed in a net of suffering.

Patients with *shinkeishitsu* vainly aspire to an ideal standard of life. In clinical treatment, it is first necessary to allow such patients to learn that the higher the life standard they set for themselves, the greater the effort they must make to attain it–and the more they will need to experience painful anxiety. To alleviate their actual condition, patients must learn to complete whatever needs to be done, one item at a time, in the course of daily activities, and with the mental attitude of accepting whatever unpleasant feelings and worries that may arise.

Through such clinical training, patients become accustomed to affirmative mental reactions. Again, as Morita says, "the patient must live on facts not on feelings" and, further, "should live as naturally as he is." Success and satisfaction in living cannot be achieved without this kind of day-to-day behavioral exercise. Positive mental attitudes are cultivated from direct, active experience.

Aoki states that our most important attitude toward reality, the most essential feeling we associate with the motivation of human action, always has the dominant role among a variety of feelings. Therefore, if the more important attitudes associated with motivation provoke affirmative emotional experiences, the less important feelings of discomfort that occur simultaneously will not be heeded. We will not respond to those lesser feelings.[8]

Morita therapy provides a method for emotional coordination through the reformation of attitudes toward day-to-day activities. Morita remarks that no patient is obligated to love other people or even to be sincere in attitude during therapy, but in the course of treatment, a patient tends to become affectionate toward his or her parents and friends and even toward lesser living things like cherry blossoms or the fresh green leaves of the zelkova (*keyaki*) tree.[9] This process is indicative of human growth patterns and the development of human sentiment.

---

[7] Kondō, A.: Shinkeishō ni kansuru seishinbunseki gakuha (Freud and Horney) no riron to koreni taihi shite mitaru Morita no shinkeishitsushōron (Morita theory of nervosity compared with the psychoanalytic theories of Freud and Horney on neurosis) (in Japanese). *Tōkyō Jikeikai Ika Daigaku Zasshi* 73(10):2077–2123 (1958).

[8] Aoki, S.: Morita ryōhō ni okeru kanjō no mondai (The problems of feeling in Morita therapy) (in Japanese). *Seikatsu no Hakken* 129: 2–5, Hakuyōsha, Tokyo (1970).

[9] Morita, S.: op. cit.

Attention and Consciousness

Much of the time, we will not remember a sensation or an idea if it escapes our direct notice or if we pay no special attention to it. However, if we cling to it firmly, we will have a subjective fixation on our vision of it, regardless of the stimuli that we actually receive.

This subjective fixation is experienced as being the same in nature as the actual stimulus. This is why symptoms of *shinkeishitsu* are, in the final analysis, subjective and false. A sensation that is fixated in our consciousness will intensify if it is experienced as unpleasant and if we struggle to get free of it. (This point will be discussed in more detail in Part III.)

Physical and Mental Activities and Natural Phenomena

Our physical and mental activities are natural phenomena, and most of them do not depend on the exercise of our will. Nevertheless, it is commonly believed that all these phenomena can be controlled by willpower. This notion is especially prevalent in the instance of mental activity.

Only one type of physical activity is controlled by will: the movement of voluntary muscles. The only mental activity subject to willpower is that of selecting thoughts for objective ideas, when our attention is active and our thoughts are willed.

Natural thought associations occur by a passive process. We cannot foresee or precisely anticipate what kinds of idea will crop up in the ordinary stream of consciousness, always affected by time and circumstance. It is not possible to control this natural, incessant thought process freely by an effort of will. Our individual sensitivities to external stimuli, moods, emotional reactions, forgetting and so forth cannot be selected by willful option.

Feeling and Knowledge

Fear of death, anxiety concerning illness or disease, the worries that may arise from consideration of future prospects–all of these feelings are spontaneous human feelings. We may attempt to exert control, to suppress these feelings by means of informed intelligence, to put aside fears and anxieties by instructing ourselves that "men cannot bring their lives to full completion because they live in fear of death" or that "this snake at my feet is not fearful because it is not venomous." However, natural feelings, the fear of death or reptiles, will not evaporate by simply invoking intellectual suppositions or even actual knowledge.

We tend to adopt a stance of defying the threat of death. However, the fear of death is real, a subjective rather than an objective recognition and an emotional fact of life. Any attempt we make to set aside that recognition or to suppress it will not resolve the matter. It simply does not work. We are, in fact, afraid.

To take a lesser example, most of us do, in fact, feel uncomfortable, even "creepy," when we encounter a large caterpillar. This reaction is a natural spontaneous feeling. Our acquired knowledge may inform us that the caterpillar is not, in fact, venomous and that it will not leap at us. Our emotional reaction, however, is to back away and run off as soon as we see it in front of our eyes. We are, with the resource of acquired knowledge, able to approach the caterpillar, even to pick it up and remove it if necessary. Our capability of making tactile contact with the creature, despite our feeling of discomfort, comes from a harmonic interaction, a compromising compatibility, between our knowledge and our natural feelings. We can behave in accordance with what we both know and feel. This mental attitude is natural, experienced and acted on exactly as it is.

If, however, we attempt to approach the caterpillar with a forceful denial or suppression of our unpleasant feelings, with a grim insistence on "keeping calm," we fall prey to the artificial mental attitude that Morita calls *shisō no mujun* (contradictoriness in thinking), and that is the attitude that can lead to the development of an obsession.

These facts of mental and emotional activities are, of course, indicative of general psychological phenomena, not just special cases. However, because we usually consider such psychological phenomena as quite matter of fact, we are inclined to overlook the salient fact that they are universal human phenomena. We are then apt to make the mistake of behaving too intellectually or of acting in rebellion against these psychological facts. From Morita's perspective, any attempt to control psychological functions that are essentially not controllable by willpower can give rise to anxiety and other complications, leading to the gradual development of preoccupation, obsession, fixation.

Morita declares that "our objective and subjective views, our feelings and knowledge, our understanding and our learning from experience are often contradictory and inconsistent with each other. Each of these factors is different. They are not one and the same thing. If we consider them all identical, what I call contradictoriness in thinking will occur."[10]

[10] Morita, S.: op. cit.

6

Human Persona Goal of Morita Therapy

It is apparent from the history of the advances, setbacks and continual development of humanity that we will persist in working for endless progress and that we will follow the most promising routes to that end.

What is the key to continual advancement? It is none other than the creation of harmony. In the past, human beings have experienced hundreds of varied fortunes as members of the different races and peoples in human history, but it is the capability of adapting to live in harmony that has enabled human beings to achieve cultural development anywhere in the world.

Considering this historical reality, Shōma Morita never ignored the importance of human dignity as a vital force or the human capability of adapting to live in harmony. At present, as in the past, we live with ceaseless struggle and with the complications of life and death, peace of mind and anxiety, production and destruction, harmony and hostility, peace and war, good and evil, beauty and ugliness, truth and falsehood, love and hatred, all of which confront each other as polar extremes.

Continual advances in human activity have been attained by human wisdom supported by vital strength and the capability of adapting to live in harmony. Bearing in mind human history, Morita says that "human life is hope,"[1] with the implication of a positive and promising view of human life that sees each human being as seeking to live by his or her effort.

The basis for this affirmative view of life is that it is, indeed, a genuine way of life, so that all of us take into account anxiety and pain positively as inevitable companions along the way. Pain is part of the process of living with all our power. That is, the only genuine way to live as human beings is with the *jikaku* (self-awareness)[2] that we innately possess and to live as we are naturally endowed to do. To live as we are is one thing, but to come into accord with that sense and style of life is quite another. To that end, Morita therapy consists of therapeutic measures to put us in touch with our natural selves. Morita therapy is intended to create a human persona that functions effectively with self-awareness and without self-deception.

---

[1] Morita, S.: *Shinkeishitsu no Hontai oyobi Ryōhō* (The Substance of *Shinkeishitsu* and Its Therapy), 1928.

[2] This expression means that one learns one's position, ability, value, responsibility and purpose through involvement in situations: the situations are opportunities to discover oneself. The term "self-awareness" is apt to be preferred in Japan. The Japanese may be a people who value an attitude of self-awareness, as pointed out by Ushijima. (Ushijima, Y.: *Seiō to Nippon no Ningen Keisei*, Character Building in Western Europe and Japan. Kaneko Shobō, 1964). It is true that self-awareness is always solicited in Japanese society, although Western peoples do not require it in ordinary daily life. As one reason, we may note that the Japanese, in general, attach importance to belonging to a community and are extremely afraid of being placed in isolation. Therefore, they need to make evident their positions as individuals within the community to which they belong. Because the Japanese do not have a list of religious commandments to subscribe to, as Europeans do, and because they do not experience the judgment of God in respect to divine commandments, a Japanese citizen seldom acts as a sole individual with responsibilities to a deity apart from social context. Individuality is immersed in the community as one attribute of it. For this reason, each Japanese citizen may be anxious to have a worthwhile life as a contributing member of his or her local community, as well as his or her national or natural environment, and needs to be constantly aware, in situations, of his or her position within the community.

This concept is expressed by Morita: "This is not to say that we remain exactly as we are, but that we behave as naturally as we are." What needs to be emphasized here is the disposition of a patient with *shinkeishitsu* who is the object of Morita therapy.

As was discussed in Chapter 1, an inclination toward weakness and asthenia is characteristic of *shinkeishitsu.* Before Morita, it was thought that this inclination was a congenital predisposition, in other words, one that was genetically programmed. For this reason, *shinkeishitsu* was considered an incurable neurosis, subject only to superficially symptomatic treatment.

On the contrary, Morita insisted that *shinkeishitsu* is never characterized by asthenia but, rather, that it is literally *shinkei* (nerves) and *shitsu* (temperament) consisting of such psychological components as timidity, apprehension and vigor, with a pronounced tendency toward introspection and idealism, manifested as a hypochondriacal trait and as an attitude of searching for absolute perfection in all things.

The fact that persons suffering from *shinkeishitsu* exhibit such characteristics signifies the possession of a strong vital force, a powerful "desire to live."

Kōra also insists[3] that *shinkeishitsu* does not imply a tendency toward asthenia but, rather, that it indicates a complex mental constitution embedded in a powerful disposition with sufficient mental *sthenia* to resist the inclination toward asthenia. This character gives substance to the existence of that "desire to live" posited by Morita, revealing the essential strength of the ego in a person with *shinkeishitsu.*

A number of neo-Freudians, such as Horney,[4] as well as some existentialists, such as Frankl, have switched their interest in neurosis from the pathological aspects of each neurotic symptom to the whole personality of the neurotic patient. These therapists show a marked inclination to recognize a patient's creative and constructive abilities and the mental dignity and freedom with which the patient struggles for self-improvement.

Morita paid keen attention to the essentially sound personality of a patient with *shinkeishitsu* and used therapeutic measures designed to point the patient's persona toward genuine self-discovery and self-realization through day-to-day experience. Morita's understanding of *shinkeishitsu* is that such patients do have an essential desire to elevate and improve themselves assiduously.

Morita expresses this desire as the "desire to live," with the principle of Morita therapy being that of gaining a developmental realization of one's desire by first attaining the mental state of *arugamama* (leaving the symptoms as they are and leading life as it is).

With that in mind, we must examine certain problem areas closely related to that principle of Morita therapy in terms of the type of persona that is the goal of the treatment program.

Means of Release from Contradictoriness in Thinking

Contradictoriness in thinking (*shisō no mujun*) is a mental state identified by Morita, and it indicates a human psychological situation of opposing the actualities of human mentality and, instead, fantasizing what one supposedly should be or could be. Morita explains that, in this state,[5] thought is essentially construed as consisting of concepts based on description or inference of facts, and an idea is a mental symbol of the situation. Thoughts are somewhat like

[3] Kōra, T.: Shinkeisuijaku oyobi shinkeishitsu to seikaku (*Shinkeishitsu* and its character) (in Japanese). *Tōkyō Iji Shinshi* 2659(60, 61) (1930).

[4] Horney, K.: *New Ways in Psychoanalysis*, London (1939).

[5] Morita, S.: op. cit.

images reflected in a mirror. In themselves, they have no objective substance, no concrete reality.

If one does not know the difference between idea and substance, and if one intends to materialize a fact in accordance with an idea, or to manipulate the fact to change it, a situation of contradictoriness in thinking will often occur.

In general, our subjective and objective views, our feelings and knowledge, our understanding and learning are frequently inconsistent with one another. Each element of the combination should not be viewed as identical. If each one of these disparate elements is not clearly distinguished from all the others, the result will be contradictoriness in thinking. There are, however, no genuine differences among any of them if we respond in the manner of setting aside any unnatural, antagonistic mental reactions. Because immense discrepancies can arise in the process of our mental development and as our thought patterns become firmly set, a thousand centimeters of discrepancy first begin with a mere millimeter.

One feels pain when receiving a medical injection or feverish when suffering from influenza. Both the stimulus and the reaction respond to each other. Subjective and objective views are consistent with each other.

The symptom of *shinkeishitsu* is a type of mentally captivating phenomenon (*toraware*) that includes obsession, with indications of strong adhesion to fixed notions of sensation. The actual nature of *toraware*, and of *arugamama*, can be grasped through Morita's concept of contradictoriness in thinking, which in essence is the complication that intrudes between the thoughts and ideas of a person with *shinkeishitsu* and the actual facts of his or her psychological situation.

This complication may bring about the condition of captivity and may consist of no more than the mental material that obtrudes between a person's actual self-consciousness (the consciousness of what Kōra calls inadaptibility anxiety)[6] and that idealized self-consciousness for which the person endlessly yearns and searches (an ego ideal projected from negative thoughts or ideas). The latter mental construct of an ideal self, a type of idealistic dogmatism, is objectively considered to set a high standard for one's persona, but it is subjectively by no means a high standard. It is the standard of being an ordinary, healthy human being.

However, a person afflicted with *shinkeishitsu* believes that his or her image of his or her actual self, in reality, is subnormal or subaverage or that it might even be abnormal. Such a person never notices that he or she maintains an erroneous standard for his or her behavior, which may give rise to contradictoriness in thinking.[7]

In Morita's words, a story in a dream is an illusion, null and void. Discrimination between right and wrong in a state of delusion is likewise null and void. A complicated mental condition of this kind can be construed as an obstacle, a sort of mental static that "jams" a person's intellectual attitude.[8] At one time, Morita classified this mental condition as one variation of *shinkeishitsu* that he called "hypochondriacal misconception." This obstacle of intellectual attitude is, in itself, a secondary mental phenomenon, however, not a primary phenomenon.

The condition that Kōra calls inadaptibility anxiety, a mental condition in which a person suffering from *shinkeishitsu* will evaluate his or her mental and physical situation as disadvantageous to day-to-day life, is ordinarily considered a mental block. However, it is a secondary mental phenomenon.

---

[6] Kōra, T.: Shinkeishitsu no mondai (The problem of so-called neurasthenia) (in Japanese). *Psychiatria et Neurologia Japonica* 42(10): 755–796 (1938).

[7] Kōra, T., et al.: Zen no igakuteki shinrigakuteki kenkyū (The medical and psychological studies of Zen). In *Essays in Commemoration of Takehisa Kōra's Appointment as Professor Emeritus*, 1964. (Printed in Japanese)

[8] Ikeda, K.: Morita shinkeishitsu to ryōhō (Morita *shinkeishitsu* and treatment) (in Japanese). *Seishin Igaku* 1(7) (1957).

The idealistic, perfectionistic attitude that Kondō (cf. Chapter 5) examines is not, then, a phenomenon of primary mentality but, rather, a resultant epiphenomenon. If contradictoriness in thinking occurs because of a primary intellectual obstacle, the problem could be resolved by theoretical persuasion and intellectual instruction given to a patient with *shinkeishitsu*, as postulated by Dubois. In actual practice, however, any such approach directed primarily to the intellect will result in further aggravation of the patient's symptoms of neurosis.

Contradictoriness in thinking is, after all, a secondary phenomenon developed out of the emotional attitude of the *kizukai*-type hypochondriacal basic tone identified by Morita. The psychopathological mechanisms of the development of the symptom of *shinkeishitsu* will be discussed later. In this chapter, we wish to define the process of extinguishing contradictoriness in thinking, which develops as a secondary symptom stemming from the hypochondriacal basic tone, to inculcate the mental state of *arugamama* (cf. Part VI).

A patient with *shinkeishitsu* cannot attain the mental state of *arugamama* through a process of intellectual comprehension. Freedom from contradictoriness in thinking is acquired by means of a new manner of cognition cultivated through day-to-day practical exercises that serve to induce the mental state of living in *arugamama*, with a cumulation of mental experiences that give daily living both interest and stability.

As a result, the patient begins to feel that living is worthwhile and experiences a sense of satisfaction. The intuitive understanding that a profoundly serious "desire to live" is characteristic of a patient with *shinkeishitsu* clearly underlies our expectation of the efficacy of Morita therapy. What Morita expects from a patient, by means of the psychotherapeutic program, is nothing other than full recognition of that desire to live.

Return to Nature

Morita often advised a patient to "be obedient to nature or the environment" or to "return to nature." This nature does not signify an external environment outside the ordinary context of human life and culture; rather, it indicates the internal human nature in which normal psychological phenomena occur naturally in any given situation.

Because it is essentially impossible for us to contend against our spontaneous mental reactions, we must come to accept them and to live for the sake of self-realization, and we also must desire to live in *arugamama*, that is, to live as naturally as we naturally are.

Morita describes the state of *arugamama* as "pure mind" bereft of self-deception and misguided management. This state is not one of sentimental self-indulgence or of relinquishment of wants and needs. It is not a negative state of mind characterized by lack of independence. It is positive, a state of mind in which we exert effort to live in concord with our naturally self-assertive human spirit. We cannot simply eliminate contradictoriness in thinking by wishing it away or by any willful intellectual process. Likewise, we cannot quickly achieve the mental state of *arugamama* simply because we are instructed to behave in alignment with that type of mentality.

The acquisition of the state of *arugamama* is an eventual rather than an immediate benefit. In that connection, Morita says that "since we become stuck to something due to certain reasons for doing so, we had better stay stuck to it as we are, without struggling to become unstuck. The adhesion will gradually disappear, because we are bound to respond to external stimuli and to adapt ourselves to them."

It is of no use to contend against the mental reactions that occur when we are stuck to something. That attitude of contrariness can intensify the adhesion. A patient afflicted with *shinkeishitsu* attempts to escape from troubles concordant with the contradictoriness in thinking that is caused by his or her internal struggle and, consequently, falls into a state of captivation with a deficient mental flexibility.

For instance, such a patient cannot concentrate on reading. Sounds around the patient disturb his or her reading. The noisier the surroundings, the harder the patient struggles to shut out the noise. This struggle induces an acute sensitivity to sound and produces nervousness. The patient makes one effort after another not to listen to sounds but does not know how to shut them out. A last resort might be stuffing cotton in the ears and then listening all the more intently. The patient's attention is fixated on noise, whether or not he or she actually hears sounds. At this point, the patient is much too nervous to continue reading. The cotton in the patient's ears becomes another distracting nuisance. The patient's original intention of reading is now remote from his or her center of attention.

It is true that noises heard while reading can be an irritant, but it is of no use to do battle against the sounds. The natural *arugamama* state is to continue reading without the distraction of manufacturing internal contention. In the natural state, the reader gradually becomes accustomed to the noise, can continue to concentrate on reading, develops increasing interest in the content of the reading matter and finally becomes wholly absorbed in the function of reading.

Morita comments on this point: "One's mind will move according to circumstances, and the mental reactions are quite subtle and profound. If one accepts and learns what nature is, one will reach a heightened level of perception without anxiety."

In other words, one's mind changes as circumstances change. This process is both profound and delicate because the incessant flow of the mind is smooth, natural and unrestricted, like a bell that rings faintly when struck gently or that peals out when struck forcefully. It is like an image reflected in a mirror, when standing in front of the mirror, but there is no image to be seen when it is not reflected.

We can experience our natural existence as we are if we live in accord with the natural motion of our minds. Anxiety, when it occurs, is accepted as anxiety. Delight is delight. There is no need to be intentionally anxious. We cannot control the natural flow of our mental reactions with the imposition of thoughts or ideas.

Morita's synonym for the state of *arugamama* is *jijitsu-hon'i*.[9] We will discuss the meaning of the latter term later. For the moment, we need to examine the problem that crops up from the mental attitude of "obedience to nature." We have explained what obedience to nature signifies: an attitude of positive intention to accept our human nature and our surroundings. However, we must deal with the objection that such obedience or acceptance is a matter of "Oriental mentality" that is not possible for other, non-Oriental peoples to induce and experience. Let us point out, in that regard, that many Japanese neurotics find it extremely difficult to gain access to the *arugamama* state of mind. The problem of becoming natural is, in fact, universal.

Morita therapy eases the way for patients suffering from *shinkeishitsu* to perceive the importance of obedience to nature, through their experience of absolute, isolated bed rest. This topic is described in more detail in Part IV.

We have, of course, considered the so-called fundamental spiritual differences between Oriental peoples and Occidental peoples, and we do not believe that non-Oriental peoples are per se excluded from coming into a state of obedience to nature. Occidental peoples tend to subscribe to a view of life that stipulates that human dignity is based on the possibility of

---

[9] Morita divides the attitudes of the mind in living into three types: *kibun-hon'i*, *richi-hon'i* and *jijitsu-hon'i*.

exerting human control over nature and the environment by an effort of human will and by expanding the sphere of human activity.

The basic Oriental view of life is that human beings can attain their subjective potentials and become noble-minded through a process of coming into accord with nature, adapting to the environment and learning to live in harmony with their surroundings.

European philosophy has placed human beings in opposition to external nature and analyzes any object of cognition from a rational, objective point of view. This mental methodology has formed the underpinnings of European thought since Bacon first proposed it. In fact, it originated in the ancient Greek civilization, where it was called positive humanism. According to Hegel, the ancient Greek spirit is one of a noble, beautiful persona mentally created to reform nature in the pursuit of human self-expression.

This sense of cognition was transmitted from the Greeks to the Romans and later resurfaced to spur the Renaissance. It has continued to hold sway to the present. It vanished only during the Dark and Middle Ages in Western Europe.[10]

The Oriental cognitive methodology does not place human beings in opposition to nature in the Occidental manner but tends, instead, to seek for harmonizing of the human self, to exercise intuitive perception of natural beauty and the essence of things and to cultivate a cognitive faculty integratively by fusion and unification with nature.

These differences in the view of life between Oriental peoples and Occidental peoples are clearly recognizable in historical developments. This is specifically true of the development of psychotherapeutic systems. For example, the differing standpoints are strikingly contrasted by comparison of psychoanalysis and Morita therapy, in both theoretical and technical content. In psychoanalysis, Freud constructed a topological segmentation of the nonconscious mental realm, introduced a concept of mental apparatus that Oriental peoples call depersonification and attempted to elucidate, in a rational theoretical manner, the realm of human mental phenomena within a construct of general principles.

Further, Freud tried to have a patient gain human freedom and creativity by a temporary extension of self-consciousness and thus to bring whatever involuntary impulse that was the motivating factor of the patient's symptoms under the patient's control.

This Freudian methodology arose from Freud's view of life: that the human self has, in itself, an identity and that identity has the same type of existence as any other objective substance. On that point, Binswanger[11] comments that Freud's psychoanalytic theory could be deduced from the theory of *homo natura.* The view of life based on the *homo natura* notion is that a human being is a mechanical apparatus, with its interior hidden in deep shade.

Morita therapy is different in that it is based on the life-affirmative standpoint that a patient with *shinkeishitsu* does not have a pathological personality. Accordingly, a patient undergoing Morita therapy learns to tolerate anguish and anxiety, to accept those feelings as they are and then to live in the mental state of *arugamama.* Thus, any comparison between Freudian psychoanalysis and Morita therapy reveals striking divergences in the life views of the two men, the Occidental in contrast to the Oriental, particularly in the management of *shinkeishitsu.*

Morita therapy imbues a patient with a mental attitude of enduring and accepting pain as it is. Wendt and one other group of therapists point out the distinction in principle between Morita's approach and those of the Western world's schools of psychotherapy.[12,13]

---

[10] Higashiyama, K.: *Fūkei to no Taiwa.* Shinchōsha, Tokyo (1967). (Printed in Japanese)

[11] Binswanger, L.: Erinnerung an Sigmund Freud und Mein Weg zu Freud (published in *Der Mensch in der Psychiatrie*); Translated into Japanese by N. Takeuchi and M. Takeuchi. Modern Psychoanalysis Series; Iwasaki Gakujutsu Shuppansha, Tokyo (1969).

[12] Wendt, I.Y.: *Zen, Japan und der Westen.* Paul List Verlag, Munich (1961).

[13] Kumasaka, Y.: Discussion of Morita therapy. *International Journal of Psychiatry* 1(4) (1965).

Wendt also comments that Morita therapy will never be replaceable by the psychoanalytic technique and that it is likely that Morita therapy could have the role of affording someone who does not find life worth living an opportunity to exhibit his or her inner creative vital force.

Wendt recognizes, too, that it is immensely difficult to apply Morita therapy to Occidental patients because of the disparities we have discussed. It is still, however, worth examining the possible application of Morita therapy to the treatment of non-Japanese patients. The obstacles may not, after all, prove to be insuperable because any factor that draws a person into *shinkei-shitsu* captivity can be considered a universal human psychophysiological phenomenon.

For instance, we all feel that filth is filthy, any one of us can be suddenly panic-stricken when standing on a lofty height or feel anxious about the possibility of illness when we hear news of the sudden death of someone we know, we are all afraid of breaking a fragile and valuable object when we handle it or worry about whether or not we shut and locked the door when we left the house.

These mental reactions are fundamental and universal in human beings. It is not possible for any of us to live volitionally in contention with such mental reactions by the exercise of will-power, even if the reactions make us feel uncomfortable. It is inevitable that we feel lonely or anxious about aging. And nothing is accomplished by trying to defy those reactions.

A healthy person can behave in a way that will concretize his or her desires in life by accepting those mental reactions as they are. Morita often mentions that the correct form of acceptance is equivalent to nonacceptance. If we acknowledge our concern for aging as it is, and continue to live with all our strength, we will feel as though we do not have a fear of death and will thus live as though we were free of it. Morita says that our desire to live and our fear of death are two faces of the same coin, having the interrelationship of either the subject or the background of a painting.

It is obvious that the various mental reactions that originate from the desire to live and the fear of death cannot be voluntarily controlled by will. This is true of all human beings. When we consider this, we begin to see that it is incorrect to suppose that it is possible only for the Japanese to come into obedience to the dictates of nature.

The Western world's view of life and the world, constructed on the foundations of positivism and the speculative philosophy developed in the nineteenth century, beginning with the rationalism of the eighteenth century, construes the call for obedience to nature and the environment as a concept that denies the dignity of the human rational faculty.

According to that Western viewpoint, nature should be controlled by human reason because reason is the basis for creating the human world and for the pursuit of eternal truths. Even if we say, in imitation of Pascal, that rationalism of that genre is no more than a comedy of thought, we can still admit that the ability to think is humanity's basic asset. However, we should not forget to think, first, of what it is to be human and to learn the lesson of Pascal that man is a reed, the weakest reed in the world.

Some people go through life without perceiving that fact of human life. As a result, those people lose their human sensibility and simply attempt to live in accordance with concern for other people's opinions, behaving out of a need to be appreciated, glossing over the unnatural character of that kind of fictitious human existence but living under the pressure of it all the time, disregarding the very real imperatives of a genuine human life.

We need to acknowledge within ourselves the anxiety that we experience about the meaning of our existence. In Morita's interpretation, we continually live with certain feelings of unease. Therefore, from the outset, we should bear in mind that man is a weak creature and learn to behave as naturally as we can. By doing so, we can develop our sensibility of a real and natural existence without resorting to self-deception.

Implications of Morita Therapy

In Morita therapy, we expect the natural manifestation of the human desire to live to emerge in the natural attitude of human beings, in the state of *arugamama*. This includes the state of mind of the Morita psychotherapist. It is the attitude that Morita calls *jijitsu-hon'i*. The concept of the hypochondriacal basic tone, which is an intuitive concept, is the basis for Morita's concept of the desire to live, a concept that has directional valuation.

When Morita mentions living as naturally as one is, or the desire to live, he is not referring to any instinctive impulse but, rather, to a manifestation of human mentality that lies beyond instinct. The essence of this concept is not analyzable because it rests in the primary, nonconscious mentality. However, it does exhibit a variety of phenomenal orientations that are identifiable.

Occidental people often have an attitude toward God that makes them say: "There is nothing other than the existence of God that can ordain the value of the human spirit and the significance of human life." In other words, the self has a God-given destiny, and even "If a man were not created by God, why couldn't he still be happy simply by being together with God?"

In Japan, there is no comparable concept of absolute subjection to an all-powerful deity. The Japanese have a religious or ethical system composed of filial piety, with obligations that arise from a system of ancestor veneration. This traditional system hardly seems workable as a basis for modern-day ethical standards needed to guide and regulate the private and social conduct of a human being.

The spirit of death in Japan is conventionally called God or Buddha and is an active presence in day-to-day mentality, so that it is possible to feel that happiness is due to the protection of the spirit of the dead. In fact, this conviction sometimes serves as a sort of standard for living.

Because the contrast between the nature of God in Japan and in the Western world is not our major subject of consideration, we will not delve too far into it. However, when we consider what to do and how we intend to realize the true nature of the self, there is a need to establish some sort of criterion, a basis for spiritual civilization.

Questions relating to human spirituality have been considered, first and foremost, as the problems of living human beings, but we are also sometimes apt to examine the general subject in itself, isolating it from the specific problems of each person.

To avoid generalization of concepts as much as is possible, we need to take a look at the image of a human being living in modern society. For the moment, however, we will examine the general subject without reference to specific examples. More concrete and specific descriptions will be given in Part VI with regard to therapeutic procedures and patient improvement.

Morita's conception[14] of the three factors he calls *kibun-hon'i*, *richi-hon'i* and *jijitsu-hon'i* is touched on in Footnote 9 of this chapter, but the author will now examine this conception in more detail. What Morita calls *hon'i*[15] indicates a certain value orientation: the way of life that any person values most. It is, in other words, a mental attitude for the conduct of life.

Morita calls the attitude of *kibun-hon'i* one in which a state of mood is, at any moment, assigned more value than the facts of any situation. The key point lies in whether the mood is

---

[14] C. Buhler's concepts of the basic tendencies in human life were deduced theoretically from a combination of biological and psychological ideas, whereas Morita classified human value orientations on the basis of his clinical experience in psychotherapy. Morita's conception seems to be based largely on observation of the value orientations of his neurotic patients.

[15] *Hon'i* expresses one's fundamental attitude.

positive or negative, whether or not one feels an intention to press forward, whether or not self-confidence and courage are present. With this attitude, human life must be interesting, pleasant and substantial. If everything is not to our liking or in our favor, life does not seem to be worth living and has no value. Morita describes this attitude as the hysteria type, and it is observed in some patients with *shinkeishitsu*.

In Morita's words, the alternative attitude of *richi-hon'i* is one in which we make meaningful evaluations of human life as being right or wrong, good or evil, with a determination not to conform to our superficial knowledge or notions, or to be captivated by a mental "desk plan" influenced by mere abstractions, or to live at a great mental distance from the facts of reality. This attitude is observed in most patients with *shinkeishitsu*.

The attitude of *jijitsu-hon'i* is one of striving to live as one is, in accordance with the actual facts of any situation. Morita expresses this attitude as "obedience to nature and the environment." It is an attitude of pragmatism or naturalism[16] in the genuine sense of those words. We have already explained that "nature" in this instance indicates the changes of mind that continuously occur in human life, with the mental content originating in all the reality norms of life.

Morita says "be obedient to nature" but does not explain his meaning of nature in sufficient detail. It is probable that he considered human conduct in its actual manifestations from a creative and progressive standpoint and that he took that conduct to be the true measure of one's way of life. In a thoughtful person, "nature" is the reflection of a longing to succeed in life and to be respectable, but this desire does not include thoughtless and irresponsible actions out of whim or simple impulse.

Morita insists[17] that we will not have idle lives if we know our true character and behave in accordance with our natural mental reactions; his *jijitsu-hon'i* attitude toward living is the mental state of *arugamama*, the self-realization of what we, in fact, are from a naturalistic point of view.

These three basic attitudes toward living, defined by Morita, include the *jijitsu-hon'i* attitude as the anticipated goal in the management of *shinkeishitsu* with Morita therapy.

We will next consider the issue of value orientation in psychotherapy. This issue raises complicated issues of patient and therapist valuations, which depend on their personalities and a range of sociocultural considerations. For this reason, it is difficult to go into this subject at great length, but it is obviously impossible to discuss the problems of therapeutic cure without considering a therapist's influence on a patient's value orientation.

In Morita therapy, each therapist understands the varied aspects of the three basic attitudes toward life, but in the therapist's attitude as well as in his or her position of leadership, there is, of course, a definite value orientation that the therapist perceives as the objective of his or her professional work. A therapist's influence on a patient can be extremely strong, in both direct and indirect terms.[18] Because a therapist's personality also plays a part not only in Morita psychotherapy but also in other systems of psychotherapy, the influence exerted by his or her leadership of a patient cannot be disregarded.

The problem of value orientation in psychotherapy is acute, as Buhler[19] points out; a psychotherapist inevitably brings certain normative convictions into the conduct of therapy. Such

---

16 What Morita calls naturalism is a matter of accepting reality as it is from a scientific standpoint. It is different from the naturalism discussed in C.M. Lowe's classification of value orientations.

17 Morita, S.: Ningensei no jijitsu (The facts of human nature) (in Japanese). *Shinkeishitsu* 1(5) (1930).

18 In Morita therapy, it is likely that a psychotherapist's view of life will have a strong effect on a patient. Most patients who undergo Morita therapy seem to acquire a similar view of life and to perceive their therapists as pioneers of a sort. For this reason, a Morita therapist must be properly qualified to practice (Sakurai, T.: On the limitations of the various psychotherapies (in Japanese). *Seishin Igaku* 7(2) (1965)).

19 Buhler, C.: *Values in Psychotherapy*. The Free Press of Glencoe, New York (1962).

convictions may or may not be specifically communicated to a patient, but they underlie a therapist's activity and to some extent determine the goal set by the therapist for himself or herself and for the patient as well. Those values are consciously or unconsciously reflected in the therapist's questions, statements or reactions.

Bearing in mind Buhler's conviction concerning value orientation in psychotherapy, the Morita normative standpoint is that self-realization of the self *as it is* must be considered the most meaningful and fundamental outcome of the therapeutic program and of the patient's subsequent way of life. This conviction will contribute to determining the goal that a therapist will set for himself or herself and for a patient; the therapist's firm conviction will assist the patient to learn the basic principles for an efficacious way of life.

If is useful to compare Morita's conception of the three basic attitudes with some of the other conventional conceptions of value orientation. A separate comparison between value orientation and anthropological findings will be discussed in Part VII. Our discussion here will be independent of that comparison.

In 1956, Morris[20] studied seven types of religious valuation and found 13 conceptions of the "good life." These conceptions represent 13 ways to conduct one's life that are, in varying degrees accentuated in different religions and culture. Morris says that these various ways of life are manifested in three principal patterns, which he calls the basic components of human personality: Dionysian, Promethean and Buddhist.

The Dionysian way of life is defined in terms of tendencies to release and indulge stimulating desires. In Greek myth, Dionysus is the god of wine and drama; he is thought to govern human life in terms of biological impulses. The Dionysian concept also refers to the essence of life; Nietzsche considers it a musico-artistic impulse characterized by spiritual intoxication. Morita's notion of *kibun-hon'i* is, of course, different from Morris's definition of Dionysian because the two men do not have the same standpoint. However, Morita's *kibun-hon'i* is derived from a notion of vital force or source of human action, with an inclination to pursue sensuous pleasure.

The Promethean way of life is defined in terms of active tendencies to manipulate and remake the world. The Buddhist way is defined as tendencies in the self to regulate the self by holding desires in abeyance. Both the Buddhist disposition and the Promethean disposition represent intellect-directed life-styles that are characterized by active attempts to reconstruct the world, with a strong will to eschew the unrestrained pursuit of materialistic desires and to maintain a spontaneous sense of order.

Prometheus was originally thought of as a "forethinker," and the life-style named after him may seem remarkably similar to what Morita calls *richi-hon'i*. However, the basic attitude of *richi-hon'i* is so heavily slanted toward exercise of intelligence that it tends to be deficient in freedom of action. Morita's *richi-hon'i* and *kibun-hon'i* can both be considered patterns of value orientation in neurotic patients, but they also can be viewed in a different light as processes of human personality development.

In 1959, Lowe[21] attempted to categorize value orientation into four different types. One is naturalism, with an orientation toward obtaining physical comforts. This type agrees in many respects with Morris's Dionysian and Morita's *kibun-hon'i* orientations. *Jijitsu-hon'i* is a value orientation toward self-realization as one is. It seems to have elements in common with Lowe's humanism, defined as value orientation toward self-sufficiency and self-realization, or with Buhler's expansive creativity, defined as an orientation toward expansion, creativity, self-realiza-

---

[20] Morris, C.: *Varieties of Human Values.* University of Chicago Press, Chicago (1956).

[21] Lowe, C.M.: Value orientation and ethical dilemma. *American Psychologist* 14(11): 687–693 (1959).

tion and an upholding of internal order directed toward integration, self-sustenance and peace of mind.

Lowe's theism is defined as value orientation toward submission to God and love of God, and Morris's Buddhist orientation has love of God and acceptance of Buddhist commandments adopted as standards of value.

It is difficult to align these concepts with Morita's *jijitsu-hon'i* because of differences in spiritual and cultural bases. Some of the concepts may have something in common with one another if they are considered from a standpoint of highly refined mentality, but reservations must be exercised for interpretation of Morris's notion of "Buddhist."

Morris's concept of "Buddhist" signifies self-control by the control of desires, whereas Morita's concept includes an attitude of self-realization by living in accordance with one's desire (the desire to live) as it is. These two concepts obviously spring from extremely different viewpoints of the desire to live. Morita's concept of the desire to live not only is biologically based but also holds a reflection of a higher mentality. Morris sees tendencies in the self to regulate the self by holding desire in check. Morita views the self as the true subjective existence of living naturally in accordance with the desire to live. This way of life is almost identical to Buhler's upholding of internal order and Lowe's theism, which is related to Allport's extensive transactional commerce with the environment.[22] In this orientation, there is an attitude of naturally adapting the self to the future and to the commonplace world.

This type of attitude may bring one into an encounter with another person who assumes the same attitude. What Morita sought in treatment with Morita therapy was to have a patient acquire exactly that attitude and to live in accordance with the desire to live. In Morita's view of human life, the process of therapy cannot be considered a mere scientific process but, rather, as a situation of existential negotiations from a future-oriented standpoint.

The mental state of *kibun* (humor, mood, frame of mind) in *kibun-hon'i*, which Morita considers a value orientation of neurotic patients, is closely related to the original phenomenon of "being there" (from the German *Dasein*) in the tenets of existentialism, provided that the "there" of "being there" includes something suggestive of the *Geworfenheit* and *Entwurf* of (human) "existence," which is the so-called being there and in which what we call "mood" or "humor" functions as a motivational trigger.

Kierkegaard divides the process of human self-development into three stages of existence. He calls "aesthetic existence" a primary stage in which we live without awareness of the meaning of our existence. In this stage, we seek to explore all sorts of possibility and to pursue our desires without any sense of restriction. This stage is, in other words, one of "physical" existence regulated by "actuality" and "temporality" states of mood and humor.

It is interesting to compare this concept with the attitude of *kibun-hon'i*. In fact, Morita's *kibun-hon'i* is a "direct" way of life. "Authentic existence" cannot be experienced by the self in the state of *kibun-hon'i* because one is alienated from the self by filling day-to-day life with all sorts of mental diversion.

The *kibun-hon'i* persona is apt to minimize the meaningfulness of daily living and to disregard the value of authentic human experience. Such a person is usually unaware of self-alienation. The person shrinks from responsibility and attempts to live by depending on other persons. Heidigger calls this persona a state of decay (*Verfallen*) from genuine existence. In this state, there is no attempt to live an existence with awareness of individual responsibilities, as M. Boss points out, and this persona falls into the mentality of an incognito community.

Kierkegaard's secondary stage of existence is that of ethical existence. In this stage, there

[22] Allport, G.W.: *Pattern and Growth in Personality*. Holt, New York (1961).

is awareness of the meaning of one's existence and responsibilities and an acceptance of humanistic and ethical order as an obligation.

The human persona usually arrives at this secondary stage of ethical existence after experiencing discontent and frustration in the primary stage of aesthetic existence. Living in the ethical manner is an indication that one becomes what one should be, and this stage of existence is the same as Morita's understanding of "humanity," but it cannot be regarded as natural self-realization.

Morita states that "it is still unreal forces that cause one to search for an idealistic image that one should be thus and so." The ethical way of life corresponds to the recovery phase in Morita therapy, during which time a patient becomes aware of the meaningfulness of community participation through repeated practice.

The realization of belonging to a community will give one a sense of responsibility and can also arouse fears of one's sinfulness. Following this stage of ethical existence, one proceeds to a higher stage of religious existence. At this stage, one is concerned with God through a dialectic process of debate within oneself. This type of existence, in Christianity, is much the same as the process of internal debate that precedes the attainment of *pāramitā* (nirvāna).

This struggle is indicative of authentic existence and has aspects similar to Morita's understanding that manifestation of authentic humanity lies in the internal struggle of a patient with *shinkeishitsu* to live in accordance with the desire to live.

Sartre, who denies the existence of God, sees this essential aspect of existence to lie ultimately in the act of denying God and one's conscience, although this type of existence cannot be compared in parallel with Morita's concept because it is appreciably different.

The human ordeal is to realize that one is responsible to make choices for oneself and for mankind with a sense of responsibility. Morita seems to see this ordeal in human mentality expressed as the desire to live. The processes by which the self is moved from aesthetic to ethical and then to religious existence are manifestations of self-development from a non-authentic to an authentic existence; they can form an existentialist backdrop to Morita therapy, with a patient gradually progressing through *kibun-hon'i* and *richi-hon'i* to *jijitsu-hon'i*.

K. Jaspers defines human existence as *In-der-Situation-Sein*. Human beings exist in a context of situational possibilities that surround each and all of us anywhere, anytime, and that have close ties with our actual lives. These situations can include natural, historical, social, political, economic and cultural factors. However, we need not be passively influenced by these situations; rather, we can take positive steps, in some instances, by decision and choice, and attempt to find out, in situations, the meaning of our existence.[23]

This is a distinctly human quality that emerges in the mental state of *jijitsu-hon'i* as a natural manifestation of the desire to live. Morita, as a psychotherapist, tried to communicate this concept to a patient in a therapeutic context of human relationships. In their encounters with one another during the course of Morita therapy, the therapist mentally communicates with a patient in a manner of vital response to each other, and both persons are bound together in subjective existence. At the same time, the patient experiences and learns a new way of life.

Jaspers[24] says "be obedient to oneself but not to others" and tried to identify the psychotherapeutic process by which one can develop oneself by accepting one's actual existence as it is, through self-enlightenment. Concerning psychotherapy, Jaspers comments that in counseling and instructing a patient regarding how to look at his or her real situation, personal world and

---

23 Jaspers, K.: *Philosophie; Existenzerhellung.* Translated into Japanese by M. Kusanagi and S. Nobuta. Shōbunsha, Tokyo (1964).

24 Jaspers, K.: *General Psychopathology* (Allgemeine Psychopathologie). Translated from the 7th German edition by J. Hoenig and M.W. Hamilton. Manchester University Press, Manchester (1962).

himself or herself, the important thing is that the patient should implement a decisive yes and no. It is of no real help to the patient merely to learn something; the learning phase has to be followed by a certain vision of things. Learning must be mastered. There must be a recognition and taking over of what has been learned. It is a patient's responsibility to decide what he or she will assimilate and what he or she will reject. The patient's existential decision ultimately determines his or her actual way of life.

It is beyond the power of any psychotherapist to make a patient achieve this goal. The most a therapist can do in communication with a patient is to afford some unpredictable opportunities for an awakening.

This statement seems to suggest the future pathway that psychotherapy should take.

We have discussed the human persona that we hope to form during the process of Morita therapy and have stated that a psychotherapist engaged in such therapy helps a patient learn his or her distinctive way of life, in which the patient accepts the fact of humanity as it is and realizes himself or herself with a new set of aspirations.

We intend to cultivate a better understanding of the benefits of Morita therapy from a number of different standpoints. This can raise a certain specter of contradiction; for example, the more that Morita therapy becomes ambiguous, the harder we struggle to explain it with lucid precision.

Verbal explanations of Morita therapy do not, in the final analysis, hold much substance, frequently drifting into abstract discussions remote from the actual case in point. We seem to gain a deeper understanding of the problems of each patient when we do not attempt to explain the matter with a dense screen of words.

7

Morita's Status in Japanese Psychiatry

The author would like to discuss two subjects before we proceed to the main topic of this chapter. The first subject is Morita's childhood and its correlation with his later academic inclination (an outline of the latter subject was given in Chapter 3). The second subject is the general academic trend in psychiatry in the nineteenth and twentieth centuries.

Morita's Childhood and His Academic Inclination

In order to assess Morita's achievements, including the therapy that bears his name, it is useful to first review the events in his life that helped shape his interest in psychiatry. The events of Morita's early life will be reconstructed according to his personal records.

Morita writes that his interest in psychiatry dated back to his youth. When he was about ten years old, he saw a depiction of Hell in a Buddhist temple near his birthplace. It was a richly colored, carefully detailed painting that showed the spectacle of a flaming Hell, including a mountain of needles and pools of blood, all vividly drawn. A strange odor of incense had drifted into the hall where this picture was hung.

The boy felt intensely shocked and frightened. He said that the painting made his hair stand on end. The impression it left on him was so strong that he was frequently assailed by a fear of death in later life. He sometimes thought about life after death and the world of supernatural spirits. And he suffered from nightmares.

Because of those experiences, the issue of life and death was always on his mind during childhood. Even after he had entered middle (junior high) school, he took a frequent interest in fanciful mysteries and miracles. He studied religious phenomena associated with Buddhist temples and Shintō shrines, investigated various superstitions, prayers and charms and had a reputation among his friends of having become absorbed in fortune-telling. During his high-school years, he showed intense interest in phrenology and physiognomy, while also being engrossed in studies of Buddhism and Christianity.

Morita had a considerable interest in various popular therapies based on folk remedies, to the extent of experiencing them himself. He also had a strong interest in Oriental philosophy and psychology and for a long time read numerous magazines specializing in those subjects. He had a vast intellectual appetite and curiosity but did not become a devotee of any specific religion. He was seriously absorbed in his diverse private studies without becoming addicted in a generalized, amateurish manner. In the instance of fortune-telling, he studied and commented on it with an attitude of calculating the rate of correct predictions in a scientific manner.

With the issue of life and death constantly on his mind, his consequent interest in metaphysics, philosophy, religion, logic and views of life was considerable.

During Morita's university studies, his interest turned toward empirical science, dealing with concrete, practical topics. Morita explained this shift of interest by saying that "the most correct course of thought is to make note of the fact that visionary ideology is insufficient; it is first necessary to know what the body is, and then to study subjects from both physical and mental points of view."

This conception bolstered Morita's interest in the study of psychiatry. Another reason that Morita devoted himself to studies of neurosis and psychotherapy in his later life was that he had suffered from neurosis (of the type that he later came to call *shinkeishitsu*). Morita had a weak physical constitution but also a strong spirit of inquiry and an aggressive bent of character. It is apparent that his constitutional nervosity, which he referred to as "a congenital mentally weak character," included a chronic *enuresis nocturna* that had not completely stopped even when he had reached the age of 12.

Morita also suffered from such symptoms of *shinkeishitsu* as palpitation, hyper-fatigue and feelings of illness, beginning at the age of 13 or 14. He began to experience severe headaches at the age of 16 or 17, and the headaches continued to plague him until his sophomore year at the university. His family doctor frequently told him that "everyone has headaches to about the same extent," and his mother accused him of "causing the headache by thinking 'I have a headache'."

He contracted typhoid fever in his fifth year of middle school. One day, when he was riding a bicycle while recovering from the fever, he experienced severe palpitation, physical tremors and a convulsive fit, and that night he was struck with an acute fear of death. After this episode, similar fits, of variable intensity, occurred several times each year, and, frequently, two or three fits followed one another in rapid succession. This condition continued until Morita graduated from the university. One physician told Morita that he had heart trouble, but the Internal Medicine Department of the University Hospital diagnosed the condition as neurasthenia and placed him on medication for about one year.

Morita thus suffered from symptoms of *shinkeishitsu* when he was young. However, his thoughts about the neurasthenia changed fundamentally about one year after he had entered the university. The symptoms that still plagued Morita had been preventing him from concentrating on his studies. Even when examinations were imminent, he could hardly study. To aggravate matters, remittances from home did not arrive for two months.

He continued to suffer, plunged into worry and felt driven into a desperate loneliness and a problematical "bitter feeling toward other people building to a peak of wretchedness and desperation." He considered suicide, to spite his parents, but thought better of it. He stopped taking medication and gave up caring about his health; instead, he plunged into his studies without sleeping at night. As a result, his examination scores were better than expected, and the symptoms from which he suffered had vanished.

Through this experience of self-extrication, after he had felt driven into a corner, then consigned himself to fate, he had experienced the disappearance of fear by plunging headlong into fear as if hoping against hope.

It is believed that this experience had a deep influence on his thought in later years. Thus, the basic thinking underlying Morita's *shinkeishitsu* therapy of "fear the fear itself" and "let everything exist as it is" was acquired from his personal experience.

Morita considers this experience the "underlying cause of devoting myself to studies of *shinkeishitsu*" and also comments that "my study of psychiatry was the opportune cause." These early experiences were the motivation for his numerous achievements, including the psychotherapy of his later life.

As mentioned by Frank,[1] the author considers that Morita's experience is one of the

---

[1] Frank, J. D.: *Persuasion and Healing.* Johns Hopkins University Press, Baltimore (1961).

epitomes of the development of modern psychotherapy, which has two historical traditions: the magico-religious tradition and the naturalistic, or scientific, tradition. In Morita's work, the principles of traditional cultural values, expressed in Oriental philosophical, religious and ethnic ideas and activities, are incorporated into scientific thought structures and thus are made useful for modern-day clinical application.

Psychiatric Trend in Morita's Time

The dawn of modern psychiatry came in 1789 when P. Pinel (1755–1826) released psychotic patients from their chains at Salpêtrière. Pinel was interested in the psychiatric theory, which had its origins in English empiricism and also in the descriptive method. He enunciated the belief that psychosis is an illness. His pupil, G.E.D. Esquirol, likewise laid stress on amiable communication between physician and patient and subscribed to a sociopsychological school of thought. It is said that the term *psychiatry* was first used by J.C. Reil in 1808 in his "Contribution to Therapy by the Psychologic Method."

What Reil stipulated by that term is similar in content to any modern-day school of psychotherapy, which has the sense of psychotherapeutics as a discipline that deals with psychological salvation or spiritual welfare. Reil's psychiatry was intended for application to all mental patients. Consequently, in his thinking, psychopathography is strictly a treatment nosology.

The primary objective, at the beginning of modern psychiatry, according to at least Pinel and Esquirol, was the treatment of psychopaths. Heated discussion of nosology occurred as a direct result. For example, there was controversy during the first half of the nineteenth century in Germany, emanating from the institutional psychiatric school of Heinroth and Beneke, who insisted that psychosis is an illness of the mind, and the somatology school of Friedrich and Jakobi, who considered psychosis a physical illness.

W. Griesinger ("Pathology and Therapy of Psychopaths," 1845) asserted while this debate was under way that "psychosis is a localized illness of the cerebrum and can be cured only on the basis of material changes in the nervous system." Griesinger was the most famous psychiatrist of the time and later became the pioneer spirit of so-called university psychiatry.

With progress in the natural sciences during the latter half of the nineteenth century, C. Wernicke and T. Meynert defined somatology in terms of explaining mental disorders in a mechanical fashion as originating in localized functions of the brain. Changes in the social attitude concerning treatment of people with mental disorders also took place during this time. It was emphasized that such people should be isolated from their homes and hospitalized in specialized institutions as quickly as possible. Treatment of mentally disordered patients became more impersonal, and priority in treatment was given to biological viewpoints.

Since the first mention of *dementia paralytica*, there had been a trend toward consolidation of all mental disorders as entity psychosis, in accordance with the somatological mode of thought. K.L. Kahlbaum attempted a classification of psychosis in 1863, explaining his concept of entity and furnishing a compilation of observations on catatonia. His pupil, E. Hecker, had already done a compilation of observations on hebephrenia. (In France, the concepts of J. Falret's *Folie Circulaire* (1854) and F. Morel's *Démence Précoce* (1856) had appeared.)

A comprehensive study of these trends was completed by E. Kraepelin, who made an effort to consolidate the classifications of the various mental disorders under the "entity" principle. The result was published as the first edition of *Psychiatry* in 1883. The two concepts of dementia praecox and manic-depressive psychosis were fully clarified by Kraepelin in 1896, and a nosological system of psychiatry with this pair of entities as its principal supports was then established. This epochal achievement was eventually accepted all over the world. There was some dissent and a number of suggestions for modification of Kraeplin's theory, but in essence it has remained intact to the present.

The Kraepelin school can be considered the final representative somatological school based on the biological position, when examined from the standpoint of historical trends in psychiatry. It could also be called a predynamic school, with reference to the dynamist school that developed later.

Importance is placed on hereditary disposition as the foundation of Kraepelin's system, which is based on pathoanatomical, nosological and clinical interpretations of the human brain. Psychiatry might even be considered a separate, independent branch of medicine from that point of view because priority was given to nosological classification and because there was considerable criticism of the Kraepelin school's passive attitude toward therapy.

The concept of dementia praecox was replaced by the concept of schizophrenia, first advanced by E. Bleuler in 1911. Later, the concepts of loosening of associations and of autism (which became the basis of a new psychological theory) were introduced.

Kraepelin's system came under fire from the psychological school and the advocates of dynamic theory. If the school of Kraepelin, who can be designated the founder of modern psychiatry, is considered the orthodox school, Sigmund Freud, who originated the school of psychoanalysis, could be called the fiercest critic of this orthodox school. Freud's psychoanalysis, advocated after 1895, is based on a psychogenic theory of therapy with psychotherapy as its main constituent. This was in opposition to Kraepelin's system, which rests chiefly on somatological diagnosis. In view of that, psychoanalysis was rejected by the orthodox school in the psychiatric field in Germany but was adopted in Switzerland, England and the United States.

In Japan, Dr. Baelz, a German professor of medicine, delivered a lecture on psychiatry in 1879 to the Faculty of Medicine at the University of Tokyo. Later, in 1886, Professor H. Sakaki established the Psychiatric Department in the Faculty of Medicine at the same university. Following Sakaki's sudden death, he was succeeded by S. Kure.

Residing in Europe from 1897 to 1902, Kure had studied under both Kraepelin and Nissl in Germany. What he brought back to Japan was the descriptive and nosological classification system of psychiatry of the German orthodox school, along with its brain pathology.

Kure exerted great effort to popularize and develop that orthodox school of thought in Japan. He also worked to promote the application of psychotherapeutics and mental hygiene in psychiatry and took part in various activities of a humane nature, such as reformation of mental hospitals for treatment of psychopaths.

Kure had a great interest in psychotherapy as well. He accumulated information on all types of scientific psychotherapy and published this material in volume II, number III, of the Japanese Internal Medicine Compendium (1916). Morita read this material carefully at a later date, and there is no doubt that he used it as a reference. He was officially appointed the assistant to Kure in February 1903, when he was 28 years-old.

In December of the same year, Morita was granted admission as a graduate student with the qualification of assistant. The subject Kure assigned Morita to major in was psychotherapy. (That year, 1903, was 17 years after the first lecture on psychiatry had been presented in Japan.)

Morita was soon entrusted by Kure to take charge of work therapy for schizophrenics confined to a mental hospital. This clinical experience probably provided important comparative information that gave Morita the clues for his discovery of the "desire to live" in *shinkeishitsu* patients in his later years. Morita was directed toward studies of psychotherapy and neurosis from an early period, in this manner, but it was also his good fortune to have so superior an instructor as Kure to work with at the beginning of his career in psychiatry.

Around the same time that Morita was taking his first steps as a psychiatrist, the foundations of modern psychiatry in Japan were being laid down by Kure. Both Morita and the entire field of psychiatry in Japan had the same instructor at the same time.

The seeds planted by Kure in the field of Japanese psychiatry began to sprout in the specific areas of university and hospital psychiatry and mental hygiene. Growth, however, was not harmonious. The most rapid growth occurred in the biological point of view in university psychiatry. Much slower growth took place in the other two areas.

Genuine interest developed from psychological and social viewpoints mainly after 1945, more than 40 years after Kure's era. The mainstream of Japanese psychiatric thinking in Kure's time was the somatological view, based on the Kraepelin system, with histopathological, heredoembryological, biochemical and electrophysiological studies being done with greatest fervor.

In the field of psychopathology, most studies were focused on the narrow image of psychosis centered on schizophrenia and manic-depressive psychoses, with use of the descriptive phenomenological method. Indications of future development of the psychogenic theory were present but chiefly peripheral. Studies relating to mental hygiene and social factors received little attention.

By contrast, remarkable progress took place in the natural sciences and in technology, which made more detailed studies possible, particularly from the somatological viewpoint. The methodology gained great precision, but the major objective remained unclear.

The original notion that mental phenomena can be reduced to material factors might have been modified in character to a subsequent notion of a biochemical nature, but there was no essential change in the basic postulate. The therapy applied to psychopaths was mostly a matter of manipulation by materialistic techniques.

Since satisfactory therapeutic results were not forthcoming, the patients were labeled incurable. Patients, as a result, did not receive psychogenic-based treatment and were accommodated in completely sealed institutions, to prevent them from disrupting public peace and order, with total isolation from society.

The idea of social rehabilitation and cure of psychopaths, initially proposed by Kure, became an obscure academic notion that ignored the human being, with the field of psychiatry led by the so-called university school of thought.

Morita's Status as a Psychiatrist

Morita was educated with studies of modern psychiatric concepts and the scientific methodology of the Western world immediately after those elements had been introduced in Japan by Kure. Morita accordingly became a psychiatrist of the orthodox school. His professional nature, interests and abilities were enhanced by the attitude he took as a clinical physician who placed emphasis on observation and description of clinical facts by developing methods that incorporated a humane approach to patients.

Because the general trend in the academic field at the time was biological (somatogenic), it was hardly remarkable that Morita subscribed to the academic mainstream. He did, however, depart somewhat from the mainstream in selecting neurosis and psychotherapy as his major fields of study, and this departure was not due only to his attachment to the studies that Kure had assigned him in graduate school.

Morita had a great personal interest in the psychological, or psychic, phenomena of human existence, as we have mentioned, and this interest also directed him toward the field of psychiatry. To limit himself to learning what deviations occur in the pursuit of human nature was, for Morita, an exercise devoid of meaning, even if done with naturalistic scientific methodology.

His interest gradually shifted toward the constitution, predisposition and psychogenic problems of mental disorders. The term *neurasthenia*, first introduced by Beard in 1868, had become a general description in popular use, although its pathological basis was obscure. The number of people suffering from neurasthenia was not inconsiderable. Morita had been one of them. He did not accept the theory that an irritable weakening of the central nervous system, as advanced by Beard, was the cause of neurasthenia. Morita substituted the expression "pseudo-irritant weakness" because he did not consider the condition a genuine nervous disease. To avoid misunderstanding, he proposed, in 1919, use of the term *shinkeishitsu* instead of neurasthenia to identify the disorder.

Beard had stressed that physiological fatigue is the sole cause of the evolvement of that fatigue into so-called chronic neurasthenia. In Morita's opinion, however, a specific condition, a fixed psychological mechanism, also comes into play. He insisted that the symptoms of *shinkeishitsu* were not somatogenic but, rather, psychogenic.

At that time, the irritable constitution theory proposed by Matsubara was considered the causal explanation of what was called neurasthenia in Japan (see Chapter 8). Morita believed that the condition was psychogenic in origin because a number of people who had severe somatic states of irritable hypersensitivity did not exhibit symptoms of neurasthenia. On the contrary, a number of people who were somatologically healthy complained of complex symptoms of neurasthenia.[2] It is worth noting, as an aside, that Freud attempted a classification with the nomenclature of actual neurosis that included independent syndromes called neurasthenia, anxiety neurosis and hypochondriasis, in contrast to psychoneurosis, because he considered Beard's concept of neurasthenia to be much too inclusive.

Like Beard, though, Freud thought that the phenomena were due to somatic factors that arise from sexual life rather than to psychological factors. It is well known that Freud first proposed the theory that a psychogenic factor is the cause of psychoneurosis, although actual neurosis has a somatic foundation. It may be said that Morita's concept of neurasthenia originating from psychic factors was, in a certain sense, one step ahead of Freud.[3]

Morita adopted the term *shinkeishitsu* to replace neurasthenia because he considered the former to be due to psychic factors, but the presence of a disposition that can easily give rise to a mentally hypersensitive condition appears to be the premise. This mentally hypersensitive disposition was later categorized as one type in Morita's classification of degenerate conditions,[4] but he still called it *shinkeishitsu* (i.e., not a disease).

What the author needs to stress here, however, is Morita's view of degenerate conditions. In a thesis titled "Comments on Kraepelin's Classification of Degenerates,"[5] he does not take any fixed position that such people are on the verge of psychosis and that they have a strong, inherently abnormal personality, in line with Kraepelin's definition of degenerates.

Morita insists that the degenerate condition of *shinkeishitsu* changes and is fluid. As it changes in a highly complex manner by correlations with disposition, the environment and

---

[2] This topic is explained in detail in Part I. It appears that Morita divides neurasthenia into two types, that due to a somatic irritable disposition and that due to a psychological irritable disposition, for the sake of convenience.

[3] Kondō, K.: Ōrigin of Morita therapy. In *Gendai no Morita Ryōhō: Riron to Jissai* (Present-day Morita Therapy: Theory and Practice), edited by K. Ōhara. Hakuyōsha, Tokyo (1977). (Printed in Japanese)

[4] Morita calls this disposition "abnormal personality" or "abnormal personality reaction" (1927).

[5] Morita, S.: Kenkō to henshitsu to seishinijō–Kraepelin gakuha no henshitsusha bunrui no hihan (Comments on Kraepelin's classification of degenerates; healthy individuals, degenerates and neurotics). In *Morita Shōma Zenshū*, Vol. III (edited by K. Ōhara under the supervision of T. Kōra). Hakuyōsha, Tokyo (1974). (Printed in Japanese)

circumstance, the condition cannot be viewed as one that is fixed. Further, Morita advanced the idea that the problem of good or poor adaptability for improvement and development or for preservation of the species will crop up readily in a person of degenerate or abnormal character as an issue of existence.

In many cases, abnormal personality reactions occur as a result of certain changes made for the purpose of survival. These reactions can be excessive or insufficient, but they do not always indicate that a person will become morbidly abnormal, both physically and mentally, on the one hand, or asocial or antisocial, on the other. Sometimes, the condition leads the person to excel in some way or to become an important contributor to society.

Together with acquired and environmental factors, Morita includes disposition as a causal factor in *shinkeishitsu*. His basic view of *shinkeishitsu* could not depart from the standpoint of placing emphasis on disposition. There were delicate differences in what he stressed throughout his career, but he always places his major emphasis on disposition.

Morita's theory of neurosis differs from the dynamic theory because it is based on the premise of dispositional theory. It reflects the extent of the influence wielded by the orthodox German psychiatric school of the time, represented by Kraepelin.

Although the psychiatric field did place the greatest priority on the biological view, Morita pointed out the relevance of the mental factor in mental disorders and, further, rejected the fixed view of degeneracy by electing to understand it dynamically and from a holistic point of view. He made a collective correlation between human beings and the environment, which he refers to in terms of the life reactions of human beings. It is the human beings who work out life relationships with the environment who are at the center of Morita's concern, so that his viewpoint is fundamentally practical rather than academic.

Morita's Major Achievements

Morita's *shinkeishitsu* theory and his system of therapy were his greatest achievements. Nevertheless, his work in the field of invocational psychosis[6] and superstition,[7] which has not received much attention, is also noteworthy.

Invocational psychosis can be induced by prayers, incantations and similar activities. The chief symptoms include character transformation, religious delusion and the delusion of possession by a spirit. These symptoms are special mental conditions that may continue for several days or even several months. Most often, the disorder arises from an emotional experience, with autosuggestive reinforcement either acutely or subacutely.

Morita mentions the hysterical tendency in a personality receptive to this type of mental disorder, but the condition can be generated by incantation if circumstances exist in which the autosuggestive mechanism is accelerated in correlation with the environment. In other words, certain relics of primitive religious mentality that come into correlation with the basic life assumptions of a person give rise to the disorder.

This condition is akin to superstitious mentality, but there is a preliminary phase in which a certain type of psychogenous reaction occurs readily through impressions made by environmental factors on a person's personality. The disorder will then be ignited by one or more profound emotional experiences induced by prayer and incantation or by the conviction of

[6] Yo no iwayuru Kitōsei seishinbyō ni tsuite (On Morita's clinical experience of the so-called invocational psychosis) (in Japanese). *Psychiatria et Neurologia Japonica* 14:286 (1915).

[7] Meishin to mōsō (Superstition and delusion) (in Japanese). In *Morita Shōma Zenshū*, 1974; ibid.

being accursed. The most important factor is, of course, the conviction of personal inferiority, which readily accelerates the autosuggestive process or the emotional experience.

However, Morita also stresses the factors of the social and the cultural environment that contribute to the condition, as well as a person's basic mental state. The same factors can also lead, at length, to the development of *shinkeishitsu*. Psychopathological schema of psychogenous disorders had probably been elaborated by Morita at the time he wrote about invocational psychosis.

Morita's views of superstition are also illuminating. In 1904, after becoming a psychiatrist, he wrote his first thesis on superstition, titled the "Dog God of Tosa."[8]

Morita saw superstition as having an opposite relationship to genuine spiritual faith. Both forms of belief are motivated by a need to attain peace of mind through dissolution of fear and anxiety, and they are similar in consisting of a conviction that seeks to appeal to a supernatural power. However, superstition differs from genuine faith in not having a systematic, universal and traditional form and in lacking social solidarity. It is strictly a personal matter. It resembles delusion, but the latter occurs suddenly and is characterized by a morbid condition.

Morita examined superstition as one element in what he calls the "life mode of the human being" and sought to understand it as a form of correlation between disposition and the environment. He seems to have applied a psychiatric scale to the phenomenon of the friction that occurs when folkloric customs of an older culture are threatened by a new, more sophisticated culture. His concept could probably be considered the forerunner of such studies as "folkloristic psychiatry"[9] and "culture-bound reactive psychosis"[10] if we substitute present-day terms and expressions for Morita's original language.

Other Interests

Morita directed attention to abnormal child psychology and mental disorders by successively writing "Children's Superstitions" (1904), "Children's Psychosis" (1906), "Education of the Feeble-Minded Child" (1914), "Parental Affection Toward the Feeble-Minded Child" (1917), "Education of the Delinquent Child" (Imitative Nature of Children) (1917) and "Fears of Children" (1917).

He also commented on family environment, on the importance and present attitude of parents concerning education and on methods of education and educational therapy.

During the same period, he apparently began to investigate human psychology from the point of view of developmental psychology, but it was probably his strong interest and detailed clinical observations of child psychology that laid the foundations for his view of the "desire to live" in terms of developmental psychology in the *shinkeishitsu* theory of his later life.

In 1917, Morita founded the Japanese Society of Psychiatry together with K. Nakamura and began publication of the periodical titled *Ijōshinrigaku* (Abnormal Psychology). He wrote numerous papers spanning a broad range of subjects—"Superstition and Delusion," "Mind Reading," "Shinkeishitsu," "Suicide," "Hysteria," "Psychotherapy," "Subconsciousness," "Degenerates," "The Concept of Neurosis," "Study of Dreams" and "Jealousy Delusion"—

---

[8] This thesis was published in *Neurologica Japonica* (1904). The *inugami* (dog god) religious persuasion was common in Tosa (Kōchi Prefecture) from early historical times.

[9] Oda, S.: Minzokugaku to seishinigaku (A review of folkloristic psychiatry) (in Japanese). *Seishin Igaku* 18 (10) (1976).

[10] Yap, P.M.: The possession syndrome—A comparison of Hong Kong and French findings. *Journal of Mental Science* 106: 114 (1960).

before he consolidated his *shinkeishitsu* theory in 1920. Only a few of these papers dealt with the narrow issue of mental disorders.

Morita carried out psychopathological studies with a narrow focus on psychosis until around 1910, as is evident from such published reports as "Delusion," "Paranoia" and "Monologue," but he almost completely discontinued such studies afterward. Reports on organic psychosis (e.g., toxication and infection) and methods of neurological diagnosis were also published in that early period, but such reports lack special interest because they reflect the mainstream field of investigation.

It is more noteworthy that he wrote a series of articles called the "Appearances of Dolls," which was published in an art magazine in five installments in 1905, but there was no further development of the subject, except for attempts to examine consciousness of beauty in terms of personality differences.

Detailed reports on Morita's lifelong interest in hypnosis are available;[11] we have also discussed this matter in Chapter 1. Morita learned hypnosis almost entirely by self-study and wrote on the technique in 1904. The following year, he reported a case of obsession cured by hypnosis therapy. Hypnosis had been used by Morita for the management of neurosis for several years, before he developed Morita therapy. The concept termed obsessive-compulsive neurosis had only just come under discussion in Japan, and there were only a few case reports. Therapy had not even been considered. Setting aside the effectiveness of hypnosis as a therapeutic approach, it can be said that Morita's report was important at that time. However, Morita gradually lost interest in the use of hypnosis, finding that temporary improvement could be induced by hypnosis but that such therapy could not prevent recurrence of a disorder.

Work Therapy

The position of work therapy in modern-day psychotherapy is far from unimportant. In fact, it now has major importance. There had been little application of intensive work therapy in Japan until Morita took an interest in it. There is no doubt that Morita was a pioneer in systematic work therapy in Japanese psychiatry.

Morita started out by assigning simple manual tasks of an indoor nature to patients with chronic schizophrenia who were confined to mental hospitals, but he gradually expanded the scope of the program, adding outdoor work, including practical and productive activities in farming and animal husbandry.

His chief objective, at the outset, was to afford such patients some relief from their wearisome hospital confinement. In present-day terms, this therapy was a form of recreation. Morita eventually applied this work therapy to the treatment of patients with *shinkeishitsu* because he had found that the physical labor involved in work therapy was useful for diversion of moods, training the will or concentrating attention.

The essence of the work therapy that Morita finally refined was an awakening of spontaneous activity in the mind and of experiencing harmony with nature (in the *arugamama* condition of experiencing one's own mind and body as they are) and of becoming "one" with the surrounding environment by involvement in ongoing work.

---

[11] Nomura, A.: Morita Shōma: Sono hito to sakuhin (The human figure and its personal achievement and later publication). In *Gendai no Morita Ryōhō: Riron to Jissai*, edited by K. Ōhara. Hakuyōsha, Tokyo (1977). (Printed in Japanese)

Impact of Morita's Work in Psychiatry

Morita's major achievements were the product of his consistent direction, as a psychiatrist, toward the original objective of psychiatry: giving relief to patients. For Morita, this objective was not a matter of inspecting the static, fixed phenomena of the patient's inner mental world; rather, his interest was directed toward an academic illumination of the "life modes" of human beings who live dynamically in social, cultural and interpersonal situations, and his goal was to understand those life modes.

Morita's field of practice was thus not restricted to the narrow confines of so-called university psychiatry; rather, he studied the wide range of the whole of human life. He did not attempt a definite systemization of the numerous human phenomena that he studied. Many such attempts had ended in a sorry state of academic grasping at straws, which was probably inevitable, given the level of psychiatric practice in Japan during Morita's lifetime. His academic intentions were quite the opposite of the mainstream and represented the efforts of a pioneer spirit engaged in exploration of unknown territory.

Morita's work culminated in his theory of *shinkeishitsu* and its management. He ventured into the unknown and undeveloped region of neurosis therapy and theory, a field of study almost completely ignored at the time, and produced his original theory and system of therapy by trial and error methods carried out for more than ten years.

The theory of *shinkeishitsu* and Morita therapy represented a staggering achievement in the benighted academic field of his era. The true meaning of his work was not fully recognized until 30 years or more after his death. Its importance will continue to grow in the future because the foundations of Morita's thought and philosophy will not be abandoned. His professional work and his writings were full of a loving affirmation of human life that serves to nourish the principles and practices of Morita therapy.

Part II

Symptoms of *Shinkeishitsu*

8

Characteristics of Morita *Shinkeishitsu* and Its Symptoms

When the author examines the process of thinking that Morita pursued for psychopathological clarification and nosological positioning of so-called neurasthenia or nervosity, which was considered a composition of a different kind at that time, the author realizes that the strenuous efforts Morita exerted can be perceived clearly, even by an outsider.

The author believes it is essential to make a macroscopic, comprehensive survey of the transition in thinking that led Morita to attach importance to the presence of constitution or traits, while also directing attention to the factor of a patient's life history (the mode of the patient's human relationships and nurture in the home), which has an important role as a basis for the development of *shinkeishitsu.*

In this chapter, the nosological positioning of Morita *shinkeishitsu*, its classification and the symptoms that characterize it will be described. Further, Morita's thinking, based on his clinical experience up to that time, will be traced. This information will serve as an introduction for understanding Morita's mode of thought in regard to disposition and environment, which we will examine in Part III.

In Chapter 9, the features of one representative type of Morita *shinkeishitsu*, that is, so-called anthropophobia (of a type in conformity with Japanese culture) will be described.

Morita's Concept of *Shinkeishitsu* as an Entity Disorder

The title of this chapter will be explained by taking a macroscopic view of the process of Morita's thought up to the time that he consolidated *shinkeishitsu* into a single disorder.

According to Jaspers,[1] the wholeness (unified mind-body) that is clinically grasped is ideological and represents a clinical entity, an *eidos* or *bios.* Personality becomes an issue when an attempt is made to grasp the whole field from a basis of comprehensible relationships in a psychopathological study that aims at a clinical entity as an idea. This is indicative of the idea that something that has a similar personality trait is coupled to one unit, on the basis of a hypothetical viewpoint of degenerate personality, which is one method for supporting this idea in the process of investigating basic psychological structure.

For example, this mode of thought maintains that, in the instance of *shinkeishitsu*, any data that cannot be understood in psychological terms, even when directly traced further than this point, must be construed as the constitution or trait of *shinkeishitsu* and that *shinkeishitsu* occurs as one pathological unit stemming from this condition.

---

[1] Jaspers, K.: *Allgemeine Psychopathologie*, Vol. II, translated by U. Uchimura, S. Nishimaru, T. Shimazaki and K. Okada. Iwanami Shoten, Tokyo (1958).

Also, the wholeness that is clinically grasped is ideological, and it represents a clinical entity, an *eidos* or *bios*. Initially, Morita considered hypochondria a pathological condition, but during the process of investigating its basic psychological structure, he began to think that the hypochondriacal trait is essentially derived from *ki-zukau* (to become concerned about something). He also determined that this trait is one expression of the human desire to live. He concluded that this trait appears most frequently as one feature of the psychological trend in the trait called *shinkeishitsu* (including development of the life history).

Morita also thought that a hypersensitive constitution (Matsubara) and, mentally, a hypersensitive psychological trait determine the hypochondriacal trait. Consequently, the wholeness that Morita tried to grasp clinically is a whole that is expressed as one unit, and it cannot be severed from the *eidos* of constitution and temperament.

The wholeness indicates that an entity, that is, the phenomenon of developing psychogenetically on the basis of a hypochondriacal trait, is a form of *bios* referred to as *shinkeishitsu*, and this *bios* is also an idea, as a disease entity.

Morita *Shinkeishitsu* and Degeneration Theory (Abnormal Personality Theory)

In summarizing the features of the mental structure of Morita *shinkeishitsu*, we can term it a sensual or ideological phenomenon that is developed psychologically, with the hypochondriacal trait as its nucleus. The contradictions and inconsistencies that arise between the desire to live and the fear of death accelerate a further degree of ego-consciousness into an introspective disposition and a strengthening of psychological sensitivity. As a result, consciousness converges toward a focal point of sensual and ideological phenomena, leading to a condition in which the fluid function of life-adaptability reactions is difficult to rouse in the ego. In fact, the efforts of the ego to resist fluidity are formed by internal conflict.

What motivates this? According to Morita, the conflict arises between the "desire to live," for improvement and development of the self, and a basic desire for the safety and constancy of the self (the desire for existence or survival, which is a hypochondriacal trait as well).

These two desires share the same roots, but one can be understood as a phenomenon of centrifugal self-manifestation, and the other as a phenomenon of centripetal self-preservation. A harmonized life adaptation for human beings is possible by achieving an equilibrium between the two desires.

If that equilibrium is lacking, it signals a time of danger in the path of life.[2] Facing that loss of equilibrium, human beings will show various reactions in defense of life adaptation. In the instance of *shinkeishitsu*, self-consciousness indicates a condition with the hypochondriacal trait cited by Morita as its basis.

Including *shinkeishitsu*, which has those characteristics, Morita takes the position that a positive or negative functioning for life adaptation is rooted in constitutional theory (or trait theory). This condition is determined by the features of a psychological disposition based on the natural constitution or trait of a person.

[2] According to an investigation of consciousness by Mashino in regard to the introversion that occurs before the onset of *shinkeishitsu*, about 73 percent of his subjects became conscious of their condition at 13 or 14 years of age, with early adolescence as the peak period. Mashino, H.: Shinkeishitsushōsha no personality kenkyū (A study of the personality of "nervosity") (in Japanese). *Shinkeishitsu* 4(2): 69–85 (1963).

From around 1919, Morita worked out his concept of degeneration (abnormal personality) in terms of contrast with a condition of functional excess or deficiency of life adaptability and clarified its classification. Morita's original concept of degeneration actually dates back about ten years earlier.

Morita's Concept of Degeneration and Its Classification

Although this is only an assumption, since there is no accurate record, Morita seems to have considered *shinkeishitsu* a kind of nervous or mental degeneration until 1919. He considered it an excess or deficiency of faculty rather than an essential change. Further, he referred to something less serious than this as a mental trait or disposition. The feature of this trait, in the instance of *shinkeishitsu*, is, for Morita, a form of mental sensibility.

Morita not only thought of *shinkeishitsu* as a condition developing from a mental sensibility type of mental trait or disposition but also attempted to classify other types of degeneration on the basis of other respective mental traits. At first, apart from *shinkeishitsu*, he thought hysteria to be an emotional sensitivity type of mental trait. He also grouped together several types of degeneration in a strict classification that included weak-willed persons having emotional insensibility as a mental trait. He considered these three types as degenerative in a broad sense.[3]

One salient point of Morita's concept of degeneration is that he thinks of mental trait or disposition as the basis of the development of mental degeneration.[4]

Degeneration is readily caused by an excessive or deficient mental trait with respect to adaptation as a life reaction, with reference to the outside world. The features of the mental trait can generate either a sensibility reaction or an insensibility (degenerative) reaction, even with a minor cause of any such reaction.

As its second feature, quite apart from *shinkeishitsu* and hysteria, degeneration is related to sociopathological phenomena in human beings, including those who are essentially criminal, the sexually insane, the morbidly querulent and those who have an impulsive inhibition deficiency. These sociopathological conditions are included in degeneration of the strict definition falling under type 3.

Morita classifies degenerates (abnormal personalities) as persons who consider themselves defective and suffer within themselves and who are, apart from this category, not truly aware that they are, in fact, abnormal. Society suffers from that lack of recognition (as the author will explain later). He classifies degenerate between the categories of healthy and sick, in line with the academic trend of the time.

Still, Morita's degeneration is different in purport from the ordinary opinion when we note that there is no strict differentiation of the various categories, and there are cases of mutual transfer or merger, because they are classified on the basis of factors of trait or disposition, observed from a viewpoint of character and ability with respect to a person's life.

Morita's degeneration is not limited to persons of a low level, physically and mentally, or to those of a morbid abnormality, including persons of genius as well. However, few persons of the latter group become patients in clinical practice.

---

[3] The terms trait, disposition and degeneration as used by Morita seem to resemble the classification of psychopathic inferiority used by J. L. A. Koch (see Chapter 1). However, the content expressed by these terms is different from that of Koch's terms.

[4] Morita, S.: Shinkeisuijakushō no hontai (The substance of neurasthenia), 1921. In *Morita Shōma Zenshū*, Vol. I. Hakuyōsha, Tokyo (1974). (Printed in Japanese)

The author has discussed Morita's viewpoint of degeneration as a sort of preface to a full understanding of the nosological positioning of *shinkeishitsu*. The question of how and when Morita first worked out his concept of degeneration will now be considered. In correlation with this question, Morita's thoughts on constitution and temperament, and the period of time when he began to form his opinion of the mutual shifting of stereotypes of degeneration, are of considerable interest.

The first paper in which Morita clarifies these matters, from a bibliographical standpoint, is a thesis titled "Neurasthenic-Psychopathic Constitution."[5]

In this thesis, Morita clearly explains his opinion, acquired from his clinical experience, and also describes his thoughts on the neurasthenic condition. According to Morita, the neurasthenia of his era is, in fact, nervosity combined with hysteria. A condition of mutual shifting between these two elements is frequently observed. He had encountered two cases (a patient with a hypochondriacal neurasthenic state and one with an obsessive neurasthenic state) that correspond to those factors. His observations are that:

1. Most cases of a neurasthenic-psychopathic nature are constitutional and indicate a condition that is different, or somewhat abnormal, from that of other children, beginning in infancy, and there is a tendency for this condition to develop as such children grow older.
2. This condition can be observed in many people, but most of them do not complain; rarely do their doctors listen to them if they do complain.
3. The younger the patient, the more effective the therapy for this condition will be; good results may not be obtained, and treatment will be more difficult, as such patients grow older.

The content of this thesis will be examined in detail because it is considered the beginning of the future concept of Morita *shinkeishitsu*.

Both of these cases involved persons who were deemed constitutionally weak, with problems encountered from a child-rearing standpoint. Symptoms of *shinkeishitsu* began during infancy. Morbid sensations and other phenomena became more pronounced, physically and mentally, as the persons grew older.

In addition to the condition of ordinary neurasthenia and obsession, an inclination toward suffering had become more marked by autosuggestive exaggeration of the morbid psychological condition that anyone may normally experience in childhood.

With this clinical experience, Morita explains the features of neurasthenia. He identifies the causes of neurasthenia as inborn constitution and the negative effect of child-rearing (excessive protection or excessive interference) as well as emotional experience, along with mental and physical fatigue, as the motivating elements in its occurrence.

Various mental and physical phenomena that comprise the symptoms of neurasthenia are present from infancy, and such phenomena become more pronounced, as definite symptoms, from around 15 to 30 years of age, evolving into a chronic condition.

These symptoms can be classified into the categories of gastroenteric factors, motoricity, vasomotoricity, psychosexual factors, hypersensitivity, emotional factors, fatigue and abnormal thought syndromes. There are shifts of various conditions of alienation that can be classified into the groupings of hysterical, depressive, dull-brained, obsessional and hypochondriacal.

The following states are a summary of our understanding, acquired by the observation of results based on Morita's clinical experience of the so-called neurasthenic condition:

---

[5] Morita, S.: Shinkeisuijakusei seishinbyōshitsusei taishitsu (Neurasthenic-psychopathic constitution), 1909. In *Morita Shōma Zenshū*, Vol. I. Hakuyōsha, Tokyo (1974). (Printed in Japanese)

1. There was a feeling of heterogeneous composition because there was no fixed nomenclature or concept of neurasthenia or neurosis at that time. However, Morita had an understanding of a syndrome in which neurosis consists of *shinkeishitsu* disorders, on the one hand, and of hysterical disorders, on the other, with mutual shifting between the two types of disorder.
2. In terms of causation, he emphasizes inborn constitution and such life history conditions as child-rearing practices used by parents during infancy (excessive protection, excessive interference or, at the opposite extreme, a hands-off policy of noninterference).
3. Morita classifies neurosis within the scope of degeneration (later, abnormal personality) and understands it as being one type of life reaction exhibited by human beings, but it seems evident that he already had his own concept at the time; the condition, to Morita, germinates in infancy, develops with age (especially during youth), is indicatively abnormal, evolves into symptoms and then progresses into a chronic stage.
4. When this chronic stage arises, autosuggestive psychology acts etiologically, triggered by emotion, plus mental and physical fatigue, and becomes fixed in consciousness as various emotional and conceptual phenomena.
5. A solution of the condition becomes therapeutically difficult if an attempt is made to persuade a patient theoretically, on the basis of interpretation and explanation of the symptoms, when the characteristics of the abnormal psychological condition displayed by the patient are taken into consideration. A vocation in the field of agricultural production, with numerous opportunities for direct contact with nature, is encouraged.

A rough outline of Morita's notion of degeneration had already been conceived at the time he wrote this thesis. There is no doubt that he had directed his attention toward the neurasthenic-psychopathic constitution, noting the title of this thesis.

He tried to understand *shinkeishitsu* and hysteria as variants of degeneration caused by this type of constitution. Morita writes in the thesis that Kraepelin provided the category of *originäre Krankheitszustände* and included those who "suffer by themselves" from nervosity and obsession, but he did not follow Kraepelin's mode of thought. He attempted to construct his own classification of degeneration. Morita's concept of degeneration was closer to the thought of K. Schneider than to the thought of Kraepelin, as Uchimura[6] points out.

Process of Establishing the Hypersensitive Psyche Theory of *Shinkeishitsu*

At the time, around 1919, that Morita started to describe the psychopathological basis of and a method of therapy for *shinkeishitsu* to establish it as a clearly defined disorder, it is believed that the subject in which he had the most interest was the hypersensitive constitution.

It has been mentioned that Morita gives serious consideration to the possibility of a congenitally weak constitution as the cause of so-called neurasthenia, in his thesis on the neurasthenic-psychopathic constitution, but he seems to have first clearly explained the hypersensitive constitution in his thesis on *shinkeishitsu* ("Shinkeishitsu no Hanashi," The Theory of *Shinkeishitsu*, 1919). Since he mentions constitution frequently thereafter, we will cite a few of his descriptions.

---

[6] Uchimura, U.: Seishin igaku no kihon mondai (Basic problems of psychiatry: A view of the structural theory of psychopathology in psychosis and neurosis), Chapter 15: Theories of neurosis (in Japanese). *Seishin Igaku* 13(11) (1971).

"What I call *shinkeishitsu* generally includes a neurasthenia which is due to so-called congenital constitution; it is caused by a congenital trait. This trait has both physical and mental aspects. The physical aspect is the hyper-sensitive constitution described by Matsubara[7] which is due to an inborn physical and mental irritative weakness."[8]

"Although Dr. Matsubara's hyper-sensitive constitution theory, with respect to neurasthenia, differs from my own point of view, his concept is quite moderate, and I believe there will be numerous points in his theory which will be seen to agree with my theory as studies of physical and mental relations progress in future."[9]

"In regard to hyper-sensitive constitution, there is first a difference in the degree of good or poor health in our constitutions, and no clear boundary between health and weakness. From that standpoint, *shinkeishitsu* signifies that the constitution has veered away from the level deemed normal health.... *Shinkeishitsu* will occur in accordance with differences of relative rate and strength between the hyper-sensitive constitution and the hypochondriacal trait; the degree of hyper-sensitivity of the constitution may be strong even if the mental trait is weak, as Dr. Matsubara has asserted. On the other hand, complications of *shinkeishitsu* will occur when the hypochondriacal trait is strong, even if the hyper-sensitive constitution is weak, which is my own particular viewpoint."[10]

It is clear from these quotations that Morita directed his attention to the hypersensitive constitution by comparing it with his concept of the mental trait involved in the disorder, and he devoted serious consideration to it as one of the causative factors of *shinkeishitsu.* For that reason, he at first tried to classify *shinkeishitsu* from the two aspects of physical (hypersensitive constitution) and mental (temporary irritative weakness) factors.[11]

This theory of the hypersensitive constitution attracted Morita's interest for some time, but he gradually changed his point of view. Morita wrote two papers on *shinkeishitsu* ("Shinkeishitsu no Hanashi," The Theory of *Shinkeishitsu*, and "Shinkeishitsu no Ryōhō," The Therapy for *Shinkeishitsu*) in June and December 1919, before establishing this theory. In both papers, he gives serious consideration to the hypersensitive constitution, and he stresses the importance and presence of both mental and physical factors of the hypersensitive constitution as the substance of *shinkeishitsu.*

There is no mention of the hypochondriacal trait in either paper. It can be inferred that the concept of the hypochondriacal trait, which became the nucleus of Morita's later theory, had not been worked out at that time. In the latter of the two papers, "The Therapy for *Shinkeishitsu*," Morita proposed a "mental sensitivity," which we may assume to be the kernel of the concept of the hypochondriacal trait, rather than referring to the hypersensitive constitution.

"Dr. Matsubara has proposed a theory of hyper-sensitive constitution in the instance of neurasthenia, and I concur with this in general. But I consider *shinkeishitsu* a mental weakness, or a lack of resistive mental strength for living, or a hyper-sensitive constitution .... Consequently, *shinkeishitsu* is a matter of mental sensitivity, and particularly a hyper-sensitivity of the senses in respect to illness; it is subjective and does not indicate an actual physical weakness ....

"I suggest that *shinkeishitsu* is due to a trait of mental hyper-sensitivity. I do not consider

---

7 Saburō Matsubara explained his theory of the hypersensitive constitution in neurasthenia from a correlation with the endocrine and autonomic nervous systems.

8 Morita, S.: Shinkeisuijakushō no hontai (The substance of neurasthenia), 1921. In *Morita Shōma Zenshū*, Vol. I, Hakuyōsha, Tokyo (1974). (Printed in Japanese)

9 Morita, S.: Shinkeishitsu no hontai oyobi ryōhō (The substance of *shinkeishitsu* and its therapy), 1928.

10 Morita, S.: Shinkeishitsu oyobi shinkeisuijakushō no ryōhō (The therapy for *shinkeishitsu* and neurasthenia), 1921; ibid.

11 This classification was also mentioned in Chapter 1 (footnote 2). It was elsewhere mentioned by Morita (The substance of neurasthenia, 1921).

the patient to have some kind of disease. I refer to the therapeutic method as a training therapy for the personality, because, ultimately, the problem can be considered a weak personality reaction toward a state of health . . . . With reference to the marked success of therapy based on my own point of view, I wish to affirm my theory of mental sensitivity . . . ."

We may assume from Morita's statements that a complete affirmation of the hypersensitive constitution theory of Matsubara had now shifted to a partial affirmation only. (This affirmation soon recedes from the foreground of Morita's thought, and the nucleus of the pathological basis of *shinkeishitsu* shifts from a trait of mental hypersensitivity to the hypochondriacal trait.)

When the author summarizes the transition in Morita's thinking from emphasis on a physical trait (hypersensitive constitution) to emphasis on a mental (hypochondriacal) trait, the author sees that "the notion that an inborn weak constitution is the substance of *shinkeishitsu*" (Neurasthenic-Psychopathic Constitution, 1909) has changed within ten years to consideration of a constitutional trait (hypersensitive constitution) and a mental trait (mental sensitivity) as equal factors (The Theory of *Shinkeishitsu*, June 1919). However, his emphasis again shifts toward mental sensitivity in his thesis of six months later (The Therapy for *Shinkeishitsu*, December 1919), in which he proposes the "mental sensitivity" theory that formed the premise for the "hypochondriacal trait."[12]

Morita's endorsement of Matsubara's hypersensitive constitution theory continued, even after 1919, although it had receded in importance. Morita gave serious consideration to the constitution theory, as we can see in his major thesis, "The Substance of *Shinkeishitsu* and Its Therapy," in 1928,[13] although its content replicates his statements as cited above. In his words, ". . . . from the standpoint of the theory of the oneness of body and mind, it is not possible to know the degree of a physically hyper-sensitive condition in terms of the hypochondriacal trait, but since Dr. Matsubara's notion of the hyper-sensitive constitution is proposed by the relationship with the autonomic nervous system or the endocrine system, I firmly believe that my mental trait theory and Dr. Matsubara's hyper-sensitive constitution theory have an extremely close relationship, and an important contact point should be found between the two theories in future."

Morita did eventually shift his thinking to an emphasis on the mental trait (mental hypersensitivity or the hypochondriacal trait) based on his clinical experience. However, in this process he leaves, as it is, the presence of a physical trait (hypersensitive constitution) as a causative factor of *shinkeishitsu*. He looked forward to discovering the mental and physical intersections in terms of the concept of the essential oneness of mind and body.

At one time, he prepared a draft for the classification of *shinkeishitsu* on the basis of physical, mental and obsessive factors.

---

[12] By addition to this, the author notes that the "mental sensitivity theory" that Morita proposed in December 1919 was revised to the "hypochondriacal theory" two years later, in 1921. However, Morita does not offer any explanation for this revision. The author's view is that Morita proposed the "mental sensitivity theory" after considering that mental hypersensitivity is the chief factor in the substance of *shinkeishitsu*, rather than the preceding notion of "hypersensitive constitution," so that the latter concept could be left as it was. If so, what was the reason for the shift from the mental sensitivity theory to the hypochondriacal theory? It is believed that the *kizuki* or *kizukau* mentality, which is concerned with human existence, in other words, the "hypochondriacal humor," manifests, with more clarity, the factors that give rise to *shinkeishitsu*. Further, Morita had probably reached the decision that this condition could be manifested more easily in persons, like himself, who have a mentally hypersensitive "temperament." As has been mentioned, Morita considered "emotional sensitivity" as one factor of hysteria and probably wanted to differentiate the two types of sensitivity.

[13] Morita, S.: Shinkeishitsu no hontai oyobi ryōhō (The substance of *shinkeishitsu* and its therapy), 1928. In *Morita Shōma Zenshū*; ibid.

Nosological Positioning of Morita *Shinkeishitsu* and Classification According to Type of Disorder

The general concept of Morita *shinkeishitsu* can be first explained by quoting Morita's own description. "I would like to confer the word *shinkeishitsu* on the condition previously referred to as neurasthenia. The reason for this is that my opinion of its substance differs in definition from Beard's so-called nervous weakness or exhaustion; I consider it a pseudo-nervous weakness, and not a true weakness of the nervous system."[14]

"The *shinkeishitsu* I refer to is one of seven types of human temperament, or mental trends.[15] It progresses to a disorder and its precise characteristics cannot be understood unless it is accurately defined as 'Morita *shinkeishitsu*'."[16]

This specific Morita *shinkeishitsu* is caused by two major factors: taints on mental and physical sensibility and the hypochondriacal trait (or hypochondriacal mental trend). Neurasthenia had been previously classified, in general terms, into congenital and acquired characteristics, according to the presence or absence of hereditary factors, but the taints identified by Morita that give rise to *shinkeishitsu* are a mix of hereditary characteristics and a condition that causes a weakening of mind and body, owing to some type of disorder during infancy, coming into combination. Another example is that of an acquired hypersensitive constitution following oophorectomy, even after attaining maturity. Further, what Morita means by mental and physical sensibility is, for instance, a condition in which the autonomic nervous system (or the vasomotor nerves) becomes hypersensitive.

A marked demography appears, which is interpreted as physical sensibility, with a trait of excessive concern over slight changes in mental or physical phenomena. The factors of the mental trend in *shinkeishitsu* combine to increase an introspective tendency by strengthening the desire for self-preservation.

Although a patient with *shinkeishitsu* has an intellectual presence, he or she is also self-centered and easily attached to all sorts of subject matter. The patient's modes of thought and feeling cannot be naturally expressed because he or she adheres to logical analyzing and can easily become eccentric. The patient is frequently absorbed in his or her personal condition because he or she is introspective. The patient is prone to experience self-loathing or is hesitant and suspicious.

Morita describes the relationship between Morita *shinkeishitsu*, which exhibits these specific personality trends, and the prior concept of neurasthenia:[17]

---

[14] Morita, S.: Shinkeishitsu oyobi shinkeisuijaku no ryōhō (The therapy for *shinkeishitsu* and neurasthenia), 1921; Shinkeisuijaku no hontai (The substance of neurasthenia), 1921. In *Morita Shōma Zenshū*, ibid.

[15] Morita, S.: Henshitsusha no bunrui ni tsuite (On the classification of degenerates), 1927 (in Japanese): *shinkeishitsu* (mental sensibility) taint, hysteria (emotional sensibility) taint, weak-willed taint, hyperthymic taint, hypothymic taint, paranoiac taint and schizothymic taint. In *Morita Shōma Zenshū*, Vol. II; ibid.

[16] Morita, S.: The road to *shinkeishitsu* therapy, 1935. In *Morita Shōma Zenshū*, Vol. V; ibid.

[17] Morita, S.: The substance of neurasthenia, 1921 (in Japanese). In *Morita Shōma Zenshū*, Vol. I; ibid. Morita wrote a thesis titled "The therapy for *shinkeishitsu* and neurasthenia" some two months before writing this thesis and specified the following classification to clarify the relationship between *shinkeishitsu* and neurasthenia: 1) acquired neurasthenia (a. mental and physical exhaustion; b. hypochondriacal misconception; c. combination of 1 and 2); 2) congenital constitutional neurasthenia (*shinkeishitsu*) (a. physical hypersensitivity; b. psychological hypersensitivity, including hypochondriasis and obsession). Paroxysmal neurosis is not included in the subdivision of psychological hypersensitivity in *shinkeishitsu*.

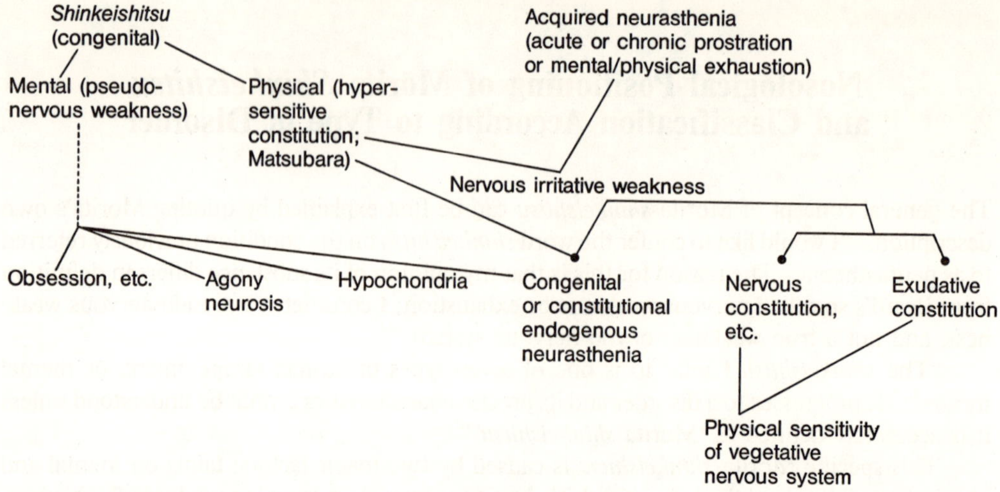

In this classification, Morita considers purely congenital neurasthenia as being due to a disturbance of the metabolic norm, the ordinary condition of human health, caused by exhaustion or other factors. It is an acute or chronic prostration, or a condition of psychosomatic exhaustion.

Morita holds that it is not especially necessary to consider this a condition of neurasthenia because the various functions of the body are in a genuine condition of nervous weakness at the time. Mental pseudo-nervous weakness in this classification indicates Morita *shinkeishitsu*; although this subdivision was frequently revised later, it seems that the basic concept had been established, after numerous clinical experiences, around 1919.

However, *shinkeishitsu* had been divided into the physical hypersensitive trait and the mental hypersensitive trait even in the thesis of June 1921; further, constitutional endogenous neurasthenia and anxiety neurosis had been included in the latter category, which differed from the subdivision in the classification. This point has been cited in the pertinent footnote 17.

In a thesis[18] dated eight months or so after the two papers of 1921, the condition resulting from the physical hypersensitive trait has been omitted from Morita *shinkeishitsu*, the congenital or constitutional endogenous neurasthenia included in the classification has been categorized as *shinkeishitsu* in a narrow sense (parenthetically) in the subdivision and agony neurosis has been revised to paroxysmal neurosis.

The following statement by Morita explains his reasons for omitting the physical hypersensitive trait from the sphere of *shinkeishitsu*:

"Even if I divided *shinkeishitsu* into a physical hyper-sensitive trait and a mental hypersensitive trait, the mental trait is a condition which is essential to the formation of *shinkeishitsu*. Although a physical aspect is present, I believe it is not necessarily related to *shinkeishitsu*."

In this instance, too, Morita does not completely negate the physical hypersensitive trait but considers it an inessential condition, in an aggressive sense, for the development of symptoms of *shinkeishitsu*.

It is clear that Morita's classification was revised, almost bewilderingly, in a short span of only two to three years, beginning in 1919, when he first proposed his theory of *shinkeishitsu*. The difficult work involved in psychopathological clarification and establishment of a unit for

---

[18] Morita, S.: Shinkeishitsu no hontai oyobi ryōhō (Über das Wesen und die Therapie der Nervosität) (in Japanese). In *Morita Shōma Zenshū*, Vol. I; ibid.

one disorder, on the basis of painstaking clinical experience, can be inferred from these frequent revisions.

The modern-day classification of Morita *shinkeishitsu* was formulated and finalized after he had written his thesis "On the Classification of Degenerates" (June 1927).[19]

The three types of *shinkeishitsu* are ordinary *shinkeishitsu*, paroxysmal neurosis and obsession.

Morita offers the following explanation of the classification of these three types: "There was a time when hypochondria was included, for a total of four types, but this has now been omitted, since it was found to be difficult to clearly differentiate it from ordinary *shinkeishitsu*. Earlier investigators paid almost no attention to this sort of classification. This is because the true substance of *shinkeishitsu* was not understood, and it was classified only by external symptoms. It is regrettable that, even now, experts in the field cannot understand that this type of obsession and common *shinkeishitsu* are of the same character. It is particularly clear from therapeutic results that the characteristics are the same, in view of complete cures achieved in the same number of days by exactly the same method . . . ."

A general description of the three types of *shinkeishitsu* is given in the paragraphs that follow.

Ordinary *Shinkeishitsu*

The most characteristic type, the common variant can probably be termed *shinkeishitsu* in the strictest sense of the definition. It is generally known as congenital, constitutional or chronic neurasthenia. The symptoms of this type are rarely increased or fixed by errors of diagnosis or therapy over a wide range that takes in internal medicine, gynecology, ophthalmology, otorhinology and urology.

It is not possible to specify all the symptoms because they are much too numerous. If an abnormality of the head is taken as an example, the symptoms include a dazed condition, a feeling of numbness, headache, a feeling of heaviness and pressure on the head. There are cases that involve the senses of vision and hearing, in which the symptoms include dizziness, swirling of the head and depersonalization.

There can be other uncomfortable feelings, such as a rise in body temperature, a feeling of blood rising to the head, hotness or coldness of the limbs, palpitation or a feeling of pulsation throughout the whole body. In cases in which the stomach and intestines are affected, there may be stomach discomfort, poor appetite, a feeling of abdominal swelling or constipation.

There are various mental symptoms, such as distraction, poor memory, lack of patience, quick irritation or fatigue and inability to understand reading matter.

These various symptoms are all subjective; there is no actual, objective abnormality.[20] The one factor common to all these symptoms is that of control by the hypochondriacal humor (temperament); they become attached to morbid feelings, and the experience of acute self-consciousness continues permanently.

Paroxysmal Neurosis

This nomenclature was first used by Morita. He reported in 1919 a case that corresponds to this

---

19 Morita, S.: Henshitsusha no bunrui ni tsuite (On the classification of degenerates), 1927 (in Japanese). In *Morita Shōma Zenshū*, Vol. II; ibid.

20 Kōra expresses this as the subjectively fabricated nature of the *shinkeishitsu* symptom. Kōra, T.: The problems of so-called neurasthenia (in Japanese). *Psychiatria et Neurologia Japonica* 42: 755–796; Morita therapy. *International Journal of Psychiatry* 1: 611–640 (1965).

type, as being cardioneurosis, but it is apparent that, until that time, there was no awareness that this variant is a type of mental disorder.

This type is characterized by a variety of symptoms, such as tachycardia, a fearful paroxysm that heart failure will occur at any moment, paroxysm over loss of strength in the hands and feet, paroxysm of dizziness, paroxysm over feelings of vertigo and fainting, unstable paroxysms, paroxysmal chills and shivers, paroxysmal pain in the internal organs (e.g., gastalgia), paroxysmal loss of consciousness and paroxysm due to a feeling of losing oneself, becoming crazed or not knowing oneself.

However, what is common to all these symptoms is an affective explosion of fear and a marked mood of anticipatory anxiety. Control by the hypochondriacal trait of this affective explosion is increased, and an affected person is captivated by the objects of fear.

The personality trend of a person with this type of disorder differs from the trends of persons with other types of neurosis because there are numerous cases in which the mental hypersensitivity and the introspective trend characteristic of the *shinkeishitsu* trait have receded into the background; such persons are extroverts, with an active, reality-oriented personality trend. However, differentiation of this disorder from hysterical, unstable paroxysm is important.

As was indicated in the classification of 1921, Morita called this disorder an agony neurosis at one time but later called it paroxysmal neurosis because he designated paroxysm on the basis of an emotional experience of fear as the major symptom.

Morita had long ago pointed out that the potential for a cure for this type of disorder is high if no error is made in the diagnosis and therapy. He reported many cases in which therapy was relatively easy and complete successes in treatment were frequently achieved by psychotherapy alone. Nevertheless, the disorder is associated with dangerous conditions and can become chronic if the diagnosis is ignored.

Obsession

According to Morita, obsession denotes a condition of conflict generated by feelings of resistance that an affected person experiences as a result of considering a certain concept or feeling as a hypochondriacal, morbid abnormality and trying not to think of or feel it. There is no obsession if this mental conflict does not arise.

The difference between obsession and ordinary *shinkeishitsu* is that the symptoms of obsession are limited to agony, discomfort, anxiety and fear, for example, headache, dizziness or insomnia in the case of ordinary *shinkeishitsu* but resistance against feeling pain as pain, shame as shame or fear as fear in the case of obsession. Further, obsession is a condition characterized by constant anticipation of future feelings of fear. Complicated mental conflict is also present.

The most important characteristic of what Morita calls obsession is that the obsession is not morbid; it is a commonplace concept and a feeling that everyone normally experiences.

The history of obsession dates back long ago. Many investigators have discussed obsession, beginning with the description by Esquirol (1838), but seemingly in terms of heterogeneous mixtures of symptoms. The issue of the composition of symptoms has given rise to differences of opinion; the points that are emphasized differ according to the manner in which the condition is observed. Some investigators have called obsession morbid or heterogeneous and, from a qualitative point of view, primitive, immature, impulsive, offensive, sadistic or masochistic in presentation, undisguised sex or squalor.

When it is explained from a chiefly psychoanalytic point of view, importance is placed on the content of the obsession, as symbolic expressions of repressed desire and of a defensive resistance to desire, indicating a compulsive character. By comparison, Morita's view is that the content of obsession does not lie outside the scope of psychological normality; he considers it a psychological inconvenience, however, an unpleasant factor, or one that generates anxiety from the hypochondriacal trait, with a naturally resistant action of the mind taking place to eliminate it. However, the more one experiences this mental resistance, the more the concept and feeling that occupy the consciousness of an affected person are reflected in abnormal character, with a simultaneous aggravation of unpleasant feelings and anxiety.

If, for example, one has the thought that the content of what one has said was mistakenly communicated to another person during a certain conversation, a mental shock rooted in the desire to correct the error or to confirm that a mistake has been made will arise, because such afterthoughts are accompanied by uneasy feelings. Nonetheless, this sort of concern is experienced on a daily basis by all human beings.

A healthy person will utilize the phenomenon as something that is socio-positive. However, it becomes socio-negative in a person with *shinkeishitsu*, who is captivated by the fear of uncertainty in speech due to anticipated anxiety. The notion that one's meanings were probably not communicated correctly to another person develops into the notion that one's words were probably incorrect, so that the other person did not grasp the meaning correctly. This reaction generates even greater captivation, with the belief that any such notion is, in itself, "abnormal and morbid."[21]

What is important, in the occurrence of *shinkeishitsu*, is that it is determined by how an affected person accepts any life reaction that is activated by actual living conditions. The decision of whether or not the consciousness of the person, and the concepts that come into mind, invite feelings of inconvenience or anxiety in life can function to fix one's attention on such disturbing concepts even more acutely. This tendency is particularly strong in a person who has a mental hypersensitive trait, such as the *shinkeishitsu* persona.

This is what Kōra refers to as the psychology of inadaptability anxiety. Thoughts or feelings that have the role of providing the fuel for personal crisis originally contain the anxious feeling. Resistance to these thoughts and feelings stems chiefly from mental (or intellectual) theorizing, and in view of this, one will naturally experience contradiction or have irrational feelings but is not aware of this process. (Morita refers to this condition as contradiction in thinking.) An affected person may become oppressed by obsession because of greater and greater efforts to eliminate contradictions and irrational feelings.

There is, for example, the superstitious fear of numerals, chiefly the numerals 4 and 9 in Japan. The cause of this fear is the notion that the numeral 4 (*shi*) can be associated with death (*shi*) in Japanese phonetics; the numeral 9 (*ku*) is associated with suffering (*ku*). Such a superstitious person fears the numerals 4 and 9 and avoids them.

The numeral 4 is only an ordinal number. The person can insist that 4 is a simple numeral that follows 3 and precedes 5, or that two times 4 is 8, with 8 considered a lucky number. However, this is intellectual theorizing. If 4 is associated with one's death or the death of family members, and some related misfortune also comes into association, it is natural to feel uncomfortable or anxious.

The emotional phenomenon cannot be understood by logical analysis, and it is not possible to control it as one wishes, simply because the emotion is inconvenient. Such a superstitious person does not become aware of contradictory notions and attempts to ignore the numerals 4 and 9 (as do other people), but the more the person tries to do this, the more his or her attention converges on the matter, so that the conflict is aggravated.

Associating one word with another phonetically is a mental activity that can occur in

[21] The patient's judgment of abnormal or morbid arises, in most cases, from a fear of feeling "different from normal persons."

anyone. Morita's position is that constitutional and mental trends must be present for this sort of mental activity to evolve into obsession.

This claim can also be made for acrophobia. Most of us can sense fear and tend to cower at a great height. Anxiety over the possibility of impulsively jumping off or falling off because of carelessness can graze the mind. (This is also a factor of mind.)

In an ordinary, mentally healthy person, the mind will also take a natural resistive action to harmonize itself and the actions of the person. The *shinkeishitsu* persona will resist this anxiety of imagining a jump or fall and will try to eliminate the notion. This persona will, on the contrary, come into confrontation with the concept. In a manner similar to previous examples, a person suffering from *shinkeishitsu* will try to eliminate the possibility of anxiety by an intellectual process of logical analysis, to assure himself or herself that there is no possibility of a foolhardy leap because there is simply no sensible reason for it, or that there is no possibility of falling off accidentally because, although it is a great height, he or she will be attentive to safety measures. However, as a result, the person will plunge into suffering because he or she cannot succeed in this mental maneuver. The conflict will be further aggravated because the person is not aware of the inherent contradiction: that emotion cannot be controlled by rational analysis.

Other investigators, for instance, Schultz,[22] take a position similar to Morita's on the subject of obsession. Schultz states that human mental activity is dialectic. For this reason, the notion of what it would be like if one jumps from a great height will occur instantaneously to anyone who is in that position. The condition of the experience in itself acts as the *thesis*, and the imaginative notion (of jumping or falling) that accompanies the experience becomes the *antithesis*. A healthy person will not pay special attention to this experience, but a mentally disordered person is frightened by the *antithesis*, falls into anxiety and thus creates a fixed symptom.

The obsession that occurs in the instance of Morita *shinkeishitsu*, the action of the ego in taking a resistant position, in rousing conflict, plays an important part in the formation of the symptom.

In contrast with the obsession characterized by such ego activity, we frequently find, in daily clinical practice, an obsession in which the action of the ego is weak, with little conflict. It appears that this is a phenomenon in which the person has entrusted himself or herself to the condition completely, by a compulsive act.

Morita clearly differentiates such compulsive action from other types of obsession and considers it as being caused by a weak-willed trait. He explains the phenomenon by stating that such a person may, for example, take an action in direct correspondence with the condition, simply because he or she is not satisfied by a certain opinion, such as an omen or a morbid love of cleanliness. The person may lack a desire for therapy to overcome the condition, preferring to return to normal on his or her own. By taking so-called compulsive action, the person will not exhibit any aggressive ego activity directed toward the anxiety caused by his or her experience, but will, instead, take compulsive action repeatedly, with little conflict.

A person who suffers from obsession may examine the household locks, possible sources of an outbreak of fire or flammable materials and furnishings by a simple repetitive procedure, day and night, until he or she is satisfied. Although these activities appear to be confirmatory actions, they deviate from the true object of the exercise and are, instead, actions taken to allay the anxiety of dissatisfaction, the entire procedure having become a mere formality or ritual that the person recognizes as being exactly that.

Morita stresses the need to differentiate a person who exhibits such compulsive behavior from one who suffers from obsession because a compulsive person has little desire for therapy

---

[22] Schultz, J.H.: *Grundfragen der Neurosenlehre.* Thieme, Stuttgart (1955).

and because there is almost no hope for therapeutic success even if the behavior is given a phenomenological classification.

The foregoing text is a general description of the obsession included in Morita *shinkeishitsu.* His opinion of compulsive acts must be kept separate.

According to Morita, obsession in Morita *shinkeishitsu* is the ready acceptance of an experiential condition as something disadvantageous or uncertain from the standpoint of self-preservation. The attitude of the ego becomes aggressive and prone to conflict. The internal attitude of the ego (an attitude that one could possibly become introspectively aware of but is not aware of at present) is characterized by suffering from the discrepancy of consciousness (which Morita calls contradictoriness in thinking) between an immediate experiential reaction (the factual state of one's mind as it is) and the desire or demand to become this or that (the ideal) instead.

Thus, obsession differs from compulsive behavior because, in obsession, the people around an affected person do not become readily aware of the symptoms by comparison with the marked internal conflict.

There are many cases of obsession indicative of Morita *shinkeishitsu* among the conditions of general compulsive phenomena in daily clinical experience. The number of cases of compulsive activity that Morita saw as originating from a weak-willed trait is far from small. Nevertheless, there are many cases in which a satisfactory result is obtained from Morita therapy, even though the duration of therapy is long, in the face of an apparently strong resistance.

Such cases represent compulsion, or a compulsive prohibition[23] set up as a secondary defensive reaction to contend with obsession, as pointed out by Ōtsuka.[24] It cannot be claimed that all cases of compulsive acts are caused solely by a mental mechanism that differs from Morita theory. There are only a few cases that indicate pure obsession, but there are many cases that are accompanied by certain compulsive acts or compulsive prohibitions. When such acts or prohibitions are compared with the compulsive activities explained by Morita, however, there is a difference, in that they are not conspicuous actions because they are not impulsive or addictive and because the willpower that attempts to suppress conspicuous speech and behavior is also operative.

Morita's mode of thought with respect to the relationship between obsession and phobia will now be examined.

Morita concluded that there is no essential difference between phobias and the phenomenon of obsession. As was mentioned previously, obsession induced as a specific reaction to an experience is not isolated but is accompanied primarily by a certain emotion or is in a close relationship with a concept represented by emotion.

For example, an obsession results from fear of the numeral 4 and the concept of that numeral and is reinforced by trying to evade it, resulting in unpleasant associations with death or an abhorrence caused by the numeral 4. The resistive action that attempts to suppress the concept of the numeral associated with death gives rise, in fact, to a condition of being captivated more and more by the numeral 4.

There is almost no point in scrutinizing whether the object of fear is emotional or conceptual. The point is that the essential basis for the obsession is the dual conflict of fear and the fear of discomfort.

---

23 In the instance of the fear of using public transport facilities, for example, an affected person gets off a streetcar before he or she reaches the destination because he or she feels bad; palpitation occurs from the moment the person boards the streetcar. This reaction subsequently develops into the anticipation of experiencing fear, and because similar symptoms occur even when the person thinks about riding a streetcar, he or she may not be able to board and ride a streetcar, or even to go outdoors. In this condition, an affected person prohibits action on his or her own owing to fear of public transport facilities and to the anticipation of fear that accompanies the experience.

24 Ōtsuka, K.: Kyōhaku shinkeishō ni okeru kyōhaku kōi to kyōhaku kinshi (Compulsion and compulsive prohibition in obsessional neurosis) (in Japanese). *Tōkyō Jikeikai Ika Daigaku Zasshi* 74: 11 (1959).

Agoraphobia, which can be considered a representative phobia, is the fear of going to a certain place, an open area, a place where people congregate or a deserted place with no one else present, but the condition actually results from fear of cardiac acceleration, dizziness, fainting, heart failure and delirium. Morita points out that there are many cases in which this condition can be classified as paroxysmal neurosis. Anticipated fear is strong in paroxysmal neurosis; by contrast, conflict is strong in obsession.[25]

In general, the characteristics of Morita *shinkeishitsu*, including obsession, are determined by the attitude of the ego in its concern with the content of the symptoms. The content of each symptom is composed of a commonplace concept and feeling. Emphasis is placed on clarification of the internal attitude of the ego, in a condition of not being aware of the symptomatic trend, by clarifying the tendency of consciousness toward the present living conditions of the patient, rather than by pursuing the pathological basis of the symptoms.

When obsession is viewed in this manner, it falls within a category that represents the mental phenomena of Morita *shinkeishitsu*. Representative symptoms are anthropophobia (discussed in Chapter 9), nosophobia, morbid fear of incompleteness, morbid fear of omens, acrophobia, morbid fear of riding in public transport facilities, claustrophobia, morbid fear of promiscuous (desultory) thoughts and aichmophobia.

This is a general description of the characteristics of Morita *shinkeishitsu* according to type of disorder, but there are also mixtures of the disorders cited in the preceding paragraph, mutual transitions and mutual interference of other mental trends, such as weak will, depressiveness, paranoia, hysteria and schizoidal factors, that cause a dilution of the essential characteristics of *shinkeishitsu*. There has been a trend over the past ten years toward an increase in the number of cases that deviate from the standard type of *shinkeishitsu*.[26,27] Although the reasons for this

---

[25] Morita, S.: Shinkeishitsu no hontai oyobi ryōhō (The substance of *shinkeishitsu* and its therapy), 1928. In *Morita Shōma Zenshū*, Vol. II; ibid.

[26] Morita *shinkeishitsu*, which has the characteristics noted in the preceding list, is classified as follows (the ICD-9 classification of mental diseases and the DSM-III classification are given for the sake of comparison):

Morita's Classification	ICD-9	DSM-III
Morita *shinkeishitsu*	300 neurotic disorders or (301 personality disorders)	
1. Ordinary *shinkeishitsu*	300.7 hypochondriasis or 300.5 neurasthenia	300.70 hypochondriasis or 300.71 atypical somatoform disorder
2. Obsession	300.2 phobic states or 300.3 obsessive-compulsive disorder (301.4 anancastic disorder)	300.21 agoraphobic with panic attacks 300.22 agoraphobic without panic attacks 300.23 social phobia 300.29 simple phobia 300.30 obsessive-compulsive disorder
3. Paroxysmal neurosis	300.0 anxiety states	300.01 panic disorder 300.02 generalized anxiety disorder

[27] Tsunetoshi Takeyama (1933) comments on this in his "Study of the Impure Type of *Shinkeishitsu*", in the *Collection of the Professor Emeritus Morita Memorial Thesis*, 1942 (in Japanese); more recently, Y. Nishimuta mentions it in: Discussion of the so-called impure type of Morita *shinkeishitsu*. *Morita Ryōhō Shitsu Kiyō* (Bulletin of the Morita Therapy Room), Vol. 3 (in Japanese), Psychoneurological Department of the Jikei University School of Medicine, Tokyo (1981).

trend are not clear, changes in the social and cultural conditions of Japan cannot be overlooked. In that connection, the conditions that comprise the standard type of Morita *shinkeishitsu* are as follows:

1. A subjectively fabricated image of the self is formed by sensitive reactions toward experiential conditions that arise from mental hypersensitivity or the hypochondriacal trait.
2. One's actions with respect to one's desires are aggressive.
3. Perfectionistic, idealistic and self-centered attitudes are simultaneously strengthened by a lowering of actual self-valuation as a result of conditions 1 and 2.
4. The mental trend of viewing all things in terms of the subjectively fabricated image is strengthened.
5. A person afflicted with *shinkeishitsu* is self-centered, but conflict occurs as a result of a strong tendency to try to control emotional phenomena by exercise of intelligence; the mental level is normal in range, and the introspective trend is strong.
6. The desire toward life adaptation is strong; there is an awareness of the *shinkeishitsu* disorder.
7. The condition is readily cured by Morita therapy; the cure rate is high.

9

Characteristics of Anthropophobia

The author believes he has good reason for taking up the subject of anthropophobia in this chapter. Although obsession best expresses the compositional features of the symptoms of Morita *shinkeishitsu*, the author believes that anthropophobia is its most specifically representative category and that this category is closely related to Japanese culture and the Japanese mentality.

As Morita points out, anthropophobia is a condition of self-conscious suffering that makes one painfully shy in the company of other persons. (At one time, erythrophobia (ereuthophobia), Morita wrote in 1925, is one representative aspect of this condition.)

In interpersonal relationships, a person with anthropophobia believes that being shy is weak-willed. The person strongly attempts not to be shy but is, instead, captivated by the condition, seized by the fear of disgrace, according to Morita. Consequently, this condition is not simply one of shyness or tension but, rather, a condition of mental conflict that arises from a "bad loser, obstinate nature" that tries to fight the feeling of tension and shame as "weak-willed."

This bad loser, obstinate nature is, in fact, a manifestation of what Morita calls the "desire to live." With its presence, Morita *shinkeishitsu* is characterized by a double structure, having not only introverted, passive and powerless features but also, in opposition, extroverted, active and powerful features.

This is the reason that obsession, particularly anthropophobia, is considered the nucleus of Morita *shinkeishitsu*, in that such features exist from a symptomatic, structural standpoint.

It is probably necessary to mention the condition of the Japanese persona in terms of interpersonal relationships because this factor is important to a discussion of anthropophobia. The bad-loser, obstinate nature has a probable association with the "curiosity" and "stubborn determination" which are considered prominent features of the Japanese mentality. When the Japanese came into contact with Western culture (which rapidly came to the fore in Japan after the Meiji Restoration in the latter half of the nineteenth century), the contact was a turning point. The cultural gap between the Japanese and Western cultures no doubt cast a spotlight on the bad loser, obstinate nature of the Japanese mentality and caused a massive "culture shock." This powerful shock, along with the influence of the enlightened thought and realism of the Meiji Period, became the driving force that accelerated the modernization of Japan. In a contrary manner, it also provided a stage on which to observe the performance of "shyness" in Japanese behavior. This shyness will be dealt with later, but the author believes its features become distinct when it is examined in conjunction with the prevalence of anthropophobia in Japan.

In this chapter, the author will first explain the general features of anthropophobia and then its correlation with such Japanese cultural and social characteristics as *kizukai* (see Chapters 2 and 3), *mi* (see Chapter 4), *hitomishiri* (anxiety in the presence of strangers) and *seken* (or *sekentei*).[1]

Anthropophobia is called *taijin kyōfu* in the Japanese language, but it is not clear when this term was first used and by whom. Kure (1865–1932), in his preface to the second edition of *Seishinbyōgaku Shuyō* (The Essence of Psychiatrics) (1915–25), referred to anthropophobia as *jinshū kumon* (social phobia) and to erythrophobia as *sekimen kyōfu*. The term *taijin kyōfu* must have come into use later. The matter is vague, owing to lack of research, but according to Morita, someone had recently used the term *taijin kyōfu* because there are many occasions in which various forms of mental suffering occur in interpersonal relationships, although Morita does not identify the person who first used the term (*Shinkeishitsu*, volume 3, number 5, 1932).

Morita encountered his first case of anthropophobia in 1919 and published a detailed description of the case in 1925. Morita initially referred to the disorder as erythrophobia, not anthropophobia, but it was indicated as a representative case of anthropophobia in his description published in 1932. *Seishi kyōfu*, which the author will discuss later, was a term coined by Morita and is considered a mental phenomenon peculiar to Japan.

General Features of *Taijin Kyōfu*

Morita refers to the condition of suffering caused by direct, sustained eye-to-eye contact with another person as being due to *seishi kyōfu*, the fear of eye-to-eye confrontation. In general, what is commonly called *taijin kyōfu* includes, in addition to *seishi kyōfu*, a number of other subtypes, namely, *shisen kyōfu* (fear of eye expression, used to mean *seishi kyōfu* in many instances), *sekimen kyōfu* (ereuthophobia, erythrophobia), *hyōjō kyōfu* (fear of one's self-expression) or *shūbō kyōfu* (fear of ugly self-expression), *shinsen kyōfu* (fear of physical trembling) and *taishū kyōfu* or *jikoshū kyōfu* (fear of one's body odor).

What is common to all these subtypes is the phenomenon of feeling tense and ashamed when confronted by other persons and the inability to manifest fully the desire for self-actualization, which is initially present within the self as *sei no yokubō*. Instead, attention is directed to an inferiority feeling of one's self or one's attributes, and a person who has this feeling is captivated by this distraction.

When one tries to achieve *kaku aritai* (something as it could be) but finds that this ego ideal is suppressed in reality, the hypochondriacal basic tone is relatively strengthened and the mental tone shifts gradually toward *kaku araneba naranai* (something as it should be) owing to the antagonistic actions of the mind. This condition is, in fact, one of *kaku aru* (something that is what it is). In other words, it is the condition of the actual self, but the normative judgment imposed on this "actual self" is low, in terms of the person's self-evaluation. The difference between "what is" and "what should be" has the effect of strongly exacerbating the inferiority feeling that the person is experiencing and indicates a condition of suffering ego. This is the basic mental condition of *shinkeishitsu* and the reason for considering *taijin kyōfu* as being in the same category as *shinkeishitsu*.

---

[1] *Seken* is a Japanese word formed by combining the Chinese ideographs *se* and *ken*. *Se* refers to era or time period and represents the phenomenon of changes from moment to moment in relation to other factors; in other words, transitions that occur with the passage of time. *Ken* has the original meaning of "space" or of being in a location, in principle, between two substances and thus indicates a sense of "placement." *Seken* can be used, in general, to mean "the world" or "society." In another sense, it is used to mean the scope of one's activities and associations, the sphere of one's reference group (which is its chief meaning in the context of our discussion). It can also mean the people who make up a society. It is consequently a term that expresses the interpersonal relationships between or among persons or human relationships in general. *Seken-tei*, one of the *seken* compound words, has the meaning of a standard faculty, of human relationships in a correlated or associated group or of personal dignity and respect within the *seken* context.

Numerous reports[2] indicate the great prevalence of *taijin kyōfu* among the various types of neurosis evident in Japan.

Seishi kyōfu is considered a particularly representative type of Japanese neurosis. There is a strong impression that it is a uniquely characteristic clinical picture of Japanese neurosis because it is not mentioned in the foreign literature. It would be of interest to undertake a comparative cultural investigation of this phenomenon.[3]

Taijin kyōfu, including *seishi kyōfu* and *sekimen kyōfu*, is considered a conspicuously Japanese neurosis not only because it is not mentioned in the foreign literature but also because it is an aspect of interpersonal relationships, particularly the attitude of having a concern for human relationships (*kizukau, ki ni suru*), that is readily bred into the feelings of Japanese life.

The culture in which the essence of *shinkeishitsu* forms pathoplastically and easily as a clinical picture called *taijin kyōfu* is the constitutional substrate of the life attitude accepted by the Japanese.

However, a mode of thought that stems from the influence of a specific recognition system in Japanese culture is present in the attitude of observers, and this mode of thought lies in the background of the reasons that a large number of cases of *taijin kyōfu* has been observed in Japan. This type of neurosis probably has a peculiarly Japanese characteristic because it is noteworthy that the nomenclature of *taijin kyōfu* was originated by the Japanese.[4]

The life activities of any person are evaluated in relation to the society or the cultural conditions in which that person lives. The neurotic condition must be considered as one of inadaptation formed within the prescribed social and cultural norms. This is readily understood in the instance of *taijin kyōfu.* A person with this condition cannot escape the restrictions of the surrounding social and cultural matrix. The matrix imposes a realization of confrontation when the person is in the presence of other persons, which strengthens the desire for self-realization and self-toleration.

Further, the matrix forms the context of the person's daily life activities. The person becomes conscious of the evaluations made by other persons (the *seken*) and cannot avoid being concerned over what those significant others (or *seken*) think about him if he is to maintain his position as he wishes within the *seken* or among other people in general.

The person strives for greater self-expression of his or her desires, or for the future fulfillment of desires, after securing the trust of other persons. The *taijin kyōfu* persona has a frame of mind that differs from the norms in dealing with other persons. Mental tension increases, and the person becomes awkward, rigid or shy and "reluctantly" avoids the realities of day-to-day life.

This reluctant feeling confers suffering due to a strong inferiority feeling toward self and the person's attributes because he or she cannot openly confront people. The person's personality, ability, visual expression, complexion, physical expression, posture, body odor and self-atmosphere become the objects of his or her concern. And each of these objects of concern becomes the nucleus that forms the clinical picture of *taijin kyōfu*. The various phases of *taijin kyōfu* are outlined in the sections that follow.

Seishi Kyōfu or *Shisen Kyōfu*

The basic symptom of this condition is that an affected person suffers because he or she cannot

---

2 Suzuki, T.: Taijin kyōfu ni kansuru tōkeiteki kansatsu (Statistical observation of *taijin kyōfu*) (in Japanese). *Seishin Igaku* 5:1013–1023 (1976).

3 Kasahara, Y.: Seishi kyōfu no rinshōteki kansatsu (Clinical observation of *seishi* (*shisen*) *kyōfu* (Fear of eye-to-eye confrontation or of visual self-expression)). *Japanese Journal of Psychoanalysis* XIV(2) (1968).

4 Kimura, B.: *Hito to Hito to no Aida–Seishin Byōrigakuteki Nihonron* (Between Man and Man–Psychopathological Comments on Japan). Kōbundō, Tokyo (1972). (Printed in Japanese)

look directly into the eyes or face of another person and thus avoids interpersonal relationships. Frequently, however, some difference in expression of the condition is observed, depending on the case.

For example, "I have an unpleasant feeling if the other person becomes aware of being looked at, and this causes a loss of composure in me."

"The other person looks the other way because I have penetrating eyes and tries to avoid looking at me."

"I try to look at the other person because I think it may be shameful not to look straight into the other person's eyes, or it may indicate to that person that I am not in earnest, so I try to look at the other person, but this becomes painful to me."

"Because the other person looks away when I look at him, I try to avoid looking at him, but even then I look at him, so that I feel embarrassed."

"As my eyes turn naturally to look at the abdomen of the other person, I become embarrassed and cannot bear it." (This comment is frequently made by female patients.)

Similarly: "My eyes turn to the breast and abdomen of the other person, so that the other person loses composure and suffers because he assumes that I consider him offensive." (This comment is frequently made by male patients.)

Also: "My body becomes cramped and stiff (or I feel ashamed), so I cannot look at the other person and instead look down and suffer because I have taken an impolite attitude toward the other person."

There is the common feature of not being able to look directly into the eyes or at the face of the other person or of being oversensitively conscious of "my own" gaze as well as the other person's, and this feeling ends in efforts to evade interpersonal relationships. However, this evasion is not easy and gives rise, at the least, to the attitude of coming into conflict with one's feelings of weakness and inferiority, which are strengthened by any attempt to overcome such feelings.

This *taijin kyōfu* (as *shinkeishitsu*) includes such oppressive sensations as feeling ill at ease, having strong tension and lacking in endurance. There are also many cases that involve fear of hurting another person's feelings, by making the other person feel uncomfortable, irritating the other person's mind or offending his or her emotions. There are other cases of persecution feelings, such as being frightened by another person.

The initial impression may be that both mental states are phenomenologically opposite, but if this condition is true of the Japanese in general, in that they are keenly sensitive to the gaze of another person, both of these mental states can be considered as phenomena that share the same roots.

Although this sensitivity to another person's gaze will be explored in more detail later, a brief explanation will be given here. In their normal psychological condition, the Japanese people generally experience a strong feeling of resistance to direct eye-to-eye contact. When eyes meet spontaneously, regardless of whether conversation is taking place, the general attitude is that one of the two persons should look aside. There is a feeling of being indiscreet or impolite in looking at another person eye-to-eye.

Sekimen Kyōfu (erythrophobia)

One becomes concerned about blushing in front of other persons and therefore tries not to blush. A person with this condition grieves about the experience of being shy or cowardly. The condition of suffering obsession and of taking the pessimistic view that one cannot live together with other persons of the *seken* as a mature person is called *sekimen kyōfu*. This condition differs from the condition of not trying, in which the person only blushes and evades the other persons who are present and struggles to contend against the condition.

What Morita means by *sekimen kyōfu* is one representative symptom of *taijin kyōfu*, together with *seishi kyōfu*, but a number of different conditions can be observed, depending on the interpretation made by the person. The face may become hot and red when the person becomes tense; his or her face may become even redder when people look at him or her; the person may feel that other persons make fun of him or her as being naive and childish. The person believes that he or she is ridiculed for being timid, cowardly, feministic. Or the person interprets his or her blushing in a self-punitive manner as though he or she is suspected by other persons of having done something shameful.

There are many contrasting cases of feeling that it is impolite if other persons adopt a sympathetic attitude toward this timidity and childishness, of making the other person pay attention to the condition or of making the other person feel unpleasant. From the fear of blushing, the person takes the attitude of wiping perspiration off his or her face, or pretends to be cooling his or her face with water because of feeling hot, and that is what makes the person blush or redden.

The person may wear a surgical mask or sunglasses, or conceal his or her face with the hair, as much as is possible, to avoid being "seen" by other people. Such maneuvers are frequently observed in cases of *taijin kyōfu*, especially in the instances of *shisen kyōfu* and *hyōjō kyōfu.*

Hyōjō Kyōfu or *Shūbō Kyōfu*: Fear of Self-expression or Ugly Appearance

This condition can show variations from case to case, but what is common to all cases is that an affected person suffers from a fear of facing people due to his or her appearance or to physical defects, such as a face that seems unpleasant, a face that becomes distorted by laughter, a face that seems to stare or twitch or a face that is greasy and offensive.

Suffering also derives from faults observed in facial features, for example, the lips, eyebrows, forehead, bridge of the nose or jaw. The faulty feature is thought to be distorted, too wide or too narrow, too high or too low. The person also suffers because his or her manner of speech, voice, configuration of the body or the way he or she walks is faulty or because his or her appearance seems unpleasant to people.

Shinsen Kyōfu

This condition is fear of suffering from the notion that people feel odd or uncomfortable because the affected person's voice, hands, fingers or whole body shows visible tremors due to the fact that the person is too tense in front of people. This shaking intensifies the more the person tries to suppress it. This condition becomes manifest when the person is writing in front of other persons, when he or she works with the hands and when he or she serves cake and tea. Consequently, writer's cramp and occupational convulsions are included in this fear.

Taishū Kyōfu or *Jikoshū Kyōfu*

This fear arises because an affected person feels that he or she cannot be presented to other persons because they will dislike and avoid him or her due to some type of unpleasant body odor–bad breath, sweat, flatulence–on the body or in facial or neck hair. Such a person tries, as much as is possible, to avoid using public transport facilities, attending meetings and going to places where large numbers of people tend to congregate, such as a workplace. The person suffers because of this fear. To conceal the foul odor, some such persons will not face people without first employing some measure to prevent body odor, such as axillary osmidrosis, washing the body excessively, constantly washing or changing undergarments or using a large amount of cologne or perfume.

The So-called *Taijin Kyōfu*

There is no specific object of this fear. The complaint may differ somewhat, depending on time and place, but an affected person does become tense in front of people. The body becomes rigid owing to feelings of stress. Palpitation occurs. The body becomes hot, and the eyes become bloodshot or clouded or tearful.

In this condition, the person cannot converse with other persons, becomes inattentive to what is heard or said and suffers complete loss of composure. Body movements become awkward due to tension, stress or shyness experienced in facing people. An attitude of trying to avoid people as much as is possible can be observed. This attitude arises from the anticipation of anxiety.

This fear of facing people is not always the same in substance, differing from case to case. There may be no reluctance toward one-to-one personal contacts, but there is considerable resistance to appear before a large number of people; when coming in contact with another person, the person may suffer because there is no subject of conversation or because the conversation is broken off.

Because the symptoms of the so-called *taijin kyōfu* can be considered the basis of several specific subtypes (subsumed under *taijin kyōfu*), conditions in which the basic fear is differentiated into specific objects of fear are frequently observed; for example, *shisen kyōfu*.

Simple explanations of the major subtypes of *taijin kyōfu* have been given in the preceding sections. They all show a common mental state: the desire to solicit approval for oneself through contact with other persons, being favorably received if there is an opportunity for interpersonal association or for being taken seriously. At the same time, the anxiety engendered by *kizukai* considerations, in terms of "Do I make people feel unpleasant, am I disliked by other persons, or am I ignored and slighted by other persons?" comes into play. This anxiety arises simply because the desire for self-realization is constantly present in the background of the *taijin kyōfu* condition.

The mental state of *taijin kyōfu* includes timidity, hypersensitivity, introversion, shyness and evasion but is also due to the Morita *shinkeishitsu* factor of contending strongly against feelings of helplessness, timidity and shyness.

Wellsprings of *Taijin Kyōfu*; *Hitomae*, *Hito*, *Ningen* and *Seken*

A general description of the various mental states has been given in the preceding sections in regard to persons who suffer from *taijin kyōfu*, including those who try as much as is possible to avoid coming into contact with people (*hitomae*) because of strong feelings of tension, shyness or anticipated fear.

Such persons also suffer because they feel helpless when they must, reluctantly, face people. What is this specific fear of *hitomae* that gives rise to the general condition of *taijin kyōfu*?

The term *hitomae* is ordinarily used to mean "in the presence of one or more other persons." Consequently, *taijin kyōfu* is not simply a matter of feeling afraid to go where people will be present. Confronting another person signifies that the other person will form certain judgments or evaluations of the fearful person. In other words, *taijin kyōfu* occurs in the relationship of "you and me."

The condition aroused by the fear of *hitomae* differs from case to case. A one-to-one *hitomae* may not always be characterized by the same degree of severity. To certain other persons, an affected person may be a total stranger who represents no special human relationship. There is only an object-to-object phenomenon of looking at that other person or of being looked at. The fear then arises that oneself (I) will make the other person (you) feel uncomfortable and cause discomfort to one or both of us during the act of mutual observation. "I" fear that I will be evaluated as odd or weird.

There are instances of suffering similar to this generalized sort of interpersonal encounter, such as the situation of meeting a slight acquaintance rather than an old friend. The other person may seem to show a facial expression or general demeanor that impresses me as injurious to my sense of self-esteem because he or she does not, perhaps, initiate topics of conversation, because the conversation is interrupted and does not fill up the entire time,or because, for some other reason, "I" feel embarrassed in front of the other person.

The feeling of embarrassment is avoided in a human relationship in which constraint and *kizukai* concern are exercised and sustained. The *tai* of *taijin kyōfu* means "confrontation"; the *jin* means *hito* (person, human being) in the Japanese manner of reading these two Chinese ideographs. Thus, anthropophobia can be defined as the fear of confronting other human beings.

The accurate definition of *taijin kyōfu* is, however, that of the obsession that arises in a person when or she is facing another person. This obsession supplants a genuine human relationship.

Why is it that "I" become tense, bashful and stricken by tension in this situation of facing another human being? In common-sense interpretaion, it comes from a concern to secure a position (for oneself) that will not run counter to the established social order, which dictates the proper standards for human relationships within the constantly shifting milieu of day-to-day human life and social customs in one's community.

Securing this position or satisfying the desire for another person's approval of oneself is not something that is strictly confined to the Japanese. Nevertheless, the author will now discuss specific reasons that *taijin kyōfu* is so conspicuously a Japanese type of obsession.

Ningen, *Hito*, and the Psychological Nature of *Kizukai*

Taijin kyōfu will now be discussed from the standpoint that the symptoms of *taijin kyōfu* indicate one type of Japanese characteristic. A certain historical facet of Japanese culture can be observed in the transitions of the meanings of words (by an unconscious mental process). Our example here is that of *ningen* (*nin*=man; *gen*=*aida*=between) in becoming synonymous with *hito*.

The original meaning of *ningen* is that of *seken*, but the meaning was eventually distorted to become synonymous with *hito*. Watsuji[5] stresses that it is important to realize that this distortion is not a simple misunderstanding of the original definition. He cites the alteration of meaning as rising inevitably out of the historical Japanese social order, with the change in mean-

[5] Watsuji, T.: *Ningen no Gaku to Shite no Rinrigaku* (Ethics as Human Learning). In *Watsuji Tetsuō Zenshū*, Vol. 9. Iwanami Shoten, Tokyo (1977). (Printed in Japanese)

ing based on the direct understanding of *ningen* in the historical life of the Japanese, even if the shift in meaning was an unconscious process.

This historical alteration of meaning indicates that *ningen*, which originally meant nothing other than *yo no naka* (the world), came to be understood as meaning *hito* (human being).

If *hito* can be construed as completely isolated from interpersonal relationships, it is probably proper to make a differentiation, like that in the German language, between der *Mensch* (man) and *das Zwischenmenschliche* (between man (*hito*) and man (*hito*)).

However, *hito* has meaning only in terms of interpersonal relationships; consequently, it is probably correct to understand that *ningen* means *hito* if we believe that *hito* in itself expresses the whole field of interpersonal relationships.

We can probably detect a direct understanding that *ningen* signifies "society" and, at the same time, an individual human being, when we examine the entire history of the word *ningen* in its transitions from originally meaning *yo no naka* or *seken* to meaning *hito.*

Watsuji considered our concept of *ningen* in his historical discussion of the word. The Japanese learned, in their initial period of cultural development, that the words *nin* and *hito* correspond most appropriately to *anthropos*, *homo*, *Mensch* and *man*, according to the usage established in ancient China (which signifies that man is the lord of creation or the champion of all living things and that man is not man because he stands on two legs and lacks a pelt but because he has a language; these two usages clearly agree with the definition that the Greeks gave to *anthropos*).

The Japanese applied the word *hito* to this definition. However, when *nin* is viewed more precisely, it differs in meaning from *homo* and *anthropos. Nin*, and particularly *hito*, mean *ta* (another person), which is differentiated from oneself. For example, taking away something from *hito* does not mean detracting something from *anthropos* but, rather, stealing someone else's personal property.

The expression "I together with *hito*" does not mean that oneself and *Mensch* (man) are placed side by side; rather, it encompasses oneself as well as other persons. Further the meaning of "other persons" is expanded to mean an indefinite number of people. The *hito* in *hito-wa-iu* (people say) or in *hito-giki no warui* (disreputable) already contains the nuance of *seken* and indicates that "I" am afraid of whether other persons will accept me. Watsuji states that the word *hito* is expanded to include the meaning of *seken* because it signifies oneself with respect to another person(s).

This meaning of *hito* must not be overlooked. For example, I say "do not make a fool of *hito*" to someone who teases me. This response comes from the understanding that, to the other person, I myself am *hito* (other persons). The concept of *ningen* is created by adding the word *gen*[6] to the word *nin.* The meaning is not simply that of *hito no aida* (between or among *hito*) but that of "between or among *hito* that include oneself as well as other persons or the *seken.*"

This makes it clear that the field of *hito* encompasses oneself and other persons, so that the word implies a preexisting basis of the "relationships between or among myself and other persons." The meaning of oneself and other person(s) is created by delimiting the field of interpersonal (person to person) human relationships.

The fact that *hito* is other persons as well as oneself simply means that it defines the limitations of the field of *ningen.* Watsuji suggests that the reason that *ningen*, which at first meant "human society," later came to mean *hito* (person) as well is derived from the dialectical relationship between the whole and its individual parts. A part exists in relationship to the whole; at the

[6] *Gen* means *aida* (between or among), that is, the space interposed between one substance and another. It is used to express time differentials as well as spatial or other relationships between one thing and another.

same time, the whole manifests itself in its parts. In consideration of this part-and-whole relationship, *hito* becomes the social *hito* meaning *seken*, and is also *ningen*, because the wholeness of *seken* is expressed with respect to each and all of its individual *hito* components.

What differentiates the human *hito* from any other animal are the factors of language and self-consciousness, but both of these factors are a product of social interaction manifested in each and every person. As long as *hito* is "one person" having a language, society is manifested in that person, and he or she is constantly deemed *ningen* as well.

When viewed in this manner, it can be said that assigning the double meaning of *seken* and *hito* to *ningen* best expresses the true essence of *ningen*. Watsuji attempts to clarify the concept of *ningen* by considering its historical background: that *ningen* is *yo no naka* and, consequently, neither exclusively *hito* nor exclusively "human society." He states that both *hito* and *seken* are dealectically unified in *Ningen*.

As a result of Watsuji's studies of *hito*, *seken* and *ningen*, the author perceives that the "I and thou" relationship in the Japanese mentality is one of "I and society" as well as the *hito* and *hito* (person to person) relationship within the field of the *seken* or *yo no naka* (the world in which we live).

In that respect, the mental state of *taijin kyōfu* can be defined as a neurotic mental attitude adopted toward the tension that occurs between *hito* and *hito* within the whole field of the *seken*. This tension is nothing other than the *ki wo tsukau* (concerned, considerate) and *ki wo kubaru* (alert, cautious, prudent, watchful) attitudes that govern and facilitate smooth interpersonal (person to person) relationships between *hito* and *hito*. This mutual attitude enables each *hito* to indicate and express his or her position within the *seken* on his or her initiative.

Terms that have solicitous meanings, such as *kizukau*, *ki wo kubaru* and *kiganesuru*, are used between one person and another person. If *ki* is eliminated, these terms become simply *tsukau*, *kubaru* and *kanesuru*, which are general terms that no longer have any direct application to the person-to-person relationship. *Ki* seems to act as a medium or catalyst that conjoins the mentalities of one person and another person. This medium is somewhat like an "atmosphere" that is circulated between the two persons.

This solicitous "atmosphere" produced by the use of the word *ki* is generated between any two persons, from self to other persons and from other persons to self, and is the manner in which mutual communication is given a groundwork for expression and development. This ki "atmosphere" has an important implication in the "meeting of minds."

There is no essential difference in the situation whether the communication is one-to-one or oneself in confrontation with the whole of the *seken*.

Because *ki-zukau* and *ki wo kubaru* have these applications to interpersonal relationships, the normal state of the *ki-zukau* mentality in operation between two persons is that of using *ki* as a major expression to indicate respect for another person. This means that "I" am careful to express myself properly to "you" by conveying the *ki* "atmosphere" in my speech, demonstrating my concern to be solicitous and not to hurt "your" feelings. This also includes mental attention and activity to protect "my own" feelings so that "I" am not hurt by "you."

When this normal state of solicitous mentality becomes distorted, in anthropophobia, an affected person is plunged into a condition of suffering, in being bashful *hitomae* (in front of other persons). When "I" am exposed to the scrutiny of other persons, I have a strong feeling of shame and tension; I feel shackled or frightened. Yet, I cannot tolerate this condition in myself, and my efforts to reject and expel it become the substance of anthropophobia.

The condition arises because when I am put under the scrutiny of another human being, I feel that I have become an impersonal object that will be evaluated as good or bad, right or wrong, beautiful or ugly. As a result I, too, have a keen concern to judge the other person, to determine whether he or she is better than I am, whether I am inferior to the average person, whether I am a person who is disliked and not accepted by people in general and the *seken*. This concern makes me feel increasingly bashful when I am placed under the scrutiny of other persons, and I become frightened by it.

Let us summarize this condition by stating that the meaning of *kizukau* (to be concerned) in its attachment to *hito* has been in daily use by the Japanese, up to the present, and that it indicates the extent to which the Japanese conduct their lives with a heavy emphasis on interpersonal relationships. This concern has become solidified into social customs, as is evident in the cultural transitions exemplified by the shifts in meaning of such words as *hito* and *ningen*, from having disparate meanings to becoming virtual synonyms.

This *kizukai* psychology was seemingly fixed in the Japanese mentality through an unconscious mental process that took place in terms of the relationship between one person and another person. It is firmly rooted in tradition, and it became an active supporting prop to regulate and facilitate interpersonal relationships.

Phenomenological Nature of *Mi* and the *Kizukau* Psychology

In this situation, a person in an anthropophobic condition cannot naturally manifest the desire to have himself or herself approved of (owing to a desire for self-realization) *hitomae* (in front of people). When this condition is viewed from the person's perspective, he or she attempts to suppress the feeling of tension rather than manifest the actual action of self-expression. This tension is due to timidity and shyness in front of people. The person's attention is absorbed by a condition that dissatisfies self to the degree that he or she canot bear to endure it when he or she must face people.

To an affected person, *hitomae* consists of the *manazashi* (gaze) of another person. The natural feeling of *kizukau* toward the other person is cut off by this self-absorbed condition.

A person-to-person relationship in which one's *ki* is closed and not shown is a state of consciousness in which the *ki* displayed by another person is received in a unilateral manner. One's *ki* of trying not to become bashful, frightened or tense has the opposite effect: I become more and more conscious of the other person's *manazashi* and *ki* and feel placed under intense observation because of my subjective consciousness.

The anthropophobia seen in the Japanese is a condition of suffering from *kyōfuteki-toraware* (fearful captivity) that emanates from a feeling of fear or shame toward *hito* and *seken*. It is questionable whether the consciousness of the individual person, in the true sense, is present in the Japanese mentality if we take into consideration that the Japanese have been raised in a culture that has no clear consciousness of the reality of *jibun* (self). The Japanese become initially conscious of *jibun* by means of the *kizukau* psychology in interpersonal relationships. The relationship between *hito* and *hito* or *seken* is excluded.

From the standpoint of the psychological basis of anthropophobia, too, this "correlation of relationships" is lost due to a feeling that insists on trying to maintain the relationship between *hito* and *hito* and ends in a condition of becoming captivated by the fear of one's personal position becoming endangered in the context of interpersonal relationships.

This also makes it clear that there is little self-determination to express one's egoistic will in the Japanese consciousness. It is, rather, a matter of each person, as the possessor of a relative autonomy, trying to maintain a unified field of relationships between *hito* and *hito*.

The self that functions in person-to-person relationships always participates with the *kizukau* psychology. One takes action to try to live while participating. In this respect, we need to discuss the concept of *mi.* We previously touched on *mi* in a footnote to Chapter 4 but will deal with it in more detail now.

The word *hito*, as we have explained, is multivocal. So is *mi.* In essence, *mi* stands for the content of external form or substance itself, but as a general term, it is used to convey the meanings of the human body; oneself or myself; the overall mind-body condition of the person; social position, status and personal standpoint; and one's personal life-style (*Kojien*, first edition, 1967; *Iwanami Kokugo Jiten*, Iwanami Shoten, third edition, 1979).

Our reason for discussing *mi* at this juncture is that one's actions in the context of the *ki-zukau* psychology can be better understood in relation to *mi.*

If *hito* is replaced by *mi*, the *kizukau* of the *hito* in the relationships between *hito* and *hito* infers that *mi*, in reference to oneself, is a matter of living autonomously to maintain *mi* in an "expansion of subjective space."

If this phenomenon is understood as a natural matter in daily life, it means that *mi* lives while taking into consideration the positioning of *mi* in that space to which *mi* belongs. This *mi* does not simply exist as oneself, which becomes an object of cognition or action, but, instead, stands for an overall condition in which one's personal position or life-style or mind-body unity continues to live while, at the same time, trying to preserve the authentic *mi* in an outward expansion of subjective space. This is the phenomenological nature of the *kizukau* psychology.

The Japanese have a strong consciousness of so-called relative autonomy, in trying to maintain a constant relationship to a place to belong to (the *seken*). Thus, an anthropophobic person is plunged into even deeper suffering by fear of the danger of losing that *mi* (position in the *seken*). To be *hazure* (left out) of the *seken*–the place for living to which one belongs–is closely correlated with a feeling of shame. (We will discuss that shame in more detail later.)

This *haji* (shame) is essentially an inferiority feeling: that one's ability, personal condition and actions are subaverage, compared to those of other persons the whole *seken*, and that they are also out of bounds (beyond the pale of the *seken*). It is believed that this sense of shame developed from the notion of "being absent from the original niche that one should occupy" or of simply "being out of place" (*Iwanami Kokugo Jiten*, ibid).

The *kizukau* psychology of seeking to keep one's *mi* in the place that one properly belongs and of trying to stress that *mi* position in that location is probably the mode that the Japanese, in the past, have used to deal with the consciousness of *mi.* In anthropophobia, however, there is a strong tendency for that consciousness of *mi* to be blocked in its proper form of assertion. In other words, *ki* does not have its original centrifugal property (see Chapter 2) and cannot travel from interior to exterior, from oneself to other persons. Consequently, it appears that *ki* is used, most often, to indicate *mi.* It refers to everything that can be expressed by the entire body and mind and contains the meaning of *mi* in all its aspects of ability, personal condition, actions, life-style and social position.

It is thus understandable that Morita's hypochondriacal basic tone is not restricted to physical considerations, encompassing the whole of the self. It is a characteristic of concern for *mi.* This is one reason that anthropophobia is considered the essential form of Morita *shinkeishitsu.*

Meaning of *Seken*

We will now turn to a more detailed definition of *seken.* The consideration of *seken* is implicated in the common use of the word *hito*, as we have seen. For this reason, probably, numerous words formed by being combined with *seken* remain in daily use.

The first appearance of the *seken* compound words is historically obscure. One meaning, for example, of *seken-tei* (personal prestige or dignity within the world) had its most widespread use during the Edo period.[7] *Seken*, in its present-day meaning, came into common use during the Middle Ages in Japan. It was originally introduced into Japan as a Buddhist word. (It is said to have been derived from the translation of a Chinese canon at around the time Buddhism was brought into Japan, in the sixth century.)

The original word in the canon is said to be the Sanskrit *loka*. It had the original meaning of "changing with time," of something that is broken or negated, and manifests a modern type of negating psychology called *kyoka* (temporary emptiness) tinged with uncertainty.

This meaning was reversed, and the word became synonymous with the Buddhist logic of searching for a higher plane of life. It appears that the Japanese accepted the latter meaning.[8] This meaning then shifted, in subsequent Japanese thought, to indicate chiefly a region of subjective presence and a position in life.[9] Eventually, in modern times, the meaning again changed, to signify "my" human relationships with "the world of people" and the social and spatial conditions in which human life is lived out.

When we compare the phenomenon of these transitions in the meaning of *seken* with the previously discussed transitions in the meaning of *ki* (see Chapter 2), we see that the *ki-zukai* of the *ki*-complex also came into daily use around the end of the Middle Ages in Japan and is still in present-day use.

The frequency of the use of these words in literary publications (especially the popular literature) increased rapidly in the Edo period.[10] The fact that compound words formed from both *ki* and *seken* came into popular use around the same time is probably coincidental if we take into account the background of the rapid progress in development of a popular culture. The culture that was created by historical process, marked by transitions in the meanings of both of these words, can be considered a materialization of the high degree of self-consciousness among the populace of the time and probably formed the foundations that set the mental structure of the modern-day Japanese.

The manner in which each *hito* lives, in the atmosphere of *kizukai* or *kikubari*, is mirrored in the daily use of these words, when the *hito* appears in confrontation with the *seken* or *yo no naka* field. A person appears in this world as an individual human being in the modern sense or in relation to the whole of the *seken*.

The meaning of *seken*, as it is used today, is that of "associating with people, living while mixing with people" when it is used in the verb form of *seken-suru*. It is clear, then, that *seken* indicates an active, fluid living condition. It includes the scope of one's daily activities, environment, society and other persons who surround the individual *hito*.

Watsuji considers the structural feature of *seken* as that of historical or climactic type of human presence that tends to change with time and to expand spatially throughout the course of a human lifetime.

The lives of the Japanese are closely related to their *seken*, to the extent that their lives cannot be considered without constant reference to their *seken*, like the relationship of drops of water to a reservoir.

For example, a young man who has only just become an adult member of society is "someone who does not know the *seken*" (he has meager experience of social life; he lacks

[7] Ienaga, S.: *Nihon Bunka Shi* (new edition). Iwanami Shoten, Tokyo (1959). (Printed in Japanese)

[8] Aida, Y.: *Nihonjin no Ishiki Kōzō*. Kōdansha, Tokyo (1970). (Printed in Japanese)

[9] Inoue, T.: *Sekentei no Kōzō; Shakai Shinrishi e no Kokoromi*, p. 280. NHK Books, Nihon Hōsō Kyōkai, Tokyo (1977). (Printed in Japanese)

[10] Nakai, S.: Ki, ke no nihongo to shite no hensen (Transformations of the Japanese words *ki* or *ke*) (in Japanese). *Teikoku Gakushiin Kiji* 5(1) (1947).

knowledge of social situations and of how to get along in the world). The extent of his *seken* is limited, at first, because the scope of his social associations is limited.

This "not knowing the *seken*" sometimes discomfits persons around him, and at times he is frowned on because he causes a disturbance in his *seken*, as a result of behavior that does not take into consideration the *seken*. At such times. members of his family feel that they dare not show their faces in public (*seken*). Also, if he resorts to putting up a "good front" to the *seken*, "showing off" or "falsely keeping up appearances" in the *seken* group, while still lacking real capability or experience, this behavior will cause the *seken* to close ranks against him, making him feel small, losing trust, in him, making him feel despised, with the *seken* becoming censurious.

Further if he exhibits conceit or sophistication, because he has obtained a certain amount of experience, he will be reproached, because the *seken* is "not easy to deal with" and "you cannot pull the wool over the *seken's* eyes."

However, his *seken* will expand (the scope of his social associations will broaden and his knowledge of the world will increase) and his reputation in the *seken* will improve, as long as he lives an earnest, honest life. If he does live in that manner, in accordance with the "logic of the *seken*," there will be occasions when he will be assisted, even in adverse circumstances, because the *seken* is "smaller than he might believe" (he will meet someone he knows to help him at unexpected times), and this will remind him that "the devil does not appear in the world in human form."

Also, at some time, his honest efforts will be rewarded. There will come a time when he is publicly recognized by the *seken*. At any rate, it is not desirable for the life activities of the Japanese to be either too conspicuous within their *seken* or too quiet so that they are forgotten by the *seken*. Therefore, living "as other persons do in the *seken*" (as other *hito*) is not a matter of keeping an especially high or low profile; considerable effort and *ganbari* (stick-to-itiveness)[11] are required to live "as other persons do in the *seken*." This *ganbari* attitude within the *seken* context can probably be considered one of the hallmarks of being Japanese.

In the life consciousness of the individual Japanese, any deviation from *seken* norms, or to be seen as an iconoclast, is sensed as a strong inward-directed pressure created out of a person's concern for a "perfect fit" within the *seken*. The mental energy demanded to "stick it out" and live as other persons do in the *seken* could be thought to be a prime mover that accelerated the modernization of Japan. This "sticking it out" persists in Japanese society.

Words in daily use that have correlations with the *seken* have been cited. The extent of placing emphasis on correlations with the *seken* and the feeling of *kizukai* in the relationships between *hito* and *hito* can be construed from the sheer number of such words. Is not the *taijin kyōfu* of the Japanese characterized by the *seken* culture as its soil? That is, in the *taijin kyōfu* background, the cultural roots of words that have acquired the meaning of *hito*, *ningen* or *seken*, or a similar series of words, have molded the thoughts and feelings of the Japanese into the *taijin kyōfu* mentality.

The meaning of *taijin kyōfu* can probably be understood, to some extent, by nothing that the phenomenon of *taijin kyōfu* is most correctly not anthropophobia but, rather, *hitomae kyōfu* or *taiseken kyōfu*. The period of time in which both phenomena of *hitomae kyōfu* and *taiseken kyōfu* came into view is not clear, but it is probable that they first appeared in the Japanese vocabulary about the same time the *seken* complex and the *ki* complex came into ordinary, daily use,

---

[11] Japanese life sentiment is not satisfied by "maintenance of the status quo" or "peace and quiet" but, instead, approves of constant effort in search of reformation. As Yuzawa points out, there is no other country in which *ganbare* (Let's stick to it) or *ganbatte imasu* (I am sticking it out) are used as greetings (Yuzawa, Y., *Asahi Journal* 22(21), 1980).

when the Japanese became individually self-conscious in the modern sense, after the end of the Edo Period.

This matter will not be discussed in detail here, but it can be sufficiently considered historical fact; that is, *seken* was ideologically understood to be a promising social mutation during the Middle Ages in Japan but then became thought of as the environment for daily life in modern times.[12]

Seken came to be considered the daily life environment because each *hito* lives in relation to the *seken*. Accordingly, *taiseken kyōfu* develops out of that *seken* situation. Here, however, the positioning of *seishi kyōfu* within the context of *taiseken kyōfu* will be discussed, as well as the implications of the *seishi* phenomenon.

Seishi means to look straightforward at another person in a face-to-face position. More specifically, it means to look directly into the eyes of the other person. There are a large number of people in Japan who experience the phenomenon of not being able to look straight into another person's eyes. Such people suffer to an extreme over this incapability, and it is probably correct to assume the presence of a mental factor that makes looking straight at the faces (into the eyes) of other persons seem awkward in the consciousness of such people.

What sort of factor are we looking for? Before we consider this question, we would like to point out that, in Japan, there are many instances in which people are advised to look directly into the eyes of other persons, as a general rule, particularly when conversing with them. It is said that when a person is newly employed, he or she is trained in this manner as one aspect of etiquette required of employees when dealing with other persons on business matters.

This practice has two implications. One implication is that looking straight into another person's eyes signifies that one is listening to what the other person has to say, fully understanding what the other person wishes to communicate and, at the same time, conveying one's sincere intentions to that person.

The other implication is that the need to train people to look into the eyes of other persons confirms that the Japanese, in general, do tend to avoid direct eye contact with other persons.

This example illustrates a certain cleavage between principle and true intention and can readily bring about a type of psychological conflict. In the individual consciousness, this sort of contradiction can recur, from time to time, in human association. The factor that accelerates the psychological process, called *seishi kyōfu*, acts contrary to the original, natural sentiment; the more one exerts an effort to look directly into the eyes of another person–in opposition to the desire to avoid doing so–the more one strengthens that internal conflict.

Finally, one reacts with hypersensitivity to the lines of sight between oneself and another person, and one becomes captivated by the conflict that rages within.[13]

This conflict can easily occur between the poles of natural feeling and acquired ideological stance (i.e., in ideological terms, looking straight into the eyes of other persons is quite natural when associating with them). The conflict that arises here, which can develop readily into *seishi kyōfu* in Japan, probably results from the fact that the Japanese have lived in social conditions that enhance their consciousness of the lines of sight in interpersonal relationships. One opinion worth citing is that of Yanagida.[14]

". . . Anything new?' has been a phrase in common use for quite a long time among people

---

[12] Hayashiya, T.: *Shomin Seikatsu to Geinō* (Life of the Common People and Public Entertainment). Iwanami Kōza, Nihon Rekishi, 12, Kinsei (4). Iwanami Shoten, Tokyo (1976). (Printed in Japanese)

[13] Essentially, the line of sight moves naturally toward the object of vision, but if one tries to control the line of sight by will, the proper line of sight immediately seems to become unnatural.

[14] Yanagida, K.: *Meiji taishō shi sesōhen* (*Meiji* and *Taisho* history, social conditions): Chapter 5, 3. Looking at Foreign Countries; 4. Eyes for Looking at the World (15th edition). Authentic Books, *Yanagida Kunio Zenshū*, Chikuma Shobō, Tokyo (1979). (Printed in Japanese)

who enjoy social intercourse. But the evolution of what is implied by this expression, which codifies a certain natural curiosity, took place long before people became aware of it."

"Needless to say, the expression of curiosity stems from recognition that the other person is similar to oneself. But this does not necessarily signify heart-to-heart contact. Consequently, it cannot be said to create a view of mutual equality, but it does at least increase mutual understanding in that all of us experience curiosity."

". . . I was able to learn more quickly and become more susceptible to influence because I tried not to overlook anything . . . ."

If a closer observation of the matter is made, one point that we become aware of is that knowing from the outside, and being known from the outside, are quite separate phenomena and not at all mutual. A man from the country who comes to the city, for the first time, is similar to a man who looks outside from inside through a slatted bamboo blind.

Yanagida goes on to comment: "I believe there are no foreign peoples who wish to know, with such exacting detail, what the kitchens and bedrooms of Western peoples look like as much as the Japanese people do . . . This sort of curiosity has increased to an extreme with the existence of opportunities to take a look.

". . . Although it is possible that a different sort of powerful motivation is at work within the Japanese mind, the one-way exercise of curiosity, in which one makes oneself a cipher while scrutinizing the lifestyles of other (foreign) people, has apparently brought about the amazing mixed bag of thoughts and sensibilities in the modern-day Japanese mentality. It has also given rise to habits of excessive self-protection, such as trying to appear, in social situations, as if one is quite alone, walking around in the dark, rather than mixing with people in the equal, free-and-easy comings and goings of an ordinary metropolitan lifestyle.

"This air of solitude is also related to that sort of compassionate sensitivity that we call bashfulness, the *waniru* of a child. (Both bashfulness and *waniru*, in this sense, mean shamefacedness.) . . . It is believed that the basic cause lies, at bottom, deep down in the fundamental temperament of the Japanese people. We must, however, admonish any attempt to explain this away by saying it is simply due to the fact that the Japanese people easily depreciate themselves, are sensitive to novelty, and recognize the quality of something superior."

Moreover, according to Yanagida, the diversity, the mixed-bag nature of modern-day Japanese culture, is the result of an incessant absorption, owing to the high level of intellectual curiosity present in the Japanese temperament. This does not constitute a situation of mutual cultural interchange but is, rather, exercised with an attitude of constant mental precaution, of trying to peep into other persons' lives while hiding oneself in the dark (a mental state closely associated with shamefacedness). Curiosity is exercised, to the utmost, by furtively peeping around as much as is possible.

The mixed bag of native and foreign cultural components produced by this attitude has not, in historical terms, endangered or uprooted the indigenous Japanese culture. Whatever was brought in from outside was carefully filtered, selected and assimilated, in an aggressive spirit, to add new polish to the cultural characteristics of Japan. It also gave birth to new forms of Japanese culture.

This high level of curiosity, accompanied by shamefacedness, which is believed to lie at the very roots of Japanese temperament, has in this manner exhibited a human life-positive orientation, on the one hand, but, on the other, brought about a phenomenon that could be called human life-negative, meaning that the Japanese have become oversensitive to their own and other persons' lines of sight. This condition has become an important factor in molding the so-called Japanese social phobias, such as *seishi kyōfu*.

Yanagida's following comments are considerably rich in suggestions for further discussion of this condition. In another section (Eyes for Looking at the World) of the same chapter of his book, he says that the "temperament of the people, which determines history, is not only *waniru* (bashfulness). . . . There is one other matter, that of *okoru* (anger) to be considered before we move on to the next topic. . . . Grimness in the expression of someone's eyes depends on the nature of that person, or the circumstances of an encounter, so that the expression cannot be said, in any impartial sense, to be truly frightful (or tender). Depending on the country one comes from, grimness can be interpreted in either way. An apparently frightful expression does not indicate the presence of a threat. It simply means that people are customarily scrutinized somewhat more sharply in another country.

"A person who has lived, to the present, among close friends will need to muster a lot of courage in order to confront the gaze of a total stranger. Even if both of them share a mutual desire to get acquainted with each other, the one who is bashful will lower his eyes and thus become the person who does not look but is looked at.

"Ordinarily, the strength of a group is greater than that of its individual members. One can look at other people with composure if the number of one's companions is large, but we sometimes come across people who are so stout-hearted that they can stare back at a large group of people with great composure.

"Since it is possible to foster this sort of courage by an exercise of willpower, our ancestors turned it into a contest called *mekachi.* This was the origin of what we now call *niramekkura* (a staring-down match).[15] In other words: I looked at him because he looked at me; that is, he believed he could not lose a contest of wills between the two of us. At first, the object was probably our mutual desire to get to know each other, since we were strangers, but his gaze was felt as rude, impudent, an infringement of privacy, because a strong gaze is needed to be unafraid of a stranger.

". . . When a person who usually does not try to look at another person, who is shy and only looked at, suddenly wishes to know another person, his eyes do not seem as gentle as those of a child. If the eyes of a large number of men who live in Tokyo seem to be grim, all this means is that those people have been awakened to a new desire to acquire more knowledge of the world around them. . . . It is never an indication of strong antagonism. . . . There was a time when there was no other way of accepting people into equal social association except by putting an end to the discomfiting resistance manifested in losing or winning a staring match. . . ."

The curiosity and desire for knowledge in the Japanese mentality are strong. When we want to know what sort of person any other person is by looking carefully at the other person, we cannot avoid looking at that person's eyes. And the other person likewise looks at us. In this situation, both persons mutually try to look carefully at each other as the whole point of the encounter. To some extent, however, an effort is made to be unafraid of the other person but also not to seem impudent, an unpleasant intruder.

We also believe that to become someone who is looked at by someone else, or to strain our nerves to look at another person, probably became a sort of social regulation for the Japanese, so that they could get along in the world. We would rather become a person who looks at another person than the person who is looked at by someone else. We want to gain public recognition or get to make some new acquaintances. We do this, even if may seem impudent or make the other person feel somewhat uncomfortable, because our motive arises from a desire to get to know that person or from a desire to be accepted by that person.

That mental attitude makes us necessarily look straight at the other person, creating a situation in which each person becomes oversensitive to the other person's gaze. However, the psychological fact that the Japanese "do not essentially want to stare at people too much, are shy, and are always putting themselves in the position of being looked at by people" is a background

[15] A game in which two children stare at each other and the one who first laughs or looks away is the loser.

factor that cannot be ignored, as Yanagida points out. The cultural background that is correlated with the phenomenon of *seishi* in *seishi kyōfu* is thus explained by reference to Yanagida's commentary.

The psychological process that took place in the people of a closed society, who were gradually awakened to modern self-consciousness, has the characteristics of the social conditions of the Meiji and Taisho Periods, when the modernization of Japan had only just begun. The point of contact between the old and new cultures is impressed with the sentiment of the Japanese, who behave with feelings of shyness and shamefacedness.

A mental stance related to looking straight into the eyes of another person is formed if the Japanese try to exercise their powerful curiosity. If *hitomae kyōfu* and *taiseken kyōfu* arise from that mental state, the phenomenon of *seishi kyōfu* is much better understood.

Hitomishiri

The *seishi kyōfu* aspect of *taijin kyōfu* can be said to be conspicuously Japanese. The importance of *seishi* (looking into the eyes) for the Japanese in the context of interpersonal relationships, along with the phenomenological nature of *mi* or *kizukai*, has been elucidated as much as is possible.

We will next discuss a phenomenon that, we believe, is closely related. This phenomenon is *hitomishiri*,[16] which indicates one type of attitude toward other persons and which is used frequently in daily speech.

If uneasiness with respect to human physical existence is one mode of the different forms of *ki*, that is, the hypochondriacal trait, uneasiness with respect to the mental or social existence of the human being is due to *hitomishiri*, which is a different form of *ki* or *taijin kyōfu* (anthropophobia).

Although *hitomishiri* is a term that indicates a certain form of relationship between persons, called "knowing other persons by sight," its meaning is not expressed only by a word but, rather, must be understood as something closely related to consciousness of oneself in the Japanese mode of thinking. As a daily idiomatic expression, *hitomishiri* has different meanings and usages at various stages of human life.

The initial appearance of *hitomishiri* is around six months after birth, and this phenomenon becomes most marked from nine to 12 months. This period is generally called the "strange age." It is believed that what Spitz[17] calls "eighth-month uneasiness" is the type of *hitomishiri* that appears during this period. An infant begins to differentiate the mother and other persons immediately around him or her from other persons he or she is not used to seeing.

This awareness is the beginning of *hitomishiri*, but the reaction toward other human beings shown by the infant indicates that his or her position in the world is being formulated by enlarging his or her life space. The infant's experience of human environmental relationships also begins to form, but this experience is disturbing. The infant feels uncomfortable, ill at ease, in recognizing the first appearance of human beings who do not belong to the immediate environmental constellation of persons who regularly populate his or her infantile world.

The infant does not show indications of *hitomishiri* when carried in the mother's arms, whatever crowd of people may be around him or her. However, when a specific person the

---

[16] Fujita, C.: *Hitomishiri* as a Japanese concept of stranger anxiety and anthropophobia. *Folia Psychiatrica et Neurologica Japonica* 25(1) (1971).

[17] Spitz, R. A.: *Die Entstehung der ersten Objektbeziehungen, Direkte Beobachtungen an Säuglingen während des ersten Lebenjahres*, Klett Verlag, Stuttgart, 1962. *Hahako Kankei no Naritachi* (Beginning of Mother and Child Relations; translated by Y. Koga). Dōbun Shoin, Tokyo (1965).

infant does not know approaches and tries to humor, talk to or carry him or her, he or she makes a "sour mouth," blubbers and then starts to cry. The formation process of that reaction, defined as *hitomishiri*, is believed to correspond to a condition of interoceptive bodily feeling instead of being related to visual or auditory perception of the unknown person.

According to Wallon,[18] this condition is due to differences in the feeling that the infant senses in his or her body, perhaps as a result of differences in the way he or she is held in someone else's arms. In a general sense, the separation of the experience of one's body and the experience of contact with someone else's body takes place in conditions in which one's self and the other person are unseparated and fused. In that condition, one's physical consciousness is born, and perception of the other person, who is in an opposing relationship, is acquired exteroceptively.

Formation of the body scheme of an infant occurs, with both of these systems having complementary effects. One system is formed by the two momentums of the infant's bodily feeling and the other person's perception. A system that works as a totality is formed. Consequently, there is a difference in the mode of reaction that appears as *hitomishiri* in correspondence with the developmental process of this system. Infantile *hitomishiri* is only a reaction in the biological dimension, due to bodily discomfort and uneasiness, but it appears as a reaction that has become emotionally separated after the first year of life has passed and the second year has begun.

For example, when a person in the *soto* (outer world) tries to talk to an infant, the infant will look downward, bury his or her face in the mother's lap or hide behind her and will not greet or reply to the outsider. There will be an attitude of trying to avoid looking directly into the eyes of the *soto* person. However, the infant will intently monitor any conversation between the mother and the *soto* person, even while hiding in that manner.

This attitude differs from the original infantile *hitomishiri*. It is a sign that self-consciousness has emerged. Social consciousness has also begun to surface. Consciousness of *hanikami* (bashfulness) and *hito-oji* (uneasiness about other persons) are apparent and are indicated by the infant's effort to hide his or her body from the eyes of *soto* people.

The activity of an infant at the peak phase of the infantile growth period is truly the "strength of life." (Morita calls this activity the "desire to live.") An infant can manifest himself or herself in a lively manner in front of the tender mother, whom he or she knows, but when the infant senses the gaze of a *soto* person, his or her actions will not seem to be his or her own. The infant's perception will change to that of confronting self as someone who acts while observing self.

Merleau-Ponty[19] notes in a lecture on the human relationships of infants: "One begins to feel that one's self is not simply as one sees oneself with one's own eyes, but is something which other people see, and when another person looks at oneself, one's attention will be diverted from the subject or what one should accomplish and instead be focused on one's own presentation while executing that subject."

When an infant suddenly becomes aware that someone else is looking at him or her, the infant will become acutely self-conscious. This condition is a transition to the *hitomishiri* experienced in puberty.

When a child reaches puberty, the sphere of his or her world becomes broader. The child's ego will also become more powerful. At the same time, his or her attitude will change.

---

[18] Wallon, H.: *Les Origines de la Pensee chez l'Enfant.* Presse Universitaire de France (1945). In *Jidō ni Okeru Seikaku no Kigen*, translated by M. Ōkubo. Meiji Tosho, Tokyo (1965).

[19] Merleau-Ponty, M.: *Les Relations avec Antrui chez l'Enfant.* Les Cours de Sorbonne, Centre de Documentation Universitaire (1962). In *Me to Seishin*, translated by S. Takiura and G. Kida. Misuzu Shobō, Tokyo (1966).

The avoidance of *soto* people will vanish, or at least diminish. The child will also try to become aware of the fact that he or she is worth being evaluated by other persons. The child will become strongly conscious of the fact that he or she cannot talk to other persons in any way that he or she wishes. The child will face *soto* people with the uneasy attitude of wondering what those *soto* people will think of him or her or, perhaps, will experience fear that he or she is making a poor impression on other persons.

A person who experiences this adolescent form of *hitomishiri* will mentally ponder, before meeting another person, the probable situation of involvement between himself or herself and the other person. The person's tension will increase, because he or she is prone to assume a defensive stance and will not be able to speak and act as freely as he or she would like to.

The desire for acknowledgment of one's self (the desire for self-assertion) will strengthen the feeling of *hanikami* (bashfulness) and *hito-oji* (uneasiness about other persons), which arises from the *kigane* (constraint in another person's presence) that he or she feels toward *soto* people and from *kizukai* (concern, solicitude). The person will be overwhelmed by feelings of frustration.

Generally speaking, there are many instances of differences in expression of the varied internal phenomena of human life, such as front and back, inside and outside. The fact that a similar phenomenon is present in the external world is recognized by all people. With this general fact as a premise, the difference in the mode of consciousness toward *uchi* and *soto*, which can be observed in the daily lives of the Japanese, will now be explained.

The *kigane* (constraint) and *ki wo tsukau* (to feel anxious about) exhibited toward *soto* people are important feelings for life in society. Although in present-day society, human beings can live more or less freely, there are many instances in which one assumes an attitude toward the *soto* world by means of gestures or forms of speech that express such feelings and that are almost automatic.

The consideration that is given to making *soto* people not feel unpleasant and the desire to be liked by other persons, that is, the desire to become a person who is worth a positive evaluation by other persons, act in a complementary manner in the Japanese character. The desire for consideration and the need for self-expression have become fixed in combination in the Japanese mentality. The disposition to search for a standard for one's decisions and actions in the minds of other persons and the disposition toward self-restriction in the face of other persons' intentions, as Benedict[20] and other authors point out, are characteristic of a culture that is based on a sense of shame.

The need for consideration of appearance, decency, display and inferiority has been cultivated in the daily lives of the Japanese, as evidenced by the fact that they are concerned in front of other persons and maintain a good appearance. There is little in the life activities of the Japanese in which *soto* is not taken into consideration. This is certainly true of activities relating to habits daily of living, such as attitudes toward other persons, speech, gestures, customs, apparel and food.

It is believed that the "front and back" difference of what is shown to the *soto* world and what is shown within the *uchi* is prominent in Japan. In other words, it is believed that the consideration to envelop oneself, or the inside of that *uchi* that belongs to oneself and is not shown openly in the *soto* world, is at the root of Japanese involvement with other persons.

This life feeling generally has an important role in restricting one's activities in relation to the outside standards of how other persons think of oneself, so that one meets another person

---

[20] Benedict, R.: *The Chrysanthemum and the Sword–Patterns of Japanese Culture.* Houghton Mifflin, Boston (1946). In *Kiku to Katana–Nihon Bunka no Kata*, translated by M. Hasegawa. Shakai Shisōsha, Tokyo (1951).

with a concern of how to associate with that person without having him or her become aware of one's inner intentions. There is also concern for how to express oneself to satisfy one's desires.

This attitude toward *soto* people results in painstaking awareness of every movement of another person, of making certain of the other person's train of thought or of gaining understanding by exercise of intuition, which is a characteristic means of recognition used by the Japanese.

The effort not to show the *uchi* (inside, home like) of oneself to *soto* people arises out of a concern not to expose the inferior aspects of oneself. This concern not only based on a standard of judging superiority and inferiority in terms of outward appearance but also derives from a feeling of shame. At the same time, consideration of the possibility of making other persons feel unpleasant, if *uchi* is shown openly in a *soto* situation, is also operative.

The consciousness of shame that is characteristic of the Japanese is, without doubt, due to restrictions placed on outward appearance. However, as Sakuta[21] correctly points out, the consciousness of shame, which becomes a standard of superiority or inferiority, controls a person from the inside in a manner similar to the consciousness of crime, which becomes the outside standard of good and bad. This is first learned by the imposition of punishment from outside oneself and is thus impressed internally. As a result, it affects the actions of the person. Together with the aspiration toward self-expression and the sense of a will to win in the Japanese metality, the *hanikami* (bashfulness) stance of puberty motivates each person to exert effort to realize an ideal self.

The excessive demand for self-expression, which can be observed during this process, will serve to strengthen consciousness of shame and a tendency toward self-suppression. At the same time, notions of consideration for other persons will be cultivated. The life feeling that arises from the difference between *uchi* and *soto* is strengthened by the basic structure of Japanese society as its foundation. It also forms correspondent relationships for regulating cultural structure.

Hitomishiri and *taijin kyōfu* are forms of human relationship that have complicated structures in Japanese society. In explaining the symptoms of *taijin kyōfu* from a phenomenological point of view, we note that its basic structure is entirely the same as that of *hitomishiri.* The psychological nature of the Japanese, who show a strong concern about sustained eye-to-eye contact, is common to both, and it is believed that this concern characterizes the forms of human relationship exhibited by the Japanese.

In Morita's explanation, *seishi kyōfu* (fear of eye-to-eye confrontation) is probably the basic form of *taijin kyōfu*, which does not have a simple symptomatological basis but which has various phenomenological types that should be consolidated and called the *taijin kyōfu* syndrome. The various symptoms, however, all have features in common. Morita[22] points out that "in *taijin kyōfu*, the patient believes that being ashamed is weak-willed, and has a stubborn, bad loser disposition which tries not to think about shame."

This tendency to feel ashamed "contains the feeling of not being disliked by people but the desire to be liked, and also not to be thought of as being inferior but to be thought of as being superior."

The three factors of shame, its suppression and self-assertion are the basis that forms the symptoms of *taijin kyōfu*, according to Morita.

The image[23] that the Japanese have of *hitomishiri* includes elements of *meiwaku-na* (trou-

---

[21] Sakuta, K.: *Haji no Bunka Saikō* (Reconsideration of the Shame Culture). Chikuma Shobō, Tokyo (1967). (Printed in Japanese)

[22] Morita, S.: *Sekimen Kyōfu no Ryōhō* (A New Treatment for Ereuthrophobia). Jinbun Shoin, Kyoto (1935). *In Morita Shōma Zenshū*, Vol. III, edited by T. Kōra et al. Hakuyōsha, Tokyo (1974). (Printed in Japanese)

[23] Fujita, C.: vide 16.

blesome), *inki-na* (gloomy), *fuyukai-na* (unpleasant), *yami* (dark), *shōkyokuteki* (passive), *yowai* (weak) and *fukappatsu-na* (inactive) mentality. These impressions are mingled with those of *wakai* (young), *junsui-na* (pure) and *surudoi* (sharp) images. This complicated psychological "landscape" is clarified in scenes of free statement of *hitomishiri* by oneself and by indications of it observed in the conduct of other persons.

While feeling that one is being ignored by other persons, and feeling uneasy because one is thus misunderstood and is suffering for the sake of other persons, one is, at the same time, engaged in self-examination to determine whether one has a defect of character. Such a defect could be unpleasant and troublesome to other persons. One will, nonetheless, have the pleasant feeling that another person, who shows indications of *hitomishiri*, is *jun-na* (pure, innocent, chaste, natural, wholesome).

This double structure of both negative and positive feelings can be observed in cases of *taijin kyōfu* as well as in cases of *hitomishiri*. Although one of these two conditions, *hitomishiri*, is a normal mental state and the other, *taijin kyōfu*, is a type of neurosis, the continuity principle is naturally applicable between both conditions. The mental state of human relationships for the Japanese is indicated by both conditions in bold relief.

Part III

Etiological Basis of *Shinkeishitsu*

10

Disposition and Nurture

The nucleus of Morita therapy in regard to the pathogenetic basis of *shinkeishitsu* can be said to be the theory of the hypochondriacal basic tone. In this chapter, we will first explain "hypochondriacal" from the standpoint of "disposition and situation." The author will then discuss its relationships to inadaptability anxiety (Kōra) and to "training by parents" on the basis of views acquired by clinical experience. Last, the author will describe the pathogenic mechanism, which is composed of such factors as condition, chance, psychic interaction and the antagonistic action of the mind–which trigger the onset of *shinkeishitsu*–in line with Morita's thinking.

There have been many historical changes in the concept of neurosis since it was first introduced by Cullen (1712–1790). Even today, there are major differences of opinion among researchers regarding the appreciation and interpretation of this concept in the realm of present-day psychiatry, so that a standardized interpretation is not necessarily possible.

In particular, there are numerous unresolved problems, such as whether the neurotic personality and the neurotic constitution according to modern definitions are determined by heredity or the environment and, further, how these two factors are interrelated.

Consequently, the time when Morita first expounded his concept of *shinkeishitsu* and its therapy, about 60 years ago, was the period in which numerous disputes on somatogenetic theory and psychogenetic theory were finally coming to an end, but it was also a period in which the concept of *shinkeishitsu* was still vague, so that there was almost no mention of the mutual relationship between the dispositional factor and the situational factor, even in psychogenetic theory. It therefore appears that, with respect to the pathogenesis of *shinkeishitsu*, the tendency to emphasize disposition or constitution was predominant.

Needless to say, Freud's theory of psychoanalysis opened up a broad new path by providing a systematic and comprehensive theory of the development of neurosis at a time when many conflicting theories were in vogue. However, Freud's theory was not widely accepted as a useful psychiatric methodology because it was new and unorthodox, rejecting the mainstream of thought in psychiatry at the time. Further, the concept of neurosis became more confused after neurasthenia was described by Beard (who, in 1868, advocated a theory of weakness or exhaustion of the nervous system) and added to the sphere of neurosis.

Under such circumstances, it should be noted that Morita made clear, from clinical experiments carried out for many years, the psychopathological basis of what had generally been presumed to be chronic neurasthenia or constitutional nervousness, a condition characterized by a type of hypersensitive constitution or asthenic psychopathia. Morita, instead, advocated his so-called *shinkeishitsu* theory.

Morita's theory, however, was also centered around temperament because he had been influenced by the widely accepted constitutional theory of the time. The most important feature of Morita's theory, however, was that *shinkeishitsu*, formerly considered degenerative in nature, was interpreted as a psychogenic disorder.

It is well known that the concept of "psychogenic" originated from Psychogenie (a mental disorder induced and influenced by concept), first proposed by Sommer (1884) and widely interpreted as a general phenomenon induced by mental influence.

Noting the changes in neurosis theory since then, it appears that there were differences of opinion among researchers. However, this concept had been introduced into the field of research on neurosis quite early. Even with the circumstances noted in the foregoing text, it is presumed that the importance of life history situations was not questioned. The psychopathological basis of neurosis was solely an affected person's natural disposition and constitution, these factors being the preeminent concerns. The mode of thought departing from the concept of Sommer's psychogenie was the mainstream, particularly in Germany. For example, Kraepelin[1] explained that abnormal personality characteristics have a pathogenic basis in hysteria and that even if the hysteria was related to a psychogenic factor, it should not be considered psychogenic in nature because the relationship between the two factors was not known.

Although the effect of the "psychogenic" factor was not considered in nervousness and obsessive neurosis because the basis of the disorder was ascribed to the personality characteristic, it was thought to be included in the original state of the disease.

In France, Janet explained neurosis as a lowering of psychic tension and psychic energy. It is well known that this condition has been classified as psychasthenia and hysteria. However, his teacher, Charcot, considered hysteria and neurasthenia as being due to a certain type of hereditary constitution, and Ballet[2] considered obsessions variants of constitutional psychosis.

Thus, there was a strong tendency at that time to consider neurosis as being due to a type of abnormal personality or constitution.

As was explained in Chapter 1, Japanese psychiatrists at that time had been influenced considerably by the introduction of descriptive and phenomenological methodology from Germany, and this methodology formed the mainstream of thought in psychopathology. Consequently, most Japanese psychiatrists of that period ascribed neurosis to abnormal disposition or constitution.

In Germany at that time, a large number of researchers had been classifying mental degeneration midway between psychosis and normality on the basis of constitutional aspects. This condition is indicative of a continuing mental inferiority. There is no obstacle to intellectual function, but the condition has a characteristic emotional disorder, readily manifested by antisocial, maladjusted behavior.

This mode of psychiatric thought originated from Koch's concept of *Psychopathische Minderwertigkeiten*, which he classified into three stages: Disposition, *Belastung* and Degenerant. Koch's attention was directed primarily to the second and third stages because affected persons in these stages readily cause social problems. This concept of abnormality was studied in further detail by Schneider.[3] Almost all of what Koch categorized as "disposition" is believed to lie within the scope of psychogenic disorders as they are currently classified, but such neurotic disorders were not taken seriously at that time because they were considered vague concepts.

Such views of mental degeneration, generally accepted in Germany, were naturally introduced into Japan and became fixed notions. Under those circumstances, Morita adopted Koch's concept of disposition but directed his attention to the neurotic condition among the antisocial, psychopathic inferiorities and studied this concept in detail.

At about the same time, large numbers of psychiatrists in England and the United States placed little importance on the condition of neurosis from the standpoint of psychopathic states. This attitude differed from the general trend in Germany and Japan. Further, on the prescript

---

1 Kraepelin, E.: *Psychiatrie*, 8 Aufl. Bd. IV, Barth, Leipzig (1915).

2 Ballet, G.: *Traité de Pathologie Mentale.* Octare Doin, Paris (1903). In G. A. Ladee: *Hypochondriacal Syndromes*, Elsevier, Amsterdam (1966).

3 Schneider, K.: *Die psychopathische Persönlichkeiten*, IV. Aufl. 2, Wien (1940).

innate constitution and chronic duration did not receive an equal amount of emphasis, and these concepts had features that resembled Morita's mode of thought.

The pathogenetic basis of neurosis, centered around disposition and constitution at the time, was called neuropathia, a neuropathic constitution, *nervöse Diathese* (Möbius) or *neuropathische Diathese* (Nonne), with emphasis being placed on the constitutional features of the neurotic phenomenon. When emphasis was placed, instead, on the mental aspect, it was called psychopathy, a psychopathic constitution or *nervöse Psychopathie* (Bumke), *asthenische Psychopathie* (Lange, Bostrom) or *endogene Nervosität* (Cramer).

At any rate, if neurosis is determined by disposition and constitution, it may be considered, in many cases, to show some correlation with psychic degeneration or endogenous psychosis. Actual case histories revealed only occasional instances of observation from the standpoint of inherited disposition. For example, Hoffmann[4] considered it difficult to clarify the relationship between neurosis and heredity owing to "alloying of complex dispositions" because persons with various types of mental disorder were observed in the family trees of those exhibiting obsessive neurosis. Hoffmann later clarified the problem, explaining obsessive neurosis by placing emphasis on disposition and taking into consideration the confrontation between the obsessive neurotic character, which is sensitive, and the sexual impulse, which has developed into considerable perversion.

Several years later, Schultz[5] included a type of neurosis in the concept of psychopathy and stressed the hereditary point of view. What Schultz called constitutional nervousness is actually hereditary and constitutional in nature.

However, psychiatrists in Germany did not take into consideration merely temperament and constitution. With Sommer's psychogenia excluded, Strümpell had already recognized the important relationship of a certain concept to the causation of symptoms in his study on traumatic neurosis. He called this concept desire. This dispute over traumatic wartime neurosis that occurred between Nonne and Oppenheimer in 1916 ended in a victory for Nonne, who championed the psychogenetic theory. However, the psychogenic factor or the situational factor began to attract attention with this type of neurosis as the boundary line.

For example, Bumke[6] was one investigator who considered neurosis a psychopathic state, but he also classified nervousness, hypochondriacal states, obsessive states and the hysteric mental attitude as psychogenic reactions similar to delusional development. Braun[7] classified psychogenic reactions as either personality or situational reactions and made a rough differentiation between the concepts of personality factor and situational factor.

Thus, the concepts of personality factor and situational factor, or psychogenic mechanisms, finally appeared in studies on neurosis. These concepts diverted studies from the mainstream and were gradually incorporated into psychoanalysis. A trend toward obtaining a pathogenesis reading from the standpoint of a patient's developmental psychology or life history began to appear. However, the fixed dispositional, static neurosis theory, which placed emphasis on disposition and constitution, still remained dominant.[8]

Accordingly, Freud, who advocated the psychodynamic theory, was also interested in constitution for a long time, although his consideration of it differed from the conventional theory of hereditary constitution. With regard to traumatic neurosis, Nonne, who stressed the psychogenic theory, also recognized the importance of the psychogenic factor as a direct cause, but he

---

[4] Hoffmann, H.: *Vererbung und Seelenleben.* Spamersche Buchdruckerei, Leipzig (1922).
[5] Schultz, J. H.: *Die Konstitutionelle Nervosität*, Hd, d. Geisteskrankheit, Bd. V. Springer, Berlin (1928).
[6] Bumke, O.: *Lehrbuch der Geisteskrankheiten*, 7 Aufl., Munich (1948).
[7] Braun, E.: *Psychogene Reaktion* (Bumke's Handbuch der Geisteskrankheiten), Bd. V. Springer, Berlin (1928).

noted that this factor is only the last drop that causes the water bucket to overflow in many cases; in his opinion, disposition was still the predominant factor.

What were Morita's beliefs in this regard? As the author has mentioned, Morita was heavily influenced by the German theory of hereditary disposition. However, the major difference between his mode of thought and those of other researchers is that temperament, which is congenitally determined and fixed and which also indicates a tendency toward a continuing degeneration that cannot be changed, is considered unchangeable. Further, some factor associated with the temperamental tendency provokes the onset of *shinkeishitsu* through a correlation between situational and chance factors, its symptoms are formed and developed, and it finally becomes fixed in nature but can gradually be cured by psychotherapy.

There is no doubt that Morita considered temperament theory from the standpoint of this kinetic theory as involving an emotional characteristic determined by heredity as a more inward matter, but he was not shackled by academic postulates in taking into account any such concept. That is, even in the case of a tendency that is determined by a completely hereditary factor, it is reasonable to surmise that the situation in which this tendency characteristically appears is a concrete life situation, so that it will naturally conform to the context that governs the situation. Any such experience will function to form such a tendency secondarily. This phenomenon is repeated and accumulated in the flow of life, which does not stop, with continuing interaction between the hereditary tendency and the a posteriori emotional tendency taking place.

We recognize this condition as a mental tendency that appears as a concrete phenomenon. This type of temperament theory was unable to achieve widespread acceptance at that time. However, it is an understanding obtained by perceiving the mental characteristics of a person through his or her life activities. Therefore, it is preferable to call this theory a character or personality theory rather than a temperament theory.

Another feature of this theory is that, in the series of processes in which *shinkeishitsu* occurs by interaction between temperament (interpreted in this manner) and conditions of situation and chance, the formation of symptoms and their fixation actually take place throughout the growth and development process of human existence. (Morita calls this phenomenon the manifestation of true human nature.) However, in view of the characteristic tendency that manifests this temperament (Morita's hypochondriacal basic tone), natural self-development has become distorted.

Thus, although Morita considered a person's temperament to have a hereditary component as the starting point of his *shinkeishitsu* theory, he gradually modified it to take into account kinetic theory and, further indicated that the onset of *shinkeishitsu* is induced by the interaction of this temperament with life situations through the mechanism of the development of psychogenie.

His concept is somewhat similar to the concept of the transition process relative to neurosis in the German school of descriptive psychiatry. Braun, Bleuler and Schneider, who introduced the concept of reaction–because the term neurosis is not applicable to the actual condition–stipulated that pathogenic as well as pathoplastic factors are inherent in the dichotomous relationship of personality and situation, including the personality reaction, situational reaction and abnormal experiential reaction.

---

[8] Ludwig Binswanger makes the following comment in a footnote regarding a letter of reproach he received from Freud for citing the *hysterische psychopathische Konstitution* of T. Ziehen in his book *Erinnerung an Sigmund Freud*: "Freud always continued to consider this constitutional problem with reservations even after this. I discovered this when I called on him on his 80th birthday. When I said, 'If a person is confronted with a ruinous fate, he is free to select either the path of avoiding neurosis or the path of maintaining his mental balance, isn't he?' Freud replied rather summarily: 'Constitution is everything.'" (Bern, 1956) and *Mein Weg zu Freud.* In *Der Mensch in der Psychiatrie.* Pfullinger (1957). (In Japanese, *Freud e no Michi*, translated by N. Takeuchi and M. Takeuchi. Iwasaki Shuppan (1969)).

This was the school that changed temperament, static neurosis theory into situational, dynamic neurosis theory, such as that of Kretschmer,[9] in which the process of nonagreement of matured factors and retarded factors in a person's psychosomatic constitution are correlated with the incidence of neurosis from a psychosomatic constitutional point of view. Later, Binder[10] introduced the concept of development and interpreted neurosis as a developmental disorder.

Morita's concept was entirely different. Further, the fact that his theory bore curative fruit in an early era should have led to great acclaim at the time.

Morita had not studied the concept of neurosis theoretically and systematically, having developed his theory by observation of actual case histories. According to Morita, his difference of opinion regarding Kraepelin's classification of psychogenic psychosis and mental degeneration can be explained as follows:

"... I do not consider such conditions as being fixed, as do many other researchers, but consider most of them to be changing and fluid. As I have stressed before, abnormal phenomena change in a very complex manner, in accordance with the relationship between disposition, situation and chance; consequently, Kraepelin's theory that mental degeneration is a strong, congenital character abnormality resembling psychosis actually fluctuates over a wide range.

"Everyone has experienced personality changes with age; thoughts and principles also change considerably with changes in situations. They also change with differences in various conditions, such as changes in physical obesity or relative to chronic disease, or from becoming obese due to a climacteric factor...."

Morita also remarks that it is difficult to grasp phenomena that appear on the surface, at present, by discussing differences (without considering the passage of time) or by looking at a patient's condition as one that is spatially fixed. According to Kraepelin's classification, the result will be that the number of exceptions increases when a condition is described in a more detailed and accurate form. Ever-changing mental phenomena can be understood only if the phenomena are considered as moving in time and space rather than as being fixed.

Even in regard to the classification of psychogenic psychosis, mental phenomena were categorized chiefly in terms of occasionalistic causation as observed in its adjectival expression. For example, even if the occasionalistic causation is the same, the dispositional and situational conditions differ considerably. Consequently, there will be a broad range of possible reactions and changes that follow. Various kinds of symptom, even those caused by the same sort of occasionalism, such as a hysteric reaction, depressed reaction, paranoid reaction, *shinkeishitsu* reaction or hypochondriacal reaction, are often encountered in clinical practice, but attention was not directed toward this matter to such an extent in the past.

This oversight resulted from an attempt to classify the mental tendency arising from this condition in terms of "quality" and "quantity" by interpreting disposition, situation and chance from a mutually correlative standpoint. The quality of a mental tendency remarked on by Morita is that of the mode and feature of the reaction. For example, differences appear when a mother scolds a child. One child reacts slowly and remains calm, another child becomes defiant and challenging, and still another child becomes dejected, reproaching himself or herself and becoming frightened. Also, fine, characteristic differences in this tendency appear in cases of mental retardation and simplemindedness, and the extent of differentiation in such cases is minimal.

Consequently, Morita's relationship between quantity and quality can be differentiated

[9] Kretschmer, E.: *Psychotherapeutische Studien.* Thieme, Stuttgart (1948).

[10] Binder, H.: Abnorme seelische Reaktionen und Entwicklungen. In Reschardt, M.: *Allg. u. Spezielle Psychiatrie*, 4 Aufl. Karger, Basel (1955).

clinically as ranging from a genius who has a hysteric tendency to a feebleminded person who has a depressive tendency.

From about 1918, Morita attempted a classification of mental tendency or abnormal personality[11] on the basis of differences in quantitative and qualitative disposition. He mentioned that *shinkeishitsu*, in this classification, clearly shows a hypochondriacal tendency. The author will explain this point in the following chapter.

---

[11] Classification of Abnormal Personality (1927)

I. Retardation of Mental Development (quantitative)
  1. Idiot
  2. Imbecile
  3. Moron

II. Abnormal Personality (qualitative)
  1. *Shinkeishitsu*-disposed personality (mental hypersensibility)
  2. Hysteria-disposed personality (emotional hypersensibility)
    a. Hysteric temperament
    b. Somatic hysteria
    c. Hysteric psychosis
  3. Weak will-disposed personality
    a. Simple instability
    b. Pathological vagrancy
    c. Moral insanity
    d. Innate criminal
    e. Dipsomania, alcohol dependence, other drug dependence
    f. Sexual abnormality
    g. Impulsive disorder
    h. Compulsive disorder
  4. Hyperthymic-disposed personality
    a. Constitutional excitation
    b. Hypomania
    c. Manic state
  5. Melancholic-disposed personality
    a. Constitutional depression
    b. Depressive state
  6. Paranoiac-disposed personality
    a. Querulous type
    b. Enthusiastic type
    c. Paranoiac type
  7. Schizothymic-disposed personality

11

Inadaptability Anxiety and the Hypochondriacal Basic Tone

Morita basically considers the "hypochondriacal basic tone" to be the pathogenic agent of *shinkeishitsu.* This concept will be explained in this chapter in connection with the issue of adaptability. The "basic tone" signifies a mental tendency that forms the causal foundation for the morbid condition of *shinkeishitsu.* Morita tries to pinpoint the type of temperament that provokes the hypochondriacal tendency in the *shinkeishitsu*-disposed persona in his classification of abnormal personality (refer to Chapter 8).

The concept of abnormal personality was classified between mental health and psychosis during Morita's time. A person was considered as being closer or more distant from normal according to the extent of the abnormality. Morita basically agrees with this notion, but as we explained in the preceding chapter, he considers temperament not as something that is fixed but as something that changes with experience.

The relationship between what he calls the *shinkeishitsu* temperament and what he calls the hypochondriacal basic tone is explained, first of all, in mostly his words, as follows: Morita considers the *shinkeishitsu* temperament to be congenital, indicating some form of inferiority or deviation from the capability for living, by comparison with a healthy person. However, he does not consider it a morbid condition. He explains his thinking in this regard by saying: "It is true that a person of abnormal character may appear to indicate a poor adaptability toward environmental situations and have a poor reactive facility toward stimuli received from the outer world; but on the other hand, this type of individual is so hyper-sensitive that, in fact, many different kinds of tendencies appear. In view of this, an abnormal person can easily fall into a physically or mentally morbid condition due to many sorts of minor, momentary influences.[1]

"Abnormal character comes from an excess or deficiency of situational reactivity, but it does not necessarily mean that one has an inferior character or is morbidly abnormal either physically or mentally, nor does it necessarily mean that one will become asocial or anti-social. At times, this type of person may become someone of superior accomplishment or a great contributor to society. This is the reason why both genius and insanity exist. From a clinical standpoint, however, the number of people who are being treated as morbidly abnormal is on the rise . . . .

"The *shinkeishitsu* temperament is a type of neurotic or mentally abnormal character. However, this condition should be considered as a 'too high' or 'too low' character function rather than an actual alteration of human character. A mild case should probably be called *shinkeishitsu* temperament.[2]

"For example, an abnormality in the autonomic nervous system of any such person only means that its extent is somewhat stronger or weaker than that of a healthy person. Let us ask, then, what kind of mental tendency is *shinkeishitsu*?

[1] Morita develops his explanation of this process as the chance factor in the incidence of *shinkeishitsu.*

"I consider it introspective. As a result, the person becomes rational (since it is a mental tendency entirely different from a hysteric tendency) . . . .

"This introspective person with the *shinkeishitsu* character experiences morbidity due to a certain chance causal factor which may be unrecognizable (in a form that he himself does not directly experience) and he can easily become a hypochondriac. This is the reason why I have proposed the theory of the hypochondriacal basic tone to explain the origin of this disorder . . . ."

Morita explains the relationship between the *shinkeishitsu* temperament and the hypochondriacal tendency as a stereotype of what he calls abnormal character. The hypochondriacal tendency may be considered a condition that corresponds to a preceding stage of *shinkeishitsu* as a morbid precondition.

Morita believes that the type of temperament called *shinkeishitsu* is the basic component of the *shinkeishitsu* disorder, a type of proto-morbid character. The hypochondriacal attitude shown by a person who has this tendency gradually develops into a truly morbid condition. (This point will be discussed in more depth in the latter part of this chapter.)

According to this explanation, the *shinkeishitsu*-disposed persona will readily indicate a hypochondriacal tendency in even trifling circumstances, whether or not the persona is strongly conscious of it. If this explanation is accepted, what sort of relationship will the hypochondriacal tendency have with the *shinkeishitsu* condition?

This tendency can be considered the symptom rather than a condition that exists in the prior stage of *shinkeishitsu.* If so, the importance of Morita's theory of the hypochondriacal basic tone, developed from the relationship between these two elements, will be diminished. (Some investigators doubt that there is, in fact, any such relationship.[3])

If the hypochondriacal tendency is a genuine symptom of *shinkeishitsu*, Morita's theory of the hypochondriacal basic tone will contain the flaw of confusing the symptoms with the mechanics of the onset of the disorder. This flaw would, predictably, arouse a certain amount of criticism. However, most criticisms that have arisen in the past are no more than attempts to clarify the hypochondriacal tendency from a psychodynamic point of view.[4]

Although it is possible that this could lead to a revision of Morita's theory, at present there is a real difference in position with regard to Morita's concept, which is not a major point of debate when it is discussed from different standpoints.

The hypochondriacal tendency, according to Morita, is such that a person who has the *shinkeishitsu* temperament perceives ego activity in that situation from a descriptive phenome-

---

[2] Koch mentions in his book *Die psychopathische Minderwertigkeiten*, (1891), that the mildest condition is that of disposition. This statement agrees with K. Schneider's definition of the asthenic psychopath. The person may exhibit a certain mental delicateness, although ordinarily healthy, but morbid symptoms will develop in reaction to a certain chance factor. At first, it may seem that what Morita calls the *shinkeishitsu* temperament is similar to the condition mentioned by Koch, but it actually has an entirely different mental structure, which we will discuss at the end of this chapter.

[3] For example, K. Ikeda points out in his thesis in *Seishin Igaku* (volume 1, number 7, 1959) that if there is any implication to the anxiety over the matter of whether a hypochondriacal tendency is already a symptom of Morita *shinkeishitsu*, and figuring as such in Morita therapy, it is still necessary to clarify the psychodynamic factor(s) that gives rise to this anxiety. N. Shinfuku points out in *Psychiatria et Neurologia Japonica* (volume 55, number 7, 1954) that Morita places little importance on nonconscious psychodynamics, emphasizes the temperamental tendency and considers it a result of the action of the ego, but the psychodynamics that lead up to the hypochondriacal tendency must also be clarified.

[4] Apart from the criticisms indicated in footnote 3, T. Doi explains in his thesis on "Psychopathology of *shinkeishitsu*" in *Psychiatria et Neurologia Japonica* (volume 60, number 7, 1958) that it is not sufficient to consider the hypochondriacal tendency as being merely a matter of congenital constitution. It is itself the central symptom of *shinkeishitsu*, rather than a matter of having symptoms occur because of this tendency. The feeling of not being able to be *amae* (instinctive desire for dependence) even when one wishes to be *amae* is a phenomenon common to the human relationships of persons with *shinkeishitsu* and results from creating a relationship of abnormal dependence, in which one's feelings are unduly influenced by another person.

nological point of view that indicates only confrontation and conflict within the ego. It is likely that Morita considered this issue from the perspective of a correlation between situation and a chance causal factor on the premise that the congenital *shinkeishitsu* temperament is the original cause.[5] He believes that the hypochondriacal tendency is a form of human existence that indicates the locus of a person's mental existence, with the understanding that it is a fluid substance. There are quantitative strengths or weaknesses.

Morita's explanation, considered in this light, indicates that the hypochondriacal tendency is not a real symptom, eliminating any distortion of fact or any contradiction in his theory.

If the phenomenological factor called the hypochondriacal tendency is further extended, we have the condition that Kōra calls inadaptability anxiety.[6] This condition is also called a conceptual, perfectionistic or egoistic attitude by Kondō.[7] Both of these opinions are contained in Morita's point of view.

Morita points out a close relationship between the manner in which a person who has the proto-morbid character called *shinkeishitsu* indicates the way in which a hypochondriac will develop in the human maturation process. He explains that this tendency does not occur during any time of life in which mental development is still insufficient but, instead, that it appears in force from the period of puberty. *Shinkeishitsu* as a morbid condition also occurs frequently during the same period. During the process of mental development, the various aspects of living conditions will influence the formation of character of such persons, together with the factor of congenital temperament. Such persons are sometimes conscious and sometimes unconscious of the process, and they progress to a state in which it is easy for them to succumb to the disorder.

In the mental tendency called *shinkeishitsu*, there is a major difference between the vari-

---

[5] Morita explains this point to clarify his position: "I believe *shinkeishitsu* is a type of temperament in which hypochondriacy can occur easily; it is, moreover, a congenital temperament. If so, precisely what does congenital mean? I have no accurate information at present to conclude whether it means that hereditary character is derived directly from a genetic source, or that something untoward occurred during fetal growth in the womb, or that the temperament is an acquired characteristic associated with illness or upbringing after birth. All of this must be studied in depth in the future. For the same reason, too, Matsubara's sensible constitution theory of neurasthenia cannot completely explain *shinkeishitsu*. The vasomotor nerves and other physically stimulative states of sensibility are not necessarily transformed into subjective neurasthenic symptoms, due to the extent of these states. Even if the extent of the sensible state is quite high, there are people who complain of having complex *shinkeishitsu* symptoms even if they are physically healthy, and even if they do not complain of any captivating symptoms of *shinkeishitsu*. This is what I refer to as pseudo-stimulative exhaustion, the symptoms of which are entirely subjective. In view of this, I had previously classified *shinkeishitsu* provisionally into the two types of physically sensitive disposition and mentally sensitive disposition. But this classification is only for convenience's sake. Mental disposition is a condition which cannot be essentially omitted from *shinkeishitsu*; the symptoms of *shinkeishitsu* cannot be formed without it . . . ."

Marui (one of the pioneers of psychoanalysis in Japan) mentions that care during infancy has a close relationship with the occurrence of neurosis. M. Shimoda (who understood Morita's theory and was one of those who actively worked to develop it during the early period) points out that *shinkeishitsu* results from poor care during infancy. Needless to say, these factors are important and should be accepted. It may be somewhat like the difference between the natural growth of a tree and that which results from shaping and stunting it artificially to produce a *bonsai*. However, this is a difference of influence, not an instinctive differentiation or a decisive difference. We have frequently noticed that, even if cared for under the same conditions, infants exhibit differences in character naturally. Consequently, the influence of feelings colored by differences in the development of individual temperament can differ even under the same conditions.

[6] Kōra explains in his thesis, "The Problems of So-called Neurasthenia," in *Psychiatria et Neurologia Japonica* (volume 42, number 10, 1938), that inadaptability is a condition in which "one feels that one's mental and physical phenomena, in light of the condition, are disadvantageous to one's life; in other words, the anxiety that one cannot adapt oneself to present conditions," with this condition existing in a congenital form as a precondition to the occurrence of *shinkeishitsu* symptoms. This inadaptability anxiety is somewhat similar to what K. Horney calls basic anxiety.

[7] Kondō, A.: Shinkeishō ni kansuru seishin-bunseki gakuha (Freud oyobi Horney) no riron to kore ni taihi shite mitaru Morita no shinkeishitsu riron (Morita's theory of nervosity compared with the psychoanalytic theories of Freud and Horney on neurosis) (in Japanese). *Tōkyō Jikeikai Ika Daigaku Zasshi* 73(10) (1958).

able extent of the hereditary temperamental tendency and the variable a posteriori environmental conditions and life experiences. Consequently, there are cases in which the *shinkeishitsu* tendency appears in infants (those who have a hypochondriacal tendency). In such cases, there may be almost no clear indication of a phenomenological tendency, even when such infants have grown into adults, but they do become hypochondriacal due to certain chance circumstances, and this tendency indicates the onset of the disorder. This tendency often occurs in paroxysmal neurosis, which is one type of *shinkeishitsu*, as was explained in Chapter 8. The number of cases in which the disorder has a sudden onset in the fourth and fifth decades of life is far from small. In that instance, the *shinkeishitsu* tendency is not marked, but an affected person will have a hypochondriacal experience suddenly, by chance. This experience will penetrate deeply into the mind, become a controlling factor and thus set the stage to cut off escape from the resultant condition.

There is no doubt that individual differences exist in the degree to which the tendency is present in actual living. However, Morita emphatically insists that the hereditary mental temperament cannot be excluded from the factors that determine this condition.

At what point in life does a person begin to be strongly aware of the *shinkeishitsu* humor and the hypochondriacal basic tone? In general, it appears readily at the time of life in which self-consciousness abruptly arises during the process of mental maturation and, further, during a time when the person is most unstable, usually during puberty. This fact has been clinically confirmed, as Morita himself points out, but there are many cases in which this awareness indicates the period in which *shinkeishitsu* first appears as a morbid condition.

The time of life in which a person becomes conscious of having the *shinkeishitsu* character is always much earlier than the time of onset of the actual disorder. The *shinkeishitsu* tendency is indelible in one's character, but it is often not clear whether this tendency is only a matter of basic character or of an actual *shinkeishitsu* disorder. There are also cases in which the time of onset of the disorder is not well defined.

Mashimo and Tsuzura published reports on this issue independently.[8,9] Mashimo studied the period during which a person becomes subjectively conscious of the condition that Morita calls the hypochondriacal basic tone or what Kōra calls inadaptability anxiety. The time that one becomes conscious of the tendency was studied by use of retrospective and prospective testing methods. With the former method, 50 men and ten women, or a total of 60 *shinkeishitsu* patients, were selected as subjects, with 51 male university students (department of medicine) used as control subjects. With this method, detailed life histories were obtained, the Yatabe-Guilford test[10] was administered (comparison of present and past conditions extending back in time to the middle-school period) and autobiographical data (including data on family members, childhood events and postpubertal circumstances) were obtained.

By use of the prospective method, two middle schools and two high schools were selected from two districts that had appreciably different environments (one a residential district of mostly middle-class homes and the other an industrial zone of homes mostly below middle class). To determine the development of psychological change, one group in each class from the first to third grades, for a total of 12 groups composed of 519 students (134 boys and 98 girls, for a total of 232 middle-school students, and 208 boys and 79 girls, for a total of 287 high-school students) were selected.

---

[8] Mashimo, H.: Shinkeishitsu shōsha no pāsonaritī kenkyū (A study of the personality of "nervosity") (in Japanese). *Shinkeishitsu* 4(2) (1963).

[9] Tsuzura, M.: Shōni ki ni okeru fuan to shinkeishō no kankei ni tsuite (A psychiatric study of the relations between anxiety and neurosis in childhood) (in Japanese). *Shinkeishitsu* 4(2) (1963).

[10] T. Yatabe and his associates prepared a personality testing method that incorporates 160 items by summarizing and revising the first three personality items in the list prepared by Guilford and colleagues. The purpose of this testing method was to detect only the 13 characteristics that are closest to Guilford's factors.

What Filloux calls character and personality[11] were investigated. One objective of this prospective test method is to investigate the personality and character of the subjects, but the basic objectives are to determine how this type of personality develops and to determine whether the onset of *shinkeishitsu* as a disorder has occurred. If so, the objective is to investigate the progression of the disorder along with the development of personality. However, only the former objective was investigated in this study. With this method, the Yatabe-Guilford test was administered to identify general character tendencies, one list of 80 questions was prepared to detect any degree of variance from the norm and another list of questions was prepared to cover family environment, personality change and physical change as means to pinpoint personality. A sentence completion test was also administered.

The chief results were as follows:

1. The proportion of students conscious of the fact that "my character has changed" when compared with their condition before the onset of the disorder, or those who stated "I have become an introvert" was 73 percent, but the author of this study insists that this condition does not indicate any hypochondriacal tendency.
2. Eighty-four percent of the students had experienced the onset of the disorder within three years after becoming aware of the character change.
3. The process that leads to the onset of the disorder can be classified as belonging to one of the following four categories according to the aspect of personality:
   a. the hypochondriacal tendency was present from childhood;
   b. the student was introverted from childhood, although not especially aware of it, but became hypochondriacal due to the psychological mechanisms of puberty;
   c. the student was extroverted from infancy to elementary school age and was mischievous but became hypochondriacal during puberty; or
   d. the student became hypochondriacal because a certain motivating factor was definitely present.
4. In regard to the type of *shinkeishitsu*, category "a" indicates chiefly an obsessive tendency, "b" and "c" indicate anthropophobia and "d" indicates paroxysmal neurosis.
5. A strong inferiority complex and a hypochondriacal tendency were observed in 20 to 40 percent of the healthy students of pubertal age.
6. Healthy students tended to show signs of hypochondriacal tendency earlier than did those who had a *shinkeishitsu* disorder.

Tsuzura investigated the *shinkeishitsu* tendency in relation to increasing age during the normal development process,[12] using point scores for anxiety as indices. The subjects were 808 male and female students from elementary school (first to sixth grades), middle school (first to third grades) and high school (first to third grades), all in the same type of environment. Some differences appeared in all grades, but in general the anxiety scores tended to be lower in older students, with this tendency more marked in male than in female students.

Boys in the second grade indicated a maximal number of points for almost all the nine items used as anxiety indices, whereas girls in the third grade scored the highest point levels for many of these items. In general, scores of the elementary school pupils decreased as age

---

[11] J. C. Filloux explains the difference between character and personality as the difference between a painting created by a portrait artist and one drawn by a biographer; character is static at any given moment, whereas personality is dynamic, stressing continuity and uniformity (*La Personalitê*).

[12] M. Tsuzura conducted the test on the nine items of (a) learning anxiety, (b) interpersonal relations anxiety, (c) solitude tendency, (d) intrapunitive tendency, (e) sensitivity tendency, (f) somatic signs, (g) phobic tendency, (h) impulsive tendency and (i) neurotic conflict tendency as a lower index, using the anxiety tendency diagnostic test edited by Tanaka Kyōiku Kenkyūsho. The questions were asked in each index section, with three points scored when the anxiety response indicated by each of the questions was strong, two points when weak and one point when no tendency was shown.

increased, but the scores rose again in the sixth grade and in the first year of middle school, then dropped again. However, a subsequent increase in score levels was recorded for students in the second year of high school.

Mashimo explains that the onset of the *shinkeishitsu* disorder that occurred while the prospective testing took place in the case of healthy students differs from what happens in a retrospective investigation. More meaningful information on the relationship between the hypochondriacal tendency and the onset of the disorder can be obtained by using the prospective test method. It is thus regrettable that further studies by Mashimo have not been reported, possibly indicating the difficulty of any such investigation.

However, many students with *shinkeishitsu* who were the subjects of Mashimo's study were conscious of a hypochondriacal tendency at least three years before the onset of the disorder. The age at onset of *shinkeishitsu* in such students was 11 to 12 years, as determined by subtracting three years from the 14 to 15 years of age of the group in which the onset of the disorder showed the highest frequency. This finding is of considerable interest in that it coincides with the age at which the incidence of the anxious tendency is shown to peak in Tsuzura's study. A somewhat similar trend was observed in our investigation, carried out in 1965, in which 59 (40 male and 19 female) *shinkeishitsu* subjects were studied. Thirty-two subjects (about 54 percent) first became aware of a hypochondriacal tendency at 11 to 12 years of age. On the whole, this age range is one in which mental and physical development are rapid and one in which there is a marked degree of mental restlessness. There are strong, exaggerated ego demands and ready indications of repulsion and stimulation over controls exerted by the outer world, or readily induced feelings of distrust and anxiety, as well as difficulty experienced in attaining a satisfactory level of ability. It is also an age range when mental and physical instability can occur, giving rise to a dangerous psychological climate.

Gersild and Holmes[13] have remarked on the general feature of the appearance of fear and how it changes during the childhood maturation process. The dangerous condition observed in a child's reactions is that these varied responses appear in an initial period, then become a vague, undifferentiated anxiety. The degree of anxiety increases as the ability of the child to sense dangerous conditions continues to develop. The fear becomes entwined with imaginary dangers as the power of imagination develops. The child frequently loses prestige and is ridiculed. Fear of failure arises in the context of competition with other children, and keen awareness of the problem becomes evident.

A child begins to have frequent, imaginary apprehensions about adaptability to the outer world and doubts about self-realization as the development of intellectual facility progresses. Needless to say, these apprehensions are centered around mental and physical abilities and condition of health (fear of illness and death). Apprehension over interpersonal relationships is concentrated on considerations of other persons' evaluations and acceptance of one's ability or personality. These considerations are what Morita means by *kizukai* (worry, concern, indicative of the hypochondriacal tendency) and what Kōra refers to as awareness of inadaptability anxiety. However, as Morita points out, the composition of this condition also indicates a high degree of mental maturation[14] and a strong introspective tendency. It also has an asthenic desire to repel the introspective tendency as a prerequisite factor. Consequently, introversion and powerless humor are not the only attributes of the hypochondriacal tendency. A bipolar condition exists in which an active, vital force acts to repel the hypochondriacal tendency and gives rise to strong conflict. This is the true basis of the condition.[15]

The condition is characterized by a readily assumed intellectual, conscious tendency even

---

[13] Refer to *Jidō Shinrigaku* (Child Psychology), published under the supervision of H. Chiwa. Seishin Shobō, Tokyo (1957). (Printed in Japanese)

if sensitivity is keen. Delicate sensibility to psychosomatic phenomena serves to indicate a self-centered, idealistic tendency. Still another factor is a tendency to underestimate oneself, which is evaluated as disadvantageous to self-preservation. However, these hypochondriacal characteristics indicative of the *shinkeishitsu* persona can be observed even in the mental characteristics of healthy adolescents during the pubertal period and do not, as such, compose a specific feature of the *shinkeishitsu* persona.

In this instance, it is reasonable to examine the hypochondriacal tendency in terms of what Morita refers to as quantitative excess or deficiency. In those terms, the hypochondriacal tendency is essentially a natural feeling that human beings become aware of during a certain period of the normal growth process, that is, during preadolescence.

Morita's *shinkeishitsu* persona shows the same tendency, only to a stronger quantitative degree. Such persons are not considered morbidly abnormal in terms of personality but, instead, are accepted as ordinary human beings. Morita's treatment of patients with *shinkeishitsu* began with that consideration as the starting point.

---

[14] W. Janzarik supplements Sattes's opinion that there are many asthenic forms of what Sattes calls hypochondriacal depression in Sattes's thesis on hypochondria (Die hypochonrischen Inhalte der cyclothymen Depression in ihren Beziehungen zum Krankheitstyp und Persönalichkeit). Namely, Janzarik points out that the person who is affected with hypochondriacal depression has the over-concerned, hypersensitive, inferior fealing which is the characteristic feature of the proto- character, and moreover, has a lower than average intellect. *Arch. Psychiat. Neur.* 195:351 (1957). However, what Morita calls the hypochondriacal tendency does not mean that the person is hypochondriacal as such, but this tendency is characterized by an attempt to repel any susceptibility to hypochondria. H. J. Weitbrecht points out (Zur Psychopathologie der zyklothymen Depression. *Arbeiten Zum Psychiatrie, Neur. U. Ihren Grenzgebieten, Feslschr.* fur K. Schneider. Willsbach, Heidelberg (1947)) that the hypochondriacal symptom of having doubts about one's health is one of the possibilities that human beings develop as a compensatory mechanism for human foresight. However, the question here is not why someone becomes a hypochondriac but why someone does not become 80. According to Janzarik, the reason is that this type of person has a high level of ability in the sphere of differentiation and that such a person is aware of a sphere of values that lie higher than, or transcend, one's existence, but this explanation is simplistic and speculative; the issue is actually more complicated. Morita points out something that we can verify in our experience, that the decisive factors of the hypochondriacal condition lie in the strength of the person's introspective tendency and a mental attitude that is "intellect based" (*richi-hon'i*) and "whimsical temperament based" (*kibun-hon'i*). Refer back to Chapter 6 for a full explanation.

[15] Some comments will be added on this matter within the scope of our understanding. Morita considers the condition called "hypochondriacal" as the basis for consummating the structure of *shinkeishitsu* (as a clinical entity), but we believe he went through a number of vacillations before he reached that conclusion. Initially, Morita was reluctant to discard the idea that this condition of being hypochondriacal is similar to a type of clinical entity. (According to Morita: "Initially, I could not consider this hypochondriac condition as having the same root as obsessive neurosis.") Eventually, however, he begins to consider it simply as an image of a clinical condition and, further, expands his understanding to a thoughtful position that expresses concern not simply about human physical health but also about the various living conditions of human beings. (This condition belongs to a category that H. P. Laughlin calls the hypochondriacal personality and resembles what he terms something that is frequently manifested subclinically and subneurotically as an overconcern for personal health or as a somatic preoccupation) (see Laughlin, H.P.: *The Neuroses in Clinical Practice.* Saunders (1956)).

Morita's outlook can be expressed by such terms as care, concern, worry and trouble, and it has a thoughtful character that, in Japanese, takes in the *ki* complex, including *ki-ni-suru*, *ki wo kubaru* and *ki wo tsukeru* (see Chapters 2 and 9). in the desire for self-realization, these conditions take into consideration the condition of one's health, discretion over one's possibilities and impossibilities and concern over how another person accepts one's interpersonal relationships. However, we should not overlook the point that the feeling of *ki wo kubaru* in regard to oneself and other persons, which human beings experience in this manner, arises by way of an internal conflict over a strong desire called acceptance of self by the people of one's *seken* (reference group) and of how one actually manifests oneself within that group. Consequently, Morita believes that the most characteristic feature of this condition called "hypochondriacal," which is the basic compositional element of *shinkeishitsu*, differs from the feeling that indicates a personality of low intelligence or of a weak, powerless tendency lacking in the type of conflict based in an introvertive character in a broad sense. It is a condition in which an internal excellence of self-reflection is manifested externally. In other words, Morita's concept of the "hypochondriacal basic tone" can be said to contain a conflict of not being able to escape from the suffering of human life, which the person does struggle to avoid. Because this phenomenon is an internal conflict that is projected externally in that manner, Morita considers the features of the *shinkeishitsu* persona to be those of self-reflection (introspection) and a powerful intellect that strongly manifests a condition of internal conflict.

Morita's Hypochondriacal Basic Tone and *Shinkeishitsu*–"*Ki*" Atmosphere

To study the substance of what Morita called the hypochondriacal trait, his explanation of the hypochondriacal basic tone (or hypochondria or hypochondriacal tendency) will be dealt with first. Each of these terms will be explained separately for the sake of convenience.

In Morita's words, "I believe the so-called hypochondriacal basic tone to be a kind of psychic disposition related to Matsubara's hypersensitive constitution[16] and it may be considered a type of mental degeneration, depending on the extent of its severity."[17]

"The hypochondriacal basic tone is the individual's mental tendency or individuality, and is an inborn trait . . ."[18]

He referred to both "the emotional basic tone of the hypochondriac trend" and "the mental basic tone of the hypochondriac trend."[19]

"My theory of the hypochondriacal basic tone is that it is a mental trait which can occur *a posteriori*."[20]

"Psychic interaction does not occur if the hypochondriacal basic tone is weak (and) does not become a neurotic symptom."[21]

What can be understood from these explanations is that:

1. the hypochondriacal basic tone is an inborn (or postnatal) mentally hypersensitive nature (which can be considered a hypersensitive constitution);
2. it is the basic condition for the onset of *shinkeishitsu*;
3. consequently, this trait becomes the causative mechanism that triggers the onset of the *shinkeishitsu* disorder;
4. the basic tone of emotion and thought is hypochondriacal;
5. it is a condition that ranges from a simple mental trend to a degree of mental degeneration, depending on the depth and extent of the hypochondriacal trend. (This definition is the same in substance as the definition of hypochondria or the hypochondriacal tendency that we will discuss later, resulting in a duplication of definition.)

The above summary of Morita's definition of the hypochondriacal trait will be explained in more detail later and will be followed by Morita's explanation of hypochondria or the hypochondriacal tendency. However, because there will be considerable duplication of content, we will limit the discussion to two or three of the most important points.

"The hypochondriacal tendency is also one of the introvertive tendencies. It consists of intense introspection, and the individual becomes dispirited or self-centered . . ."[22]

"Hypochondria signifies a hypochondriac fear of disease, and is a manifestation of the authentic human desire for life. This fear exists in all human beings, but if it becomes a dominant mental trait, it can then become degenerative and begin to manifest more and more complex and tenacious symptoms of the *shinkeishitsu* disorder, depending on the extent of its

---

[16] Matsubara asserts that the causal factor of neurasthenia is a constitutional hypersensitivity of the vasomotor nervous system.

[17] Morita, S.: Shinkeishitsu no Hontai oyobi Ryōhō (The Substance of *Shinkeishitsu* and Its Therapy), 1928. In *Morita Shōma Zenshū*, Vol. II, edited by T. Kōra. Hakuyōsha, Tokyo (1974). (Printed in Japanese)

[18] Morita, S.: Diagnosis and Therapy of Neurasthenia, 1925; *vid. do.*

[19] Morita, S.: The Therapy for *Shinkeishitsu* and Neurasthenia, 1922. In *Morita Shōma Zenshū*, Vol I.

[20] Morita, S.: The Substance of *Shinkeishitsu* and Its Therapy, 1928. In *Morita Shōma Zenshū*, Vol. III.

[21] Morita, S.: *vid. do.*

[22] Morita, S.: *vid. do.*

severity. This mental trend can lead to a chronic fear of death and disease . . . according to its extent and type."[23]

"The word hypochondria originated in the meaning of becoming concerned about something."[24]

"The hypochondriacal tendency is one of numerous tendencies; when these are summarized, we can say that the fear of disease is excessive. When this fear is full-blown, the patient fears death or harmful substances, experiences intensely abnormal sensational phenomena, both physical and mental, and interprets these as pathological."[25]

In summary, Morita makes the following statements about hypochondria or the hypochondriacal tendency:

1. The origin of the term lies in *ki-ni-suru*, which means "to become concerned (about something)."
2. It is a manifestation of the desire to live, which is inherent in authentic human nature and which is an authentic feeling experienced by every human being.
3. It is one of the introvertive trends, characterized by excessive introspection.
4. According to its extent, it can become a distinct mental trend, then become degenerative and finally develop into various complex neurotic conditions.

The gist of our understanding of these statements is that:

1. The hypochondriacal basic tone, hypochondria and the hypochondriacal tendency are all types of mental temperament or trends that regulate the *shinkeishitsu* condition, which is itself one type of mental degeneration.
2. Although the hypochondriacal basic tone lies within the conditions defined as being degenerative, it extends in scope beyond those conditions.
3. The hypochondriacal basic tone is the determining causative factor that moves a *shinkeishitsu*-disposed person into the *shinkeishitsu* condition, and in Morita's *shinkeishitsu* theory, it is the prerequisite factor for deducing the pathological basis of the development of the *shinkeishitsu* disorder.

This leads to the question that, even though the concept of the hypochondriacal basic tone has a special characteristic of being self-regulating, it is also regulated by the specific substance of hypochondria. In concrete terms, the hypochondriacal basic tone is an inborn disposition of mental hypersensitivity. It includes various conditions that develop into a definite mental trait and, further, into a type of mental degeneration (abnormal personality).

Morita discusses *shinkeishitsu* in the context of degeneration. The hypochondriacal basic tone is a predisposition regulated by that context and is extended into neurosis as a concept indicative of a mental disorder. Clinically, Morita *shinkeishitsu* is a type of neurosis. When viewed from Morita's psychopathological schema, there is no doubt that *shinkeishitsu* is a type of neurosis that is psychogenically developed.

If the hypochondriacal basic tone is defined as a predisposition that lies within the confines of degeneration (located midway between mental health and mental illness), it poses no contradiction either clinically or theoretically. Morita's intent in constructing the theory of the hypochondriacal basic tone to replace the former theory of mental hypersensitivity is fully understandable.

First of all, we need to discuss the hypochondriacal basic tone as the psychological basis of the *kizuki* (become aware of) and *kizukau* (become concerned about) mental disposition, apart from the generalized concept of hypochondria, and to clarify its definition as an attribute of the

---

23 Morita, S.: *vid. do.*
24 Morita, S.: *vid. do.*
25 Morita, S.: The Therapy for *Shinkeishitsu* and Neurasthenia, 1922; *vid. do.*

mental hypersensitive disposition (intrinsic character) in line with Morita's conception of *shinkeishitsu* in the early days.[26]

Second, we need to define clearly the hypochondriacal basic tone as a type of life reaction, that is, the mental attitude of *ki-zuki/ki-zukau* within the context of mental degeneration, in other words, as a definite concept of a condition of mental disorder.

In the one definition, the hypochondriacal basic tone is literally the mental basic tone of *shinkeishitsu* (in its basic character). In the second definition, it is a characteristic method or action of the degenerative mental condition called *shinkeishitsu.*

The psychopathological schema of the *shinkeishitsu* disorder is not distorted or misconstrued by either of these definitions.

That is the author's view of Morita's theory of the hypochondriacal basic tone. Let us now discuss the *kizuki/kizukau* aspects of this topic.

Kizuki and *Kizukau*[27]

Morita understands the hypochondriacal basic tone as being a form of human life reaction. He tries to perceive the difference between a mentally healthy person and one who is mentally degenerate, from the aspect of good or poor adaptability to conditions of living. Kōra, too, seeks to understand the hypochondriacal basic tone in terms of a so-called inadaptability anxiety. In these instances, both men made a great effort to restore importance to the concept of human adaptation, that is, human involvement with the environment.

The author would like to examine critically the content of the hypochondriacal basic tone from just that standpoint of adaptability. Hypochondria has the essential meaning of *ki-ni-suru* (to become concerned) in regard to the circumstances of human life. The full meaning of human life does not lie simply in the fact of being alive but also takes in the fact that one is engaged in a form of livelihood and that one is imbued with a human life history. All this signifies that one has a full human *bios.*

Morita adheres to the psychosomatic (body/mind) theory of human identity, but this simply means that he tries to grasp the totality of the human *bios.* Because this total *bios* is interwoven with human group cooperation and human history as a whole, the human *bios* also takes in the sphere of interpersonal relationships. In other words, the human *bios* is fully revealed in terms of life situations.

We might use the word *mi*[28] to denote this extended concept of psychosomatic wholeness. If we do so, the human *kizuki/kizukau* condition simply means that *mi* stands for interpersonal relationships in a situational context. When the *kizuki/kizukau* condition, which is an attribute of the hypochondriacal basic tone, is considered, the hypochondriacal basic tone does not merely signify concern about illness but, rather, concern about the whole of human existence and includes the full human *bios* engaged in a constant process of forming adaptability. The fact that Morita considers the hypochondriacal basic tone to be present in various kinds of human phenomenon is again worth noting here. However, the fact that he confines it to mental and physical phenomena alone does leave something to be desired.

Let us now examine the definition of the word *shin-ki* (shin=mind). This word has the gen-

---

[26] Morita says that the decisive cause of *shinkeishitsu* is the mentally hypersensitive disposition. Morita, S.: Essays on *shinkeishitsu*, 1919. In *Morita Shōma Zenshū*, Vol. I. Hakuyōsha, Tokyo (1974).

[27] See Chapter 9.

[28] See footnote 3 in Chapter 4.

eral meaning of *kokoro-mochi* (experiencing sensation) and *ki-bun* (humor, mood), but the meaning of *ki*[29] carries in its hidden core a certain power that is generated outward by some implicit need to flow. When *ki* is coupled with another psychological term, for example, *ki-zuku* (to become aware of), *ki wo kubaru* (to be watchful) or *ki wo tsukau* (to worry about), the meaning contained in *ki* is that of the condition of human beings who exist in life involvement with other persons. It can be related to the etymological definition of *kan-shin* (interest, composed of inter=among and est=being) and is also related to the human condition of living in day-to-day deliberation, giving consideration to other persons and being involved with them, that is, having *hairyo* (concern). *Ki* in *kizukau* (to become aware of) and in *ki-ni-suru* (to be anxious about) has that exact meaning and stands for the basic situational concern of human beings.

Shin has a centripetal definition, for example, *chu-shin* (center) and *kaku-shin* (nucleus), whereas *ki* has a centrifugal definition. Coupling the two terms produces *shin-ki*, which is defined as a situational condition of something that is generated from a center toward an outer periphery and that returns again to the center. The *kizuki/kizukau* condition that is so characteristic of the hypochondriacal basic tone concentrates that inner-center attention assertively outward toward a certain object of concern. Even if inassertive, the flow of concentration flows outward toward an object to which inner-center attention has been directed.

The flow of consciousness, when introspective, going inward, is one method of expressing one's full human *bios. Mi* expresses selfhood in the setting of full human wholeness.

The *kizuki/kizukau* form of consciousness (*shin-ki*) that is exhibited in interpersonal relationships has the exact nature of this inward to outward to inward process of constant concern, and each of us perceives the optimal situational placement of our full human *bios* (*mi*) in terms of that life process.

A *shinkeishitsu*-predisposed person, struggling to adapt to situations, also seeks to confirm the optimal placement of *mi* while "breathing" inward and outward in the same *ki* "atmosphere" but with more than normal concern (mental hypersensitiveness).

[29] See Chapter 2.

12

Parental Training and the Hypochondriacal Temperament

Morita took the standpoint that family environmental factors, particularly the mode of child training imposed by the parents, have importance in the formation of the *shinkeishitsu* persona. He had frequently pointed this out in the course of practical therapy. But he did not pursue it aggressively in theoretical exegesis.

Since he did leave it thus undeveloped, it is bound to attract our attention. Although we can cite only a small number of cases, a certain amount of information can be provided, in order to discuss these factors in this chapter based on our own therapeutic experience. To begin with, however, past achievements in this area will be examined.

Morita had already explained[1] that some past literature did exist which pointed to childhood emotional experience as the cause of an outbreak of neurosis, but that this point-of-view had attracted almost no attention at the time.

Around 1920, for example, S. Marui had insisted that childhood education is closely related to an outbreak of neurosis, and this theory has been frequently compared to the congenital disposition-oriented theory of Morita *shinkeishitsu.* K. Shimoda also took the a posteriori position that *shinkeishitsu* develops out of poor methods of education during childhood.

Morita partially concurred with this position later on, but he still insisted that the finally decisive factor lies in differences of temperament. He pointed out that some people acquire the *shinkeishitsu* persona while others do not, even when raised in similar ways in the same type of environment.

Shimoda[2] was convinced that parental attitudes can affect the onset of *shinkeishitsu.* From his standpoint, a child brought up by strict, very interferent parents lacks self-assurance. On the other hand, when parents are exceptionally non-interferent, the child remains self-assured at home but acquires a self-seclusive character outside the household.

S. Nakagawa[3] remarked (in 1954) that the strict, feudalistic system of education in Japan, under which the rights and privileges of the family head are quite powerful, has a probable bearing on formation of the *shinkeishitsu* persona. Again, in 1957, T. Abe[4] reported the results of his study on the relations between the *shinkeishitsu* temperament and childhood environment, to the effect that problems can arise from the educational attitude taken by the parents toward a *shinkeishitsu*-prone child.

Both hypochondriasis and pathophobia can often occur when the parents have been preoc-

---

[1] Morita, S.: Shinkeisuijakusei seishinbyōshitsusei taishitsu (The neurasthenic-psychopathic constitution), 1909. In *Morita Shōma Zenshū*, Vol. I. Hakuyōsha, Tokyo (1974). (Printed in Japanese)

[2] Shimoda, M.: *Seishin Eisei Kōwa* (Lectures on Mental Health). Iwanami Shoten, Tokyo (1942). (Printed in Japanese)

[3] Nakagawa, S.: Shinkeishitsushō oyobi sono kin'enjōtai no yogo ni tsuite no kenkyū (Studies on prognosis of *shinkeishitsu* and its similar states) (in Japanese). *Psychiatria et Neurologia Japonica* 56(3) (1954).

[4] Abe, T.: Theory of neurosis and defence reaction (in Japanese). *The Japanese Journal of Psycho-analysis* 9(10) (1957).

cupied and neurotically overanxious about their own state of health during the child's training period. Parents of this kind are apt to rely heavily on medicines, and tend to buy two or three kinds of drugstore medicines for regular use.

Furthermore, they distress themselves excessively about their own state of health and about illness pitfalls that might lie ahead in the future. Overly strict training, including incessant demands that such parents place on the child about keeping things in proper order, or personal cleanliness and good manners, compels the parents to scold the child continually for many years. Admonitions about locking up the house securely with two or even three locks, or about spending money carefully, are also characteristically observed.

Cases of childhood anthropophobia may stem from parental attitudes of categorical scolding, including sudden outbursts of anger because the child is too passive, school grades are poor, the parents' wishes have not been carried out, or because the child complains about not being able to sleep or about physiological abnormalities.

In cases of inferiority complex, the parents have typically and repeatedly said, "you are clumsy;" "you have no brains;" "your face is ugly"–and the child is compared with brothers and sisters who are said to be better and brighter. Abe summed up these cases by saying that parents have characteristically belabored insufficiencies and exacerbated the considerable fears of children who are *shinkeishitsu*-prone. When excessive parental attention is directed toward "incompleteness," so that the child is driven to strive for excessive "completeness," uncertainties and fears about being "complete" come to the fore and force the child to concentrate on preventing or eliminating "incompleteness." This, he says, is the formative factor of the *shinkeishitsu* persona.

There were a few studies done in Japan during Morita's lifetime and later, up to the 1960s, on parental attitudes about life environment and childhood training–as opposed to inherited character–as the basic factors of character formation in cases of neurosis and thus the cause of outbreaks of neurosis. But this approach was far more popular in Europe and America than it ever was in Japan.

In particular, Freud emphasized the parent-child relations as the cause of an outbreak of neurosis. The conclusion he arrived at, during his early period of dealing with the process of psychotherapy for neurosis centered around the factor of hysteria, points to such parent-child relations as the Oedipus complex. If, that is, the special sentiment the child forms toward the parent of the opposite sex is not sufficiently dealt with during childhood, but left alone as it is, it becomes the basis for an outbreak of neurosis in later life. This condition is attributed to the libido as the dynamic cause of the sexual instinct.

Another representative therapist who placed emphasis on the *a posteriori* effect in which character formation is attributed to the personal and social environment of the individual is Alfred Adler,[5] who parted company from Freud. In Adler's view, we all originally possess the same innate temperament. However, social feelings are induced in us from the time we are born. These feelings provide us with a means to externalize ourselves for self-expression, with the anticipated result that we can live in social harmony with others through full development of social consciousness.

Environment and education during childhood, Adler believes, are experienced as restrictions. When an inferiority complex and a compensatory desire to show off arise from such conditions, they can be countered by fostering stronger social feeling. Personal character is formed by the imprints of these various relations and is firmly crystallized during childhood.

F. Künkel,[6] who belonged to the same school as Adler, similarly negated the importance of

---

[5] Adler, A.: Heilen und Bilden. Reinhardt, München (1974); Fischer Taschenbuch, Fischer, Frankfurt (1973).

[6] Künkel, F.: *Einführung in die Charakterkunde auf individual psychologischer Grundlage*, 1928, 15 Aufl. Stuttgart (1971).

inherited character and special qualities. He stressed the point that human character images are formed by environmental influences during childhood.

Other very limited theoretical concepts of parent-child relations and life environments in terms of character formation in cases of neurosis emerged during the same period that Morita created the *shinkeishitsu* principle. But all of these concepts were based on psychodynamics theory, completely negating and seeking to discredit the theories of congenital temperament or predisposition. Consequently, Morita's *shinkeishitsu* theory, which favored the temperament principle, became an object of criticism from that opposing standpoint.

However, it is likely that both of these opposed concepts went through a dialectical process of development in Japan. This situation needs to be objectively studied and discussed.

The Role of Environment

It remains true that Morita considers predisposition the cause of *shinkeishitsu* as a disorder and places less emphasis on the environment. However, he does take into account environmental factors in triggering the onset of *shinkeishitsu.*

He reasons that only what he calls the "*shinkeishitsu* predisposition" is the determining factor in the onset of *shinkeishitsu.* He evaluates the role of environmental factors by stating that "the patient would probably not succumb to the disorder if this environmental inducement were not present. However, even with the inducement present, the patient would remain healthy if he did not have the *shinkeishitsu* constitution."

This was later explained by Bumke[7] with use of the adjectival "reactive." Morita had considered the matter thoroughly and had taken into account the environmental motivation that becomes the direct focal point for succumbing to the *shinkeishitsu* disorder. Morita does not define *shinkeishitsu-shō* (*shinkeishitsu* disorder) with the stipulation of "reactive" or "psychogenous," but his interpretation of the process by which the symptom is developed and fixed indicates a theoretical construction from the standpoint of psychogenous development.

He recognizes a quantitative difference in predisposition, which is the most important and decisive factor. This quantitative difference can undergo phenomenological modification owing to the effect of the environment. However, Morita excludes the environment, for the time being, as one of the compositional factors of his theoretical construction. He considers the process of the acquisition, formation and development of the *shinkeishitsu* persona to be a correlative issue that cannot be immediately resolved, similar to the correlation between heredity and the "*shinkeishitsu* predisposition" in not having been clarified at the academic level.

He does not stipulate the onset of *shinkeishitsu* as being induced by the environment or "psychogenous" in nature for the same reason that he does not position *shinkeishitsu* in a hereditary category, even though he endorses the hereditary theory of temperament. He sometimes cautioned parents by noting that an overprotective and excessively meddlesome method of raising children can act as an inducement to the hypochondriacal attitude of a child's *shinkeishitsu* persona. He wished to emphasize this precaution to make patients also aware of the strong dependence (or self-centered tendency) that they exhibit, directly or indirectly, toward their parents.

This shows that Morita did not ignore the importance of parental training in the home. He metaphorically compared the a posteriori effect that occurs during the formative process

[7] Bumke, O.: *Lehrbuch der Geisteskrankheiten*, 7 Aufl., Munich (1948).

of the *shinkeishitsu* persona as being analogous to the difference between plants that grow naturally and those that are nurtured under artificial care.

The absence of an emphatic environmental element in Morita theory is due to his prudence in not heavily stressing parent-child relationships in the home, when constructing his *shinkeishitsu* theory, because the substance of these relationships is not simple enough to be perfectly clear.

Parent-child relationships in the home, and in particular the relationship between the mode of child-raising and the hypochondriacal tendency, is dealt with in a study of our own, with background reference to general findings compiled by a number of other researchers (most of them not Morita therapists) over a time span dating from the first appearance of Morita theory up to the present. The background material includes facts that were not actively employed in Morita theory, even though Morita considered them important. We will describe our study in the sections that follow.

Explanation of Data

In explaining our data, let us note that the study covered 59 *shinkeishitsu* patients, as shown in Table 1. The patients underwent therapy within the five-year period from 1968 to 1973. There were 15 (12 male, three female) patients with ordinary *shinkeishitsu* (so-called neurasthenia), six (five male, one female) patients with paroxysmal neurosis (so-called anxiety neurosis) and 38 patients with obsessive-compulsive neuroses, 28 (18 male, 10 female) patients who had anthropophobia (which has an especially high incidence in Japan) and 10 (five male, five female) patients who suffered from obsessions, such as morbid fear of the inability to be perfect, mysophobia and morbid fear of being superstitious, as shown in Table 1.

No special conditions were set up to investigate conditions in the homes of these patients. The study material was obtained mostly from their case histories or during interviews. It should, therefore, be noted that the data presented on the character tendencies of both parents and on the conditions in the home were based almost entirely on the subjective impressions of the patients.

Two expressions, "incomplete homes" and "problem homes," are used in Table 1. Incomplete homes are those in which one or both parents died or were separated when the patient was 15 to 16 years old; the missing parent(s) was not replaced or, if replaced, the foster parent(s) was not able to fulfill the missing parent's role.

Problem homes are those in which the patient is affected by ostensibly living at home with both parents, but there is no genuine parent-child communication for one reason or another. Grandparents, brothers and sisters or other relatives may act as de facto parents (for example, because the true parents may be absent from home for long periods due to business travel, because chronic illness has led to long hospitalization of the parents or because the parents, even if at home, do not fulfill the role of parents owing to a bedridden status forced on them by illness). Chronic illness among persons who form any part of the family household unit, such as arthritis deformans, neurosis, alcoholism or drug dependence in grandparents or siblings, desertion of the home or suicide by family members and emotional disharmony within the family unit caused by financial problems also contribute to the development of problem homes.

Both types of home can be classified as such, but it is, of course, difficult in many instances to make a clear-cut distinction between the two types, so a comparative discussion of these types was not attempted.

Table 1 Family Background

Cases / Item	Classification	Ordinary *Shinkeishitsu*		Paroxysmal Neurosis		Anthropophobia		Other Obsessive-Compulsive Neurosis		Total	
	Sex	M	F	M	F	M	F	M	F	M	F
	Number	12	3	5	1	18	10	5	5	40	19
	Avg. Age	23	29	47	47	26	25	24	31	28	27
Death from illness or accident	Father	1	1			4	1			5	2
	Mother	1				2				3	0
Suicide	Father										
	Mother	1								1	0
	Siblings	1				1				2	0
Divorce	Father Absent	1				1				2	0
	Mother Absent					1	1			1	1
Broken/incomplete home		5	1			8	2			13	3
Family discord	Parents		1	1					1	1	2
	Others	1							1	1	1
Shinkeishitsu	Father	1				2	2		1	3	3
	Mother									0	0
	Siblings	2		1		1				4	0
Psychosis	Father										
	Mother										
	Siblings	1		1		1				3	0
	Cousin	1					1		1	1	2
Chronic somatic disease	Father	1		1		1				3	0
	Mother	1								1	0
	Siblings	1								1	0
Economic destitution		2				1	1	1	1	4	2
Problem home		11		4		8	4	1	5	24	9

The "Incomplete Home" and the "Problem Home"

Ten of the 59 patients had homes in which the father or mother had died; one father and one mother had committed suicide. One patient had lost both parents at the same time, in an accident that occurred when the patient was three years old, and he was subsequently brought up by his grandparents. (The patient was a 20-year-old man who suffered from anthropophobia.) Another patient had a morbid fear of doing something sinful and had been raised by foster parents, from immediately after birth to the age of 15, without being aware of it. (The patient was a 44-year-old woman.)

Of the 40 male patients, 13 (32.5 percent) had incomplete homes; another 24 (60 percent) came from problem homes. Of the 19 female patients, three (15.8 percent) were from incomplete homes and nine (47.4 percent) were from problem homes. In sum, 16 patients (27.1 percent) came from incomplete homes, and 33 (55.9 percent) from problem homes.

The number of incomplete homes (six) in which the father had died was larger than the number (three) in which the mother had died. (The one case in which both parents had died at the same time is excluded in this instance.) In all cases, the surviving parent had not remarried, raising the child alone. There were four cases of divorce in the incomplete homes; in two cases, the patient had lived with the father, and in two cases with the mother. These parents, too, had not remarried and had brought up the child in the incomplete home condition.

Among the 33 problem homes, there were six cases (18.2 percent) of economic destitution (four male and two female patients), five cases (15.2 percent) of male patients only with problem homes due to chronic illness of parents or sublings, six cases (18.2 percent), composed of three male and three female patients, in which the father was said to have *shinkeishitsu* (as a clinical entity) and two cases (6.1 percent, composed of one male and one female patient, in which the father or mother had a history of psychosis according to the strict clinical definition.

In seven cases (21.2 percent), a sibling had neurosis or psychosis. In another three cases (9.1 percent), there was discord between the parents, and there was one case (3 percent) of sibling discord compounded by discord between the mother and grandmother.

In three cases (9.1 percent), composed of two male and one female patient, the child was raised from infancy to preadolescence by a grandmother who lived with the family, but these cases were not classified as problem homes.

In problem home cases that involved chronic illness, there was one case (female patient, 21 years old, morbid fear of inability to be perfect) in which the father had been bedridden for ten years because of the sequelae of apoplexy and one case (male patient, 23 years old, anthropophobia) in which the home became unstable because the father was an alcoholic and also had occasional paranoic states of mind.

Therefore, 33 of the 59 patients (55.9 percent) had experienced some type of family problem at home. However, because our information was obtained mostly from material provided by the patients, it may contain highly biased impressions. Further, some patients did not wish to discuss their family situations in detail, so it is somewhat questionable whether the data we present here can be said to convey an accurate description of actual conditions in these homes. Nevertheless, because the data base is composed of the patients' experiences, it does have certain clinical implications from that standpoint, although it may not be strictly objective in nature.

It is reasonable to assume that, numerically speaking, many more patients were raised under problematical household conditions. Family life can include feuding among household members owing to differences in their individual needs, wants and personal orientations. Even in a general sense, the home environment, economic condition, family composition or health factors can give rise to dissatisfaction or discord for one reason or another. Long-term conditions of strain can lead to trouble in the home as an effect of outside environmental influences. An examination of families in any neighborhood may indicate that life is proceeding smoothly on the surface, in the outer world, but there are certain problems, large or small, kept in concealment within the home. The number of homes that are free of problems is probably minute.

The percentages of incomplete homes and problem homes among these 59 patients do not have much statistical significance. The figures are far less important than the manner in which the parents in such cases viewed the parent-child relationship and the family atmosphere that prevailed in each home. We will thus limit our initial commentary to the factual material and then will proceed to comment on the data contained in Table 3. However, we would first like to discuss the aspect of the *shinkeishitsu* persona indicated by the parents in such cases.

Parental Personality

Thirty-four of the 40 male patients provided impressions of their fathers' character, and 37 of these 40 patients likewise commented on their mothers. Twenty-seven patients (79.4 percent claimed that the father had a *shinkeishitsu*-latent personality, and 23 patients (62.2 percent) made this comment about the mother. Fifteen of the 19 female patients (83.3 percent) said that the father had a *shinkeishitsu*-latent personality (18 of the 19 female patients discussed this aspect), and six of these female patients (33.3 percent) made this comment about the mother.

Of the total number of fathers of the 52 patients who discussed the father's character, 42 of them (77.8 percent) were said to have a *shinkeishitsu*-latent personality. Twenty-nine mothers (53.7 percent) were said to have such a personality. We might surmise from these figures only that a *shinkeishitsu*-latent personality in a patient tends to depend more on the presence of this type of personality in the father from a characterological standpoint. When this tendency is examined typologically, it is found that ten patients (76.9 percent) among the 13 patients with ordinary *shinkeishitsu* allegedly have fathers who exhibit a *shinkeishitsu*-latent personality and that eight patients (57.1 percent) among the 14 patients with this condition allegedly have mothers who have a *shinkeishitsu*-latent personality.

In regard to patients with paroxysmal neurosis, five of six patients (83.3 percent) said the father had a *shinkeishitsu*-latent personality and three of six patients (50 percent) made this claim about the mother. Among patients with anthropophobia, 20 of 23 patients (87 percent) said the father had a *shinkeishitsu*-latent personality, and 15 of 24 patients (62.5 percent) made this comment about the mother. Among patients with obsessive-compulsive neurosis, seven of ten patients (70 percent) made this comment about the father and three of ten patients (30 percent) made this comment about the mother.

It is clear from these typological figures that the percentage of fathers with a *shinkeishitsu*-latent personality is high in cases of children who in later life suffer from anthropophobia. Overall, a *shinkeishitsu*-latent personality was exhibited by 77.8 percent of the fathers and 53.7 percent of the mothers.

The *shinkeishitsu* tendency among siblings is indicated by three male and two female patients who said that all members of the same family line had a *shinkeishitsu* personality; among siblings, in particular, 32 male (80 percent) and 15 female patients (78.9 percent) said that one or two siblings had the same tendency. Again, however, these figures are not based on a clinically objective evaluation but, rather, are derived wholly from the subjective impressions of the patients. Nevertheless, the data can be meaningful from the standpoint of inferring one aspect of character tendency within the families of these patients.

Parental Training Attitude

The author will next explain the figures in Table 2, which indicate the impressions of the patients in regard to parental methods of raising and training during childhood, the main point of this chapter. It should be noted that there is some overlap of the same cases in these figures, so the totals are sometimes larger than the actual number of cases.

The words *genkakuna* (strict), *kuchiyakamashii* (nagging), *hōninteki* (noninterfering) and *kahogoteki* (overprotective) used in Table 2 will be briefly explained. These words were frequently used by the patients when they talked about the attitude and child-training methods of their parents and thus will be used for the sake of convenience. However, the author will first discuss in detail the meanings of these words.

The word *kahogoteki* (overprotective) indicates an attitude of *kamau* (to care about) and *kanshō suru* (to interfere) in all aspects of child growth. From a patient's point of view, there is a background feeling of parental *amayakashi* (pampering). Allowing a child to be self-indulgent, tolerating conduct that is not usually approved or permitting a child to act in whatever way the child wishes can no doubt be construed as *hōninteki* (noninterfering) in nature, but we consider these attitudes as actually *kahogoteki* (overprotective) in this instance. In other words, the author takes these words to signify excessive parental pampering.

There were, however, only a few cases of this nature. A *hōninteki* (noninterfering) parent is frequently unconcerned about his or her child's behavior because of being too busy with other daily life activities or is indifferent to the child, who feels left alone with almost no interference in either a positive or negative sense.

A *genkakuna* (strict) parent, on the other hand, does not neglect to instruct his or her child in the basic manners and etiquette of family life, social life and interpersonal relationships which these parents teach with incessant inflexibility.

Kuchiyakamashii (nagging, particular, nitpicking) signifies an attitude of thoughtless parental meddling that stems from a parent's feeling of anticipation, interest or uncertainty. It is difficult to make a clear-cut differentiation between the latter two words because of considerable differences in the patients' attitudes toward the feelings of their parents. Further, these words represent only a patient's impression and evaluation.[8]

The word *futsū* (ordinary) does not mean either "strict" or "overprotective," signifying, instead, that a patient accepts his or her parent's attitude as one that is "commonplace." In other words, the parent is viewed as "average," and for this reason, the parent's attitude is not aggressively imposed on the child. The general attitude of the parent, in this instance, has no special characteristic on the whole, but when this attitude is discussed more carefully, it is found to have certain partially "strict" or "nitpicking" aspects.

These elements of parental attitude are conditional and, in this instance, included in a patient's corresponding reaction. However, when the overall attitude is said to be average and not especially prejudicial, it is classified as "ordinary." The extremes of attitude can also be classified as *kōteiteki* (affirmative) or *hiteiteki* (negative), but when the patient's general impression is vague and passive, apart from positive affirmation or denial, it is classified as *chūyō* (moder-

[8] The word *kuchiyakamashii* (nitpicking) principally stands for an attitude of prudent cautiousness, being concerned even about minor matters, giving advice beforehand rather than finding fault and complaining, as well as instilling caution. This caution is applied not only to regulating training and teaching of the child, but even with respect to issues perceived by the child to be unnecessary matters. Some of the patients interpret this attitude as *genkakuna* (strict) or *kuchiurusai* (nagging). At any rate, in all cases, there is little trace of *hihanteki* (critical) or *arasagashisuru* (faultfinding) quality. Therefore, it can be considered as *kanshōteki* (meddlesome) or *osekkaina* (officious) from one standpoint or *kahogoteki* (overprotective) from another point of view.

Table 2 Mode of Parental Training

Cases / Item	Classification	Ordinary *Shinkeishitsu*		Paroxysmal Neurosis		Anthropophobia		Obsessive-Compulsive Neurosis (including phobia)		Total	
	Sex	M	F	M	F	M	F	M	F	M	F
	Number	12	3 (F10/M11)*	5	1	18	10 (F15/M14)*(F8)*	5	5	40	19 (F35/M35)*(F17/M19)*
Genkakuna	Father	4	1	1	0	4	3	0	2	9†	6
(Strict)	Mother	1	0	1	0	5	1	1	0	8	1
Kuchiyakamashii	Father	1	3	0	0	7	2	3	0	11	5
(nagging, nitpicking)	Mother	3	2	1	0	5	4	2	1	11	7
Hōninteki	Father	3	0	1	0	5	1	0	2	9	3
(Noninterfering)	Mother	0	1	0	0	1	1	0	1	1	3
Kahogoteki	Father	1	0	2	1	5	2	2	1	10	4
(Overprotective)	Mother	6	1	3	1	9	3	1	2	19	7
Futsū	Father	5	0	2	0	1	2	2	0	10	2
(Ordinary)	Mother	5	1	1	1	1	1	1	3	8	6
Kōteiteki	Father	3	0	4	1	6	1	1	2	14	4
(Affirmative)	Mother	2	0	4	1	8	4	1	2	15	7
Chūyō	Father	5	3	0	0	4	5	4	2	13	10
(Moderate)	Mother	5	0	1	0	7	3	3	2	16	5
Hiteiteki	Father	2	0	1	0	3	3	1	1	7	4
(Negative)	Mother	3	0	0	0	3	3	1	1	7	4
Shinkeishitsu-	Father	7 (76.9 %)	3	4 (83.3 %)	1	12 (87 %)	8	4 (70 %)	3	27 (77.8 %)	15
latent personality	Mother	6 (57.1 %)	2	3 (50 %)	0	12 (62.5 %)	3	2 (30 %)	1	23 (53.7 %)	6

*Figures in parentheses indicate father (F) and mother (M).
†Cumulative totals obtained by multiple responses.

ate). No patient in our study showed powerful feelings or an aggressive negation of their homes or parents.

The chief impressions of the patients in regard to their parents are described in the following sections.

Paroxysmal Neurosis (so-called anxiety neurosis)

For this impression, there is no statistical significance because the number of cases was the smallest, only one female patient. However, even the male patients were affirmative toward the parents with only one exception. The one female patient was also affirmative. The parental methods of teaching and training were varied, so that no characteristic tendency could be observed. The one case that had negative impressions toward the parents was that of a 28-year-old man. In this instance, the father had died of stomach cancer when the patient was 18 years-old. There had been eight children in the family; the patient had been the only male child. The household had been gloomy because the father had been cheerless and had a *shinkeishitsu*-persona and because the mother had been sickly. The patient's impression was that both parents, particularly the father, lacked a domestic nature, with a feeling of family intimacy missing. In general, the personal character of patients with paroxysmal neurosis is that of a *shinkeishitsu* persona, but such patients usually are active and cheerful. Many of them even appear, at first sight, to be extroverted. There were other cases in which that sort of character tendency was indicated, but a schizothymic tendency was conspicuous in only one case: a male patient who had been the second of eight children and the only boy. As such, he had not been treated with special affection or deference, as would be customary in any ordinary home. He said that his sisters, too, had a *shinkeishitsu* persona, with a schizothymic tendency.

Anthropophobia

Somewhat characteristic of this type of case is the fact that many such patients feel that training by both parents was *genkakuna* (strict) and *kuchiyakamashii* (nagging, nitpicking). Eleven of 15 male patients (73.3 percent) had relatively clear impressions of the father, and ten of 14 male patients (71.4 percent) had similarly strong impressions of the mother, as shown in Table 3.

Table 3 Contents of Training*

	Father/Son	Father/Daughter	Mother/Son	Mother/Daughter
Study	72 (%)	22 (%)	70 (%)	69 (%)
Manners, etiquette, courteous speech	43	53	58	71
Help with housework	10	50	22	72
Do not annoy other people or *seken*	66	61	62	61
Are not ridiculed by others or *seken*	64	62	57	56
Punctual in going out and returning home	28	35	38	45
Keep promises	37	33	36	34
Avoid bad company	13	20	28	35
Neat clothing, good taste, attentive to lessons	20	35	46	53
Economical, take good care of belongings	45	43	46	48
Keep things in good order, well-organized	35	39	39	58
Attentive to health	63	64	66	65
Attentive to fire prevention	30	31	35	34
Remember to lock doors	32	34	41	43

*Multiple-choice method.

Five of eight female patients (62.5 percent) had strong impressions of the father, and five of ten female patients (50 percent) had strong impressions of both parents.

Five of 15 male patients (33.3 percent) had an impression of the father as being overprotective, overcaring and excessively interferent. Another five male patients felt that the father did not care about anything the patient did and was *hōninteki* (noninterferent). By contrast, only one of 14 male patients said that the mother was completely *hōninteki* (noninterferent). Nine of 14 male patients (64.3 percent) said that the mother interfered in everything and was *kahogoteki* (overprotective). The proportion of females who complained of *kamawaresugi* (overcaring) and *kahogoteki* (overprotective) parents was less than that of the male patients. Only two of eight female patients (25 percent) made this comment about the father, and only three of ten female patients (30 percent) made this comment about the mother, so that no clear-cut tendency could be deduced. Many patients felt that both parents were strict and nitpicking, but only a few felt negatively toward both parents. Most patients were affirmative toward the parents even if the father or mother had been strict and nitpicking. Without being negative, they accepted the parents as *futsū* (ordinary) and *chūyō* (moderate). That is, 40 percent of the male patients were affirmative toward the father, and 57.1 percent felt this way toward the mother. Among the female patients, 12.5 percent were affirmative toward the father, and 40 percent felt this way toward the mother. There were six cases, three of male and three of female patients, in which the patient felt negative toward one or both parents. One male patient who felt negative said that his parents had been strict, nitpicking and excessively interferent. Two other males who felt negative gave noninterferent as the reason. The figures were quite the opposite in the female cases, with two patients who felt negative saying that their parents had been overprotective and one saying that her parents had been nonprotective.

There was no clear awareness among these patients of feeling negative, only an attempt to shift responsibility by saying that they somehow felt that "I am inferior to other people because of my father's or mother's training."

Other Types of Obsession and Phobia

Three of five male patients (60 percent) felt that their fathers had been strict and nitpicking, and the same proportion felt that way toward their mothers. None of these patients mentioned noninterferent. Two of these five patients (40 percent) had an overprotective impression of their fathers, and one patient (20 percent) had this impression of his mother. Among the female patients, two of five patients (40 percent) mentioned strictness in the father; no female patient made this comment about the mother, and only one patient felt the mother had been nitpicking. Two female patients felt that the father, and one felt that the mother, had been noninterferent. One female patient felt that the father, and two felt that the mother, had been overprotective. One male and one female patient had negative impressions toward both parents. However, a characteristic tendency, such as that observed in patients with anthropophobia, was not detectable, possibly due to the small number of cases.

Ordinary *Shinkeishitsu*

Five of ten male patients (50 percent) had the impression of strict or nitpicking with respect to the father, and four of ten female patients (40 percent) had a similar impression with respect to the mother. By contrast, only three of ten patients (30 percent) had the impression of noninterferent and only one male patient (10 percent) had the impression of overprotective with respect to the father. Even in the instance of the same impression, not a single male patient said that the mother had been noninterferent, whereas six male patients (60 percent) felt that the mother had been overprotective. Among the females, all three patients (100 percent) had the impression of strict with respect to the father, and two of them (67 percent) had the impression of nitpicking with respect to the mother. No patient claimed that the father had been noninterferent, and only one male and one female patient felt this way about the mother.

Parental Training Models

The author will now take a qualitative view of parental attitude toward child care, discussing specific points of parental emphasis in the training of children. This study will also indicate, more precisely, the growth patterns of children who receive parental training. This subject is a broad one, covering such topics as school studies, selection of friends, assisting with housework, health and hygiene, prevention of disease, clothing standards, orderliness, sense of proper arrangement, punctuality in appointments, etiquette, manner of speech, consideration for human relationships and ways of spending pocket money.

Specific comments on all these topics are heard by almost all such children from their parents every day. In general, however, differences in emotional relationships occur between the parents and such children owing to the method and frequency with which the parents give advice and admonitions. Parental approaches become factors that give rise to such feelings as mutual trust, respect, dependence, insubordination and rejection. Accordingly, the words and actions used by parents in the home to communicate with their children become the basis for the formation of each child's images of his or her father and mother, which then play an important part in the formation of individual personality.

The characteristics of the caution and interest that parents direct toward their children have an important bearing on a child's social upbringing. Emotional maturation is organically fostered in the mutual relationships that develop between parents and children, even in the simplicities of human relationships within the home, given the premise that the parent-child bond is effective and how the children (patients, in this instance) accept it is the key. How such children accept parental interest in child training, with regard to *shinkeishitsu* grouping, will now be examined in depth.

In general, there is a detectable difference between the attitude of the father and that of the mother toward a son or daughter, and this difference has been recognized in the instance of *shinkeishitsu*.

According to Table 3, a father tends to involve himself in his son's studies, as is apparent from the statistical difference seen between sons and daughters. It is not clear whether this difference between sons and daughters was clearly present in the father's mode of thought regarding education; nonetheless, a large number of male cases indicate a heavy interest in school studies as a characteristic feature of training by the father. By contrast, a father's interest in his daughter is more frequently oriented toward training in housework.

A mother's involvement with her daughter is statistically high only in terms of training in housework, similar to the involvement of the father. Generally, however, a mother's involvement with children of both sexes is greater than a father's involvement when statistically indicated. This involvement includes schoolwork, manners, etiquette, verbal expression, keeping oneself and one's clothing neat and clean, instilling good taste, pastimes and school lessons. Especially in regard to schoolwork, a mother demonstrates a greater interest than does a father in children of both sexes.

Interestingly enough, the items that both parents show equal concern for are a child's health and treatment of other people. The substance of this concern toward health differs from case to case but usually relates to sleep, meals and bodily cleanliness. A child is trained to go to bed early, get sufficient sleep, keep the body, underwear and outer clothing clean, eat proper meals and avoid dangerous activities, concerns that in all cases help shield the child from illness or injury and help ensure health and safety. Children consider the basis of such parental training to be concern for their health.

Treatment of other people is another important aspect of training by both parents. The father and mother expect their children to develop into respectful human beings who do not annoy other people (or the *seken*) and who are not ridiculed by other people (or the *seken*). This hope for respectfulness can be considered the criterion of the training given by both parents in accordance with their desire to instill, as habits, basic ways of acting in relationships with other people, such as manners, speech, ways to exchange greetings and keeping promises.

When the method of training based on parental value orientation (cultural orientation) is examined in relation to type of *shinkeishitsu*, some correlation is observed in the pathoplasticity of the *shinkeishitsu* persona or symptoms. Training with an emphasis on personal standards by use of advice and caution in regard to health and safety was characteristic of eight of ten fathers (80 percent) and five of ten mothers (50 percent) in male patients with ordinary *shinkeishitsu* neurosis and was characteristic of all three fathers and two of three mothers in female patients with this condition, such training was true of 11 of 15 fathers (73 percent) and ten of 15 mothers (66.6 percent) of male patients with anthropophobia and was also true of five of eight fathers and mothers each (62.5 percent) of female patients with this condition.

There was no clearly definable trend of parental training according to any fixed standard in patients with obsession, with the exception of advice concerning a broad range of activities, for example, studying hard or being orderly and well-organized. Other training related to social etiquette and personal manners, health, saving money and spending it wisely, locking doors and windows and preventing fires and thefts of other people's belongings. Such children also are taught not to inconvenience other people, to discriminate between social duties and matters of the human heart, to avoid associating with bad companions, not to be wasteful and to keep promises.

The parental attitude toward child training is motivated by expectations and desires in regard to the present as well as the future that parents project onto their children, compounded with an anxiety to prevent children from becoming social dropouts. The specific character of this attitude varies according to the character and life environment, or the life history, of each parent. However, in noting that many parents of such patients have a *shinkeishitsu* persona, we may assume that their mode of child training, in particular, is based on a strong sense of anxiety, which arises from the intensive self-reflection and the sensitivity that any such person tends to demonstrate. In turn, these attributes lead such parents to make their children exercise extreme precaution and anticipate trouble, which are not unrealistic requests. Consequently, the children, who share the *shinkeishitsu* persona, will have an impression of their parents as being strict and nitpicking.

Image of Father, Mother and Household

The images of their parents and homes that these patients had were investigated by Osgood's semantic differential method, as modified by Sagara, in which the four centroid factors (moral rectitude, sensory pleasure, potency and activity) are analyzed by the vector method and classified according to factor. The patients were requested to evaluate these factors by the five-stage method, and the results were reported accordingly (Table 4).

Male Patients

a. Image of father: There were positive as well as negative images, such as "old," "safe," "domineering," "pure," "gentle," "simple," "hard," "narrow," "active" and "grateful," but positive images were much more commonly reported.

Table 4 Factors of the Five-Stage Method

inferior ______	superior	soft ______	hard
inconsistent ______	consistent	likable ______	dislikable
scanty ______	ample	white ______	black
incorrect ______	correct	beautiful ______	ugly
bad ______	good	young ______	old
indistinct ______	distinct	hot ______	cold
ungrateful ______	grateful	pure ______	impure
unclean ______	clean	simple ______	complicated
low ______	high	negative ______	positive
insensitive ______	sensitive	narrow ______	wide
dangerous ______	safe	small ______	large
severe ______	gentle	weak ______	strong
gloomy ______	cheerful	antiquated ______	modern
pleasant ______	unpleasant	submissive ______	domineering
delighted ______	sad	violent ______	calm
light ______	dark	quick ______	slow
comfortable ______	uncomfortable	active ______	inactive

Table 5 Factors of Parents' Images

Factor		Father	Mother	Home
Moral rectitude	M*	+0.14 (+0.59)†	+0.86 (+0.73)	+0.06 (+0.63)
	F*	+0.51 (+0.52)	+0.57 (+0.56)	+0.45 (+0.30)
Sensory pleasure	M	−0.07 (+0.23)	+0.59 (+0.96)	+0.24 (+0.74)
	F	+0.28 (+0.48)	+0.84 (+0.84)	+0.66 (+0.79)
Potency	M	−0.18 (+0.36)	+0.23 (+0.22)	−0.17 (+0.37)
	F	+0.25 (+0.14)	+0.30 (+0.20)	+0.11 (+0.45)
Activity	M	+0.17 (+0.42)	+0.52 (+0.38)	+0.13 (+0.53)
	F	+0.57 (+0.10)	+0.53 (+0.24)	+0.23 (+0.32)

*M, male; F, female patients.
†Figures in parentheses indicate data from healthy subjects used as controls.

b. Image of mother: Positive images, such as "grateful," "superior," "pleasant," "likable," "gentle," "safe" and "calm," were more frequently reported.
c. Image of home: There were many positive images, such as "affectionate," "soft," "safe" and "bright," but also negative images, such as "inconsistent."

Female patients

a. Image of father: There were many positive images, such as "pleasant," "pure," "safe" and "calm," but also negative images, such as "old," "hard" and submissive."
b. Image of mother: Positive images, such as "bright," "safe," "gentle," "grateful," "calm" and "beautiful," were most frequently reported.
c. Image of home: Positive images, such as "calm," "grateful," "safe," "cheerful," "affectionate" and "joyful," were most frequently reported. Positive images of mother and home were reported more frequently by female than by male patients.

A tabulation of the above data according to factor is given in Table 5. The figures in parentheses represent data from 30 healthy male and female subjects, included for the sake of comparison. The average age of the male subjects was 27.7 years (range, 23 to 34), and of the female 27.4 years (range, 20 to 38).

It is apparent from Table 5 that the image of the father for male patients was negative for the factors of "potency" and "sensory pleasure" and that the image of the mother was more strongly positive for the factors of "moral rectitude," "sensory pleasure" and "activity." Also, the image of the home for male patients was negative for the factor of potency, but the positive image for sensory pleasure was stronger than that of other factors.

The female patients had no negative image of father, mother or home but did have an especially stronger positive image of the father for the factors of sensory pleasure, moral rectitude and activity; their images of the mother and home were quite similar.

It is clear from Table 5 that the male patients had negative images of the father for the factors of sensory pleasure and potency, but from an overall point of view, the image of the father is positive. The image of the mother, in particular, is strongly positive for all factors except potency.

The male patients received a more positive image of moral rectitude and activity than of sensory pleasure from the father. The general image of the father reported by female patients was similar to that of male patients, but the female patients received a stronger positive image of sensory pleasure from that parent than did the male patients. The female patients also had a stronger positive image of the home for all factors than did the male patients.

Both the healthy subject group and patient group used in our investigation had a more positive image of the mother than of the father for all factors, but from an overall point of view, the number of negative, rejecting images of both parents and the home was small (particularly in the female patients), with generally positive images. This result is much the same as the impression obtained in the interviews. The fact that about 60 percent of the families were one-parent or problem families was not a negative factor to these patients (except for some of the male patients) because a father, mother, grandparents or siblings compensated for any deficiency in one way or another. It can be concluded that the overall home function was positive for the factors of moral rectitude, sensory pleasure and activity. From this standpoint, any lack of unity in home function, or in functionally disrupted or broken homes, a factor often present in schizophrenics or juvenile delinquents, seems rare in *shinkeishitsu* patients.

Summary of Data

The study results can be summarized as follows:

1. The 59 subjects (40 male and 19 female patients) all had *shinkeishitsu*. When classified according to type, there were 15 cases of ordinary *shinkeishitsu*, six cases of paroxysmal neurosis and 38 cases of obsessive-compulsive neurosis (inclusive of 28 cases of anthropophobia).
2. The age range was 18 to 44 years of age, with the average being 28.8 years. There were three teenage patients, 33 in their twenties, 18 in their thirties and five in their forties.
3. Fourteen patients (23.7 percent) were from one-parent homes, and 35 patients (59.3 percent) were from problem homes.
4. There was evidence of a parental *shinkeishitsu* persona (on the basis of character analogy) in 79.4 percent of the fathers and 62.1 percent of the mothers in the male cases and in 83.3 percent of the fathers and 22.2 percent of the mothers in the female cases. The parental totals for male and female patients combined were 86.5 percent of the fathers and 49 percent of the mothers. This result alone indicates that the *shinkeishitsu* personas of these patients resembled the father's persona. This finding was especially conspicuous in patients with anthropophobia. Eighty percent of the siblings of the male patients and 78.9 percent of the siblings of the female patients had *shinkeishitsu* personas.
5. The patients' main impressions of their parents were as follows:
   a. With few exceptions, the patients' impressions of parents and home were positive, on the whole, according to the results obtained from the interviews and by use of the five-stage evaluation method.
   b. The patients had a stronger, more positive image of the mother and the home for the factor of sensory pleasure, according to the five-stage evaluation method.

c. Male patients had a positive image of the father for the factors of moral rectitude and activity and a negative image for sensory pleasure and potency. The image of the home was also negative for the factor of potency. By contrast, the image of the mother was positive for all factors, with moral rectitude most notable. These findings show that the male patients had a more positive image of the mother for all factors and, in that respect, indicated more affinity for and dependence on the mother than on the father.

d. The female patients had positive images of the father, mother and home for all factors, with the factor of sensory pleasure particularly strong for both the mother and the home.

6. More than half of the male patients (20 of 35, or 57.1 percent) had the impression that the father was strict and nitpicking, and more than half (19 of 36, or 52.8 percent) had this impression of the mother. This impression was reported by 11 of 17 female patients (64.7 percent) in regard to the father but by only eight of 18 female patients (44.4 percent) in regard to the mother. In male patients, an impression of overprotective for the father was reported in 28.6 percent of cases (10 of 35 patients), and of overprotective for the mother in 52.8 percent of cases (19 of 36 patients).

7. The number of patients with anthropophobia indicating an impression of strict and nitpicking regarding parental training in interviews was especially large, 11 of 15 male patients (73.3 percent) making this claim about the father, and ten of 14 (71.4 percent) about the mother, and five of eight female patients (62.5 percent) making this claim about the father, and five of ten (50 percent) about the mother. The number of patients who had the impression of overprotective was not small. This impression of the mother was especially noteworthy in male patients, nine of 15 (60 percent) reporting it. The impression of affirmative was reported by six of 15 male patients (40 percent) in regard to the father and by eight of 14 (57.8 percent) in regard to the mother. By contrast, the proportion of female patients reporting this impression of the mother was similar (four of ten patients, or 40 percent), whereas only one of eight female patients (12.5 percent) had this impression of the father.

8. The impression of strict and nitpicking or nagging in regard to the father was reported by 60 percent of the male patients with obsessive-compulsive neurosis and by 40 percent of the female patients with this condition. In regard to the mother, however, this impression was reported infrequently, particularly by female patients. However, this finding cannot be construed as characteristic, as in anthropophobia, because the number of cases sampled was too small.

9. Five of ten patients with ordinary *shinkeishitsu* had the impression of strict or nitpicking in regard to the father, and four of 12 patients had the same impression of the mother. The impression of noninterferent was reported by three patients in regard to the father but by no patient in regard to the mother. The opposite impression, overprotective, of the father was reported by one patient; six patients had the same impression of the mother. All three female patients had the impression of strict or nitpicking in regard to the father, and two of three had this impression of the mother.

10. Thirteen of the 14 patients from one-parent homes indicated that the father, mother or proxy parents were overprotective.

11. A summary of the emphasis of parental training in cases in which the parents were considered strict, nitpicking or overprotective is as follows:

a. The father's emphasis in training was in regard to schoolwork for the son and etiquette, manners and helping with housework for the daughter.

b. The mother's emphasis was directed toward etiquette, manners and housework for both son and daughter. The mother and father, however, show equal interest in the son and daughter in regard to schoolwork. In addition, the mother issues detailed instructions about activities of daily living, such as keeping things in order, playing with friends, wearing proper clothing and appropriates times for going out and returning home.

c. Other instructions given by both parents, from a training standpoint, involve ways to prevent fires, the need for locking doors and windows, proper spending habits and careful handling of objects, but the wish most common to all parents is that the children do not cause them any anxiety.
d. Special advice given by both parents involves personal hygiene as well as consideration for other people and for the *seken.*

Relationship Between Parental Training and the Hypochondriacal Basic Tone

Although the basis of the form of the hypochondriacal basic tone, which can be considered a prenosogenic condition of the *shinkeishitsu* persona, is fundamentally congenital and constitutional in nature, as stated by Morita, it is not necessarily correct to exclude an a posteriori effect that at least plastically characterizes the phenomenon of the basic tone. Therefore, the author must also examine the parent-child problem, which can be considered an important a posteriori factor, particularly the relationship between *shitsuke* (training) and the hypochondriacal basic tone. The author will look into this relationship, taking into account the pertinent social and cultural background, such as past family problems, the parent-child relationship and adolescent mentality.

To clarify the problems under study, related data are categorized as follows: home conditions at the time the subjects were in the childhood growth period[9], essential points of child training and other aspects of the parent-child relationship, adolescent mentality and the hypochondriacal basic tone and criteria of parental training and the child's reaction (particularly obedience or insubordination).

Conditions at the Time the Subjects were in the Childhood Growth Period

All subjects were patients between 18 and 44 years of age who received treatment from 1968 to 1973; their average age was 27.8 years. Three patients were teenagers, 33 were in their twenties, 18 were in their thirties and five were in their forties at the time of their first pretherapy medical examination. At the time of nosogenesis, 37 patients were teenagers, 19 were in their twenties and three were in the thirties; their average age at the time of nosogenesis was 17.8 years.

Therefore, with the exception of five patients who were born during the pre-World War II era (before 1941), all patients began their formal education during or after the war.

Most of the subjects thus belong to the post-war period. Of the five patients who belong to the pre-war era, it can be said that all of them spent their adolescence during wartime to the post-war period, with those at the maximum age of 44 having been 19 years old at the end of the

[9] This period is the time when body and mind develop rapidly, namely, from seven to eight years of age to 16 to 17 years of age; this time span corresponds roughly to the period of adolescence.

war. These subjects had a parent-child relationship during the transition from the pre-war to post-war culture; the parents belonged to a generation embedded in the traditional Japanese sociocultural system in force before and during the war, and their children belonged to a generation of change, when new cultural forms emerged, in that chaotic period during and after the war.

Almost all the older sociocultural forms in Japan collapsed during that period, with defeat in the war as the critical turning point. A new social system and cultural order appeared in their place and, at the same time, the makeup of the family and the parent-child relationship were affected considerably, in that radically transformed social condition. The major effect was a dissolution of the strong power of the family patriarch, who had perviously had the role of consolidating all life functions in the family, of unifying customs and education to confer harmony on the family as a unit of self-sufficient collective living. This role disappeared with the collapse of the legal family system. The lifelong positions and roles of all family members had been regulated by that patriarchal behavior system, and the old social order had been established on that basis.

The composition of the previous direct-line, family-centered system was changed to a home-centered structure of a core family; at the same time, the normal position of the housewife and, as a result, that of a child in the family, was transformed so that a mother/child-centered relationship was strengthened as proof that the family was normal. In other words, the systemic change took a matricentric rather than patricentric trend, from the standpoint of the new roles of the various family members.

Even if there was a general trend toward a new family system by reorganization to an urban type or democratic type, it is natural that, individually, each family had its characteristic features, stemming from the sociocultural histories of the family members, particularly the father and mother. This had a profound effect on the content of consciousness. Differences of opinion and conviction arose owing to the degree of receptiveness or acceptance of any new social trend. Changes in the consciousness of each person are important for creating or maintaining a certain form of culture, such as the life-style of the family, but such changes do require a period of time for the transition to take place.

In the instance of our subjects, only a few years had passed since the end of the war when they became grade-school pupils. Their average age at the time they received their pretherapy medical examination was less than 28 years (1968–1973), and, in this respect, it appears that enough time had passed for new cultural forms to become fixed features of life in each family.

Japan's high-growth economic policy, which made its appearance several years after this period, brought about rapid industrial development and as a result, a major change in the employment situation for family members, particularly the increased percentage of worktime the father spent outside the home.[10]

Whether employed daily or occasionally, the father became absent from the home during most daytime hours, if he were employed as a laborer. The length of time he was absent was increased by unavoidable overtime, night duty or business trips.

Thus, the amount of time the father was home decreased, and the home became chiefly a place where mothers and children spent time together. The general trend toward having the father absent from the home for long periods also caused him to be absent psychologically. The

---

[10] Families engaged in farming and forestry occupations represented 30 percent of all families in Japan in 1955, but this figure had decreased to only 13 percent 15 years later. By contrast, families engaged in nonfarming and nonforestry occupations had increased markedly. For example, the national census of that year showed that about 10 percent of families engaged in farming and forestry occupations contained children less than 18 years of age; by contrast, about 65 percent of families engaged in nonfarming and nonforestry occupations had children below this age.

reason was that the sites of productive work and the home had been separated, so that the children could not directly observe the professional activities of the father, and this change has been considered a recent problem. As a result, the children can no longer see how the father performs his work and thus cannot see or listen or otherwise concretely perceive his exercise of intelligence or his work methods. Further, various feelings toward the father, which should be fostered, fail to develop.

The image the children have of their father is that of someone who is close to them and who can therefore complain to them, for example, concerning dissatisfaction and anger about work conditions, or the image of someone who is completely exhausted and always lies down to rest at home.[11] It can readily be supposed that the trend toward loss of the father's paternalistic authority, due to his absence from the home, is gradually bound to change the structure of father-child relationships in the home. As a result, the role of the mother has become more important. The patients included in our study faced the pubertal period during the emergence of this era.

The structure of their families at that time was 49.2 percent of the nuclear family type,[12] 16.9 percent of the stem family type[13] and 7.8 percent of the joint family type; the family structure of the subjects was unclear. When the influence of the father and the mother in the homes is evaluated from the standpoint of the patients' impressions, with actual conditions set aside, the father-dominant type is found to characterize 40.6 percent of the families, and the mother-dominant type 18.6 percent. Thus, the number of patricentric families is still large. However, even in the patricentric families, only three subjects, or less than 1.3 percent, said that the father was self-righteous and despotic and that he had become completely alienated from other family members. In the mother-dominant families, seven subjects, or 63.6 percent, said that the mother managed everything in the family. More than 18 percent of the subjects said that their father and mother were considered equals in their families. More than 22 percent of the family situations were unknown in some respect (due to death of the father or mother or to divorce).

This image investigation of parents and families showed that male patients had negative impressions of the father with respect to sensory pleasure and his power. A negative impression was not shown in male or female patients for all items investigated in the instance of the mother. It is not possible to make a simple comparison of these results in regard to the proportions of influence exercised by the father and mother in the home, but the following inference can be made.

The patricentric impression is strong when a patient compares the father and mother as authoritative parents who symbolize the home, but when the parents are compared as actual parents with whom a patient has close contact, probably the mother-dominant impression will be stronger. The father-child relationship is not very close in daily life, but it is believed that the father has the final decisive power, even if the child is connected strongly to the mother by sentimental bonding.

Although parental training by the father and the father-child relationship have important roles in a child's character formation and acquisition of social skills, it appears that there was

---

[11] Satō, K.: Gendai kazoku no shitsuke (*Shitsuke* (training) of present-day families). In *Gendai no Esprit*, "*Shitsuke*," No. 113 (1976). (Printed in Japanese)

[12] The nuclear family refers to a household of husband, wife and children, or father and children or mother and children, and the percentage is derived from the results of a study conducted in 1955 by the Bureau of Statistics of the Japanese Prime Minister's Office. Only about 54.9 percent of the nuclear families of ordinary households were composed of similar family types.

[13] A stem family refers to one in which the daughter who belongs to the unit family (corresponding to the concept of nuclear family) lives with her parents together with her spouse after marriage and in which coupling of the unit family of each generation occurs. A joint family refers to one in which, in addition to the spouses of two or more daughters, the parents and brothers live together to form one large family.

only scant mention of this matter in Japan in the past. Setting aside the reason, not only is the father absent much of the time, but the scope of child training handled by the father also differs from that of the mother.[14]

There may be little direct communication between the father and a child, but it is not completely absent in all cases, since the sense of authority wielded by the father is felt when the mother says to the child, "You will be scolded by your father" or "Ask your father about that."[15] A child feels that the father represents the outside world, and he or she tends to view the father with an attitude of observing someone who is fearful and positioned at a certain interpersonal distance.[16]

In summary, very little of the father's role may be lost in line with the role and actions of the mother, even if the social structure changes. Among our patients, too, were many who had the impression that the mother supports the father's authority, both openly and covertly, and that she helps him maintain a father-dominant role.

To reiterate this matter of the roles and actions of the parents toward a child, it is probable that the power relationship of the parents in the home has been further changed in general (most probably in relation to loss of the father's authority) if we take into account the passing of more than ten years from the time our subjects were in their growth period.

If the trend toward enervation of the father's authority, as a result of his absence from the home and the shift in family structure to a mother/child-centered type, is the leading feature of the present-day family in Japan, this trend has an important bearing on the natural parent-child relationship and on the husband-wife relationship. When viewed from a child's perspective, it means that some problems were encountered by the father and mother in carrying out their respective roles and actions. Defects in roles and actions of parents, and a disharmony in their complementary roles, probably loomed as large obstacles in preventing these children in their growth period from developing poor and perhaps violent behavior in the home, or even neurosis or attempting suicide. However, the actual conditions indicate that there is no decisive explanation as to why certain persons manifest neurosis and problematical actions, whereas others do not. However, it is reasonable to assume that the feelings of anxiety and dissatisfaction in the consciousness of children can easily be increased if the present family condition is such that "expectations of what the child should be or do have increased" and that "there are many opportunities for stimulating a child's desires."

On the other hand, the actual conditions of "a society in which principles are not fixed" and "a society in which conventions have deteriorated" have made consciousness of criminal activity and shameful conduct vague.[17]

If imbalance and disharmony arise in the mutual roles and actions between the father and mother, problems will arise in the child-parent relationship because of the lack of a family structure that can help prevent such problems in the core families that are now evolving.

When the nosogenesis of *shinkeishitsu* is considered from that point of view, its basis was initially viewed as being due to personal disposition in Morita's time, and even if environmental factors were operative, they were considered incidental, and that conclusion was not refuted. That was because the pressures of the social structure (as sociohistorical flow) at that time formed the model for family life and because the consciousness of the family members could be

---

[14] Miyamoto, J.: *Miyamoto Jōichi Chosakushū*, Vols. 6 and 8. Miraisha, Tokyo (1967, 1969). (Printed in Japanese)

[15] Vogel, E.: *Japan's Middle Class: Salary Man and His Family in Tokyo Suburbs.* University of California Press, Berkeley (1963). (Translated by T. Sasaki. Seishin Shobō, Tokyo.)

[16] Hara, H., and Wagatsuma, H.: *"Shitsuke."* Kōbundō, Tokyo (1974). (Printed in Japanese)

[17] Matsuura, K., et al.: Kodomo no shitsuke to dōtoku kyōiku (*Shitsuke* of Children and Moral Education). (Edited by Nihon Kyōiku Shakai Gakkai). Kyōiku Shakaigaku Kenkyūkai, 18 (1963). (Printed in Japanese)

unified under principles and customs of living adopted as a common value model. Tension in relationships that can give rise to strong contradiction and conflict within the home did not disturb the general way of life for parents and children or between society and the individual.

In considering the nosogenesis of neurosis, there was no need to take into account any change in social background. Features of modernization, such as the so-called family pathology, which includes the lack of good human relationships in the home, or social pathology, which brings about alienation phenomena, such as loss of subjecthood in the individual consciousness or a sense of individual powerlessness, are felt more keenly at the present time. The starting point of the nosogenesis of the cases we have treated was in the interval between Morita's time and the 1980s.

Essential Points of *Shitsuke* (training) and Parent-Child Relationships

When father-child and mother-child relationships are consolidated from information relevant to *shitsuke*, the findings can be summarized as follows.

Patterns of *Shitsuke*

When classified as "strict," "nagging" or "overprotective," the patterns in which the parents are assertively involved with the child, without reference to content, are found to be 28.8 percent strict, 30.8 percent nagging and 26.9 percent, overprotective in regard to the father. The respective figures for the mother are 16.7, 33.3 and 48.2 percent. It is apparent from these findings that the strict pattern is frequently reported in reference to the father, the nagging pattern is slightly more common for the mother and the overprotective pattern is often noted for the mother. In regard to the "noninterferent" pattern, in which the parents leave the children alone, 23.1 percent of the patients felt this way about the father, but only 0.74 percent of the patients had this impression of the mother.

This finding makes it clear that there is a tendency for the father to be strict and nagging, although there are proportionately more noninterferent fathers than mothers. By contrast, the impression of overprotective is more frequently reported in regard to the mother than the father.[18]

With respect to the consciousness of how a child accepts such parental influences in the parent-child relationship by means of *shitsuke*, the proportion of patients that stated "affirmative" for the father was 34.6 percent, and for the mother was 40 percent. This finding indicates that the affirmative for the mother is somewhat higher than it is for the father. The "negative" acceptance is somewhat lower for the mother, being 20 percent as compared with 21.2 percent for the father. However, whether it is affirmative or negative, the difference of image in reference to the parents is not significant. The reasons for the large number of patients who report a negative image of acceptance in reference to the parents are widespread impressions, of overprotectiveness (particularly for the mother) and of noninterference (particularly for the father). The relationship between these findings and the results of the image investigation is not clear, but it

[18] When the figures for all cases of *shinkeishitsu* were compared according to type, there was an approximate similarity, with the exception of paroxysmal neurosis, for which the number of cases was small. This tendency was particularly marked in cases of ordinary *shinkeishitsu* and anthropophobia. The proportions of children who had the impression of strict or nagging for both parents (the figures for children with anthropophobia are indicated in parentheses) were as follows: 38.5 (30.4) percent and 30.8 (39.1) percent, respectively; the figure for overprotective was 0.77 (30.4) percent. For the mother, they were 0.67 (25.0) percent, 33.3 (37.5) percent and 46.7 (50.1) percent, respectively. The figures for noninterferent were 23.1 (26.1) percent for the father and 0.67 (0.8) percent for the mother. However, the slight difference in the overall trend of cases of ordinary *shinkeishitsu* is due to the fact that the figure for overprotective was low for the father and the figure for strict was low for the mother.

is probable that the negative image the patients have for lack of power and sensory pleasure in reference to the father is related to an image of the father as being serious-minded but without delicate sensibility and as someone who is uninteresting.

Important Factors of *Shitsuke* and the Person in Charge

The substance of *shitsuke* can be roughly classified into abstract/ideological and concrete/actual factors. The following three aspects are given importance: school activities and customs, ordinary life activities and customs, and social and public activities and customs.

With regard to school activities and customs, the need for diligence in schoolwork, efforts to improve school grades, not losing out to others and studying hard and earnestly are stressed. Various instructions concerning formal education in school are included, such as not neglecting lesson review and preparation, listening to and obeying teacher requests, asking a teacher or a friend about anything that is not understood to leave nothing unclarified, being on good terms with friends and not loitering on the way to and from school. There are various ways to express these directives, but they do include much advice regarding education. Many practical and actual instructions are voiced by mothers; the father's training concerns the basic upbringing of a child in regard to discipline, harmony and autonomy and such ideological issues as intelligence training, friendship and a sense of respect for justice. These concerns of the father are similarly observed in other phases of *shitsuke.*

Training that relates to ordinary life activities and customs centers around instructions that are practical and useful in daily life, such as "to be careful about your health," "to avoid dangerous activities," "to help out with the housework," "to learn manners and etiquette," "to try to keep personal belongings in order" and "to be careful about fire and locking up the house."

Last, training that is pertinent to social and public activities and customs consists chiefly of moral *shitsuke*, such as "not to cause trouble for other people and the *seken* (the public)," "to be responsible for your actions," "to keep promises" and "not to tell lies," and also includes *shitsuke* that appeals to a sense of shame, such as "not to show a disrespectful appearance in front of others" and "to avoid doing anything that would be ridiculed and make you look like a fool in front of other people." When the parent-child relationship is viewed from a moral standpoint of *shitsuke,* the person who provides concrete and practical *shitsuke* with emphasis on actual life activities is the mother, whether the child is a son or a daughter.

Many subjects included among the three aspects cited previously are common to the father and the mother, but the father differs somewhat from the mother in tending to be more ideological than immediately practical. The actual person in charge of *shitsuke* is the mother, but her relative importance is reduced from the standpoint of an ideals-oriented person in charge in which the relative importance of the father is increased.

The image of the father held by a child, whether positive or negative, is that he is the representative reference figure of the family, although there is a strong tendency for the mother to become a sentimental reference figure. There are many factors that place the mother-child relationship at the very center of interpersonal relationships within the family under such conditions.

The direct influence of the mother's consciousness on a child's consciousness is powerful; for the child, the mother is the reference figure who is the closest person to whom the child can express emotions directly and who functions as a spokeswoman for the child. On the other hand, in the father-child relationship, it is possible that a certain psychological distance will be formed for communication through an abstract and ideological *shitsuke*, and this relationship is placed at a more peripheral location than is the mother-child relationship in interpersonal relationsips within the family. Rather than someone to whom feelings can be expressed directly, as in the case of the mother, the father becomes a so-called symbolic, authoritative reference figure for a child. In view of this situation, however, the father can become to the child a reference figure who is necessary for ideological considerations of viewing oneself objectively.

The *shinkeishitsu* persona recognizes this symbolic, authoritative existence of the father as follows. First of all, the father is sober-minded but lacks delicate sensibility and seems dull. A child also feels that the father is distant rather than close because he is not only strict and nagging but also ideological, and these qualities give the impression that the father is not a reliable reference figure.

In the image investigation, too, there was a tendency for the father to be evaluated lower than the mother for all factors starting with power.

Second, there are cases in which a "negative" impression is given because the father is not only nagging but also overprotective, and these qualities can be excessive to the point of annoyance.

Third, the father's authoritativeness, if excessive, is characterized as strict or nagging. However, because the impression of being strict in this case can be considered as indicating unreasonableness toward the child, a feeling of fear in approaching the father closely develops in the child.

Fourth, the father's authoritativeness is indicated by a certain grimness, and he can give the impression of being unapproachable by affecting a coolness that can be interpreted as lack of interest. By contrast, the mother is generally a reference figure who is warm, active, strong and reliable[19]

However, there are mothers who are obedient to their husbands, follow his lead submissively and do not speak out as other than a spokesperson for the father. On the other hand, there are cases in which a child has formed the impression that the mother interferes in everything and is stricter than the father. One-half of the mothers were said to indicate an overprotective pattern. This impression of the mother, however, becomes a reason for the child to reject this quality if it becomes overbearing. If the relationship becomes such that overall harmony with the father is maintained in the mother-child relationship, it can be assumed that any such dynamism in the family will not become destructive to the ego of a *shinkeishitsu* persona. This can be seen to some extent in the study of image. The *shinkeishitsu* persona does not consider the family as being negative from an overall point of view, but when compared with the contrast (see Table 5), an impression of the atmosphere in the home as being passive for all factors is indicated (although there is no appreciable difference). This tendency is especially present in the factor of power and appears to be stronger in male patients (see Table 5).

Even if insufficient dynamic energy in the family is held as an impression by a *shinkeishitsu* persona, there are probably few real problems from a structural point of view. In many cases, the mother-child relationship was positioned at the center, with the father-child relationship at the periphery in the home in our subjects who were *shinkeishitsu* patients. (Needless to say, there are also cases in which the father-child relationship was positioned more toward the center than was the mother-child relationship.)

There were many cases in which the mother and father shared much in common vis-à-vis *shitsuke* in their respective roles and actions, and such parents were also cooperative. In this respect, the mother-child and father-child relationships are "concentric." When all the study data are summarized, the patterns of the parent-child relationship relevant to *shinkeishitsu* can be classified roughly into the following five aspects:

1. patterns in which the father is nervous and fastidious and strict or demanding but not talkative and in which the mother is tenderhearted but strong-minded;

[19] The proportion of subjects who mentioned that the father is a person to respect was unexpectedly high, being 37.1 percent, and the figure for the mother was 32.5 percent. Other subjects mentioned various persons outside the immediate family.

2. those in which both parents are either strict or demanding or overprotective and interferent;
3. those in which the father is gentle but gives the impression of lacking vitality and hardly interferes with the child and in which the mother is bright and active but demanding, overprotective and considerably interferent;
4. those in which the father is an extrovert and active, very nonchalant and noninterferent toward the home and children and in which the mother is overprotective.
5. Those in which the father is coldhearted and gloomy, even inaccessible, and in which the mother is usually concerned about her child being perturbed and agitated.[20]

These various parent-children relationships are exemplified by *shitsuke*, and the *shitsuke* patterns are derived from information obtained directly from these patients, but a simplistic decision on whether they are characteristic of *shinkeishitsu* patients in general is not possible. Typically, however, the parents evince a strong desire for the child to be healthy both mentally and physically, have a well-rounded personality, demonstrate good scholarship, associate with other people having good sense and are conciliatory and cooperative with society. If such is the case, it is natural that parental *shitsuke* is carried out in line with such expectations, and, as a result, there is a general tendency for the *shitsuke* pattern and the parent-child relationship to form along certain lines. The expectations that parents have tend to change gradually with changes in society and culture, but there is no change in essence because there is no change in parental desire for the happiness of the children.

Parental feelings of expectation toward a child are the same in any era and can be considered a prototype of the parents' ideas of life's worth. Because parents characteristically have such feelings, they experience strong anxiety and concern for a child's future, rather than a feeling of dissatisfaction, even when the child does not respond to parental expectations.

This parental feeling is also observed in the case of *shinkeishitsu* patients, without exception. However, the problem of the parent-child relationship for the *shinkeishitsu* persona is how that basic feeling of the parents is actually transmitted to a child. In addition, the *shinkeishitsu* persona also present in a large number of these parents (particularly the father) cannot be ignored. The fact that a parent's personality is such will make his or her attitude more idealistic and more introspectively sensitive.

A subtle atmosphere of *kizukau* (concern) can easily be engendered in a child due to that idealistic parental attitude. For example, even if the parental *shitsuke* is strict or demanding, a special difference will characterize the parent-child relationship and the atmosphere in the home if the parents are also predisposed to the *shinkeishitsu* persona. This difference could be the specific link that is common to all the above-mentioned five types of parent-child relationship. Irrespective of whether or not a parent is interfering (strict, demanding or overprotective), the parental sensibility is transmitted to a child, by all forms of expression, verbal or nonverbal, filtered through the *shinkeishitsu* persona. A *kizukau* atmosphere becomes a problem, whether or not an ideal criterion indicated by the parents is present.

These *shinkeishitsu* patients are brought up in alignment with the parental *shitsuke*, but they start to reject it as they enter the period of youth in which their environs widen. However, they cannot escape from the parents' subtle and fine *kizukau* atmosphere which they have absorbed through *shitsuke*, and they become concerned not to cause their parents any worry, even while rejecting the parents and their attitude. At the same time, they begin to experience *kinisuru* (concerned about) and suffer over their condition, which had not been anticipated by

[20] No special, characteristic connection was observed between these five types of parent-child involvement and the type of *shinkeishitsu*. However, a relatively large number of the first, second and third parent-child relationships was observed among patients with anthropophobia and ordinary *shinkeishitsu*, whereas the number of patients reporting the fifth parental combination was high among patients with other types of obsession.

their parents. This mental condition can be considered one in which its influence, at a certain stage of youth, is easily accepted.

Adolescent Mentality and the Hypochondriacal Basic Tone

Adolescence is the transitional period from childhood to adult life and often is a disruptive time in which the most profound change takes place. Adolescent mentality has unique characteristics, including exuberant vitality, overflowing sentimentality and romanticized self-confidence, inspiration and ambition. Dreams expand without bounds, and new situations are accepted and absorbed self-assertively. Actions are frequently too progressive and overly original, but self-consciousness is strong, and adolescents can easily become excessively self-assertive and self-righteous.

A skeptical attitude is taken toward existing standards and authority because adolescents are so self-centered, uncooperative, rebellious and defiant. On the other hand, adolescents have an ego that is easily bruised, worry often, despair frequently and readily show emotional instability.

Introversion is indicated by fits of depression, loneliness, self-deprecation and an inferiority complex. This mentality of hypersensitive instability is the most characteristic feature of adolescence, and it is due to rapid mental and physical changes throughout this transitional period that culminates in adult maturity. It is also a social type of reaction to complex environmental conditions encountered during the most robust growth period in the course of human life.

This reaction can be construed as a concrete indication of conflict manifesting the desire for self-expansion, a struggle for self-assertion and self-realization, in that particular environment in which adolescents are reaching out rapidly, but also the oppositional desire for self-preservation, intent on securing a guarantee for self-existence.

The relative relationship between these two disparate desires is exactly what Morita calls the twin-faced relationship between the hypochondriacal basic tone and *sei no yokubō*, and in view of this relationship, he considers the *kizukai* that springs up in the process of self-expansion as being a manifestation of the basic *kibun* that governs the conduct of human existence.

From the aspect of the intrinsic nature of *ki* (see Chapters 2 and 9), which we have frequently discussed in this context, the two desires express two faces of the lively motion of *sei-ki* (vitality). This *sei-ki* is the source of growth and expansion within oneself, but in the process of motivating *ki* in this direction, a contravening *ki* that tries to resist this process also springs up. This *ki* is *kizukai*, and it is sensed as a mental condition of tension and anxiety. The outward-bound, centrifugal motivation that is the essence of *ki* induces a counteractive, centripetal *shin* (mind, heart) directed toward basic self-preservation, manifested in a defensive and solicitous manner.

The two faces of *sei no yokubō*, namely, *ki* and *shin*, have the same root cause and represent the essence of the hypochondriacal basic tone. These side-by-side centrifugal and centripetal mental attitudes have a mutually conflicting relationship. Concretely, the functions of self-expansion and independence develop complementarily with self-introspection and harmony. As these functions come into integration, the faculty of common sense[21] in dealing with other

---

[21] *Sensus communis* is common to the various senses, and it indicates the basic sense that integrates all of them. Here, it indicates the prospective basis for a self-evident form of functioning that can be mutually shared and understood among groups of human beings without any effort required for explanation or persuasion following the acquisition of "common sense." (Nakamura, Y.: Seinenki no enchō to kyōtsū kankaku (Extension of adolescence and common sense) (in Japanese). In Iwanami Kōza, *Kodomo no Hattatsu to Kyōiku* (Child Development and Education), Monthly Insert, May 1979).

people is increased, so that the functions of cooperation and realistic self-adaptability can be acquired. However, because the latter functions are still undeveloped during the early and middle stages of adolescence, frustration in the struggle for adaptation can easily occur.

Concrete differences of mind arise during adolescence, depending on whether the *sei-ki* of the centrifugal desire for self-expansion or the *shin-ki* of the centripetal desire for self-preservation is dominant from the standpoint of taking action.

The instability of adolescent mentality, together with the powerful thrust of *sei no yokubō*, irrespective of whether it is manifested in centrifugal or centripetal terms, is one characteristic of this dual motivation in the context of social adaptation. The number of experiences of success or failure increases with expansion into unknown areas of life where there is little protection from that once protective world of childhood dominated by an uncritical attitude of *amae*, with dependence on and obedience toward one's parents.

During adolescence, the valuation of each experience becomes important to self-existence, and adolescents are compelled to go through constant self-appraisal. Acknowledgment of success generates a sense of self-confidence, conceit and self-expansion, with the intention for self-development further strengthened. On the other hand, acknowledgment of failure engenders feelings of imperfection and loss of confidence, and these feelings tend to make the mind take an attitude of cautionary self-curtailment.

When that occurs, the stance of centripetal, solicitous *shin-ki* (mind) becomes dominant, with self-deprecation, an inferiority complex or hypochondriacal apprehensions strengthened. The intense introversion so characteristic of adolescence is likewise strengthened, and inadaptability anxiety can readily occur (see Chapter 11).

This inadaptability anxiety is a self-doubtful form of life-adaptation consciousness and is, again, what Morita means by the hypochondriacal basic tone. In most cases, the feeling of self-doubt that occurs during the process of selfhood formation becomes the motivating factor for aiming at subsequent self-expansion and self-development through continual reassessment of one's self. In a few cases, however, this self-doubt reinforces a temporary or chronic dominance by the hypochondriacal basic tone.

The innate disposition of a person does have an important role (see Chapter 10), but other factors, such as self-image and past experience about one's body and mind (*mi*) (see Chapter 9), particularly in relation to the conditions that exist in the home and in human relationships, are also active.

Criteria of Parental Training and Child Reaction (specifically obedience and insubordination)

The hypochondriacal basic tone plays such an important part in Morita *shinkeishitsu* theory that it has become the central concept. However studies of the impact of parental training on the overlay development of the basic tone have been few and far between. Morita does stress the importance of this factor in a case study of methods of child education in the family, most particularly by parents, in the context of accelerating the *shinkeishitsu* tendency.[22] However, he makes no further mention of this factor, being too engrossed in emphasizing the importance of physical constitution and mental disposition. A few more papers on this educational factor appeared after Morita's time,[23-25] but there have been almost no published studies on the subject in recent years.

22 Morita, S.: Shinkeisuijakusei seishinbyōshitsusei taishitsu (Study on neurasthenic-psychopathologic constitution) (Ziehen) (in Japanese). *Jinsei* (Humanity) 5 (5,6) (1909). In *Morita Shōma Zenshū*, Vol. I.

23 Shimoda, K.: *Seishin Eisei Kōwa* (Lectures on Mental Hygiene). Iwanami Shoten, Tokyo, (1942). (Printed in Japanese)

Given that background, we wish to examine this factor of parental training and how children react to it, particularly in terms of obedience and insubordination, and will base our examination on available data concerning the overlay development of the hypochondriacal basic tone.

First of all, to study childhood attitudes toward parents, we will provide a general explanation of children's impressions of their parents on a statistical basis (see Tables 2 and 5).

The proportion of children who considered the father strict, nagging or officious was 59.6 percent, whereas the proportion who indicated the father was overprotective or interferent was only 21.2 percent. The proportions for the same impressions of the mother were 50.0 and 48.1 percent, respectively.

The proportion of children who considered the father, noninterferent was 23.1 percent, whereas only 7.4 percent of the children felt this way about, the mother, which indicates that mothers (in Japan) are rarely noninterferent. This finding shows that, in the cases we have studied, the psychological involvement of parents with children is aggressive, whether being strict, nagging, officious or overprotective. The children's general reactions to that aggressive stance show that impressions of the parents as affirmative, moderate or ordinary acceptance are more frequent than are negative impressions.

In the image investigation also, there was no minus valuation, on the average, with respect to the mother, but a slight minus valuation, on the average, by male children concerning lack of sensory pleasure and potency in the father.

Children who were trained in a positive child-parent relationship grew up in a spirit of acceptance until the pubertal period, that is, until they were about 11.2 years old. They acted in concert with, and were dependent on, the parents without exception. In the context of the home environment, father-dominant homes were more common, as indicated by an impression of the father as having power in relation to the mother according to 40.6 percent of the children; only 18.6 percent of the children felt the mother was more powerful.

However, it is worth noting that the proportion of children who rated the mother most powerful in the mother-dominant homes was 63.3 percent.

In correlation with this finding, a large number of children had the impression that the father was serious but delicate-minded and uninteresting; this impression agreed with the results of the image investigation. (In a small number of cases, the child's impression was that the father was authoritative, despotic and nondomesticated.)

The proportion of children who stated that the father has the principal role of molding the child's character was high at 67.3 percent, far exceeding the 15.3 percent for the mother. To these children, the father is the one in charge of setting ideal standards, and it is he who serves to make the child become objective and conscious of concepts. The father is also the supreme symbol of the home, whether the symbol is positive or negative.

By contrast, the general impression is that the mother has the role of being in charge of practical, day-to-day training. She also has a powerful sentimental influence and acts as a child's spokesperson.

The six patterns of a child's impression of parental involvement are as follows: both parents are strict or nagging; both parents are overprotective; the father is strict (or nagging) and the mother is overprotective; the father is noninterferent and the mother is overprotective; the father is noninterferent and the mother is strict (or hypercritical); and both parents are noninterferent.

Most commonly, a child's impression was that the father is strict (or nagging) and the

[24] Abe, T.: op. cit.

[25] Iwai, H., et al.: Shinkeishitsusha no kazoku kankei (The family relationships of *shinkeishitsu* people) (in Japanese). *Seishin Igaku* 130:781–785 (1969).

mother is overprotective or that both parents are overprotective. We found almost no cases in which the father was strict and the mother noninterferent.

This finding indicates that aggressive involvement of both parents in child training has some implication, although few instances of an overprotective father and a strict mother, even when both are aggressive, were observed in our data.

In regard to the subject matter of child training, a high proportion of both fathers and mothers displayed concern for their child's health and for diligence in schoolwork. Both parents also placed emphasis on giving instructions not to cause trouble for other people and the *seken* and on not becoming an object of ridicule by other people. The basic parental premise is that a boy should always act in a manly manner and a girl in a womanly way.

We have summarized the data obtained on parental involvement with children. There seems to be almost no difference between these data in regard to the fine points of ethics and involvement of the parents and the data derived from an investigation of youth and home life in Japan as compared to international norms carried out ten years later (taking into account that our data convey a child's viewpoint, whereas the latter data convey the parents' viewpoint). There is almost no difference in the general trend indicated ten years later in ordinary homes in regard to parental attitude and homelife awareness, viewed from the aspect of parental training of a *shinkeishitsu*-type child indicated in our data.

We also need to address the rather hackneyed question as to why large numbers of people have neglected this issue, without taking into account the neurotic defenses that can develop in a child to help him or her contend with the stresses and dilemmas of adolescence.

In Japan, the numbers of anthropophobic and hypochondriacal *shinkeishitsu* patients are considerable, even now. This situation likely results from the fact that Japanese parents fully expect their children always to adhere to the fine points of childhood training, namely to preserve health, to study diligently and to behave in a masculine of feminine manner. Such training is considered the foundation for later life and is intended to prevent Japanese children from upsetting the *seken* or from becoming ridiculed by other people. Whether or not this belief is true, it is generally thought that neurotic conduct emerges more readily in the transitional stages of the life situations of people who manifest symptoms of *shinkeishitsu*; such transitional stages include the periods of moving from middle (junior high) school to high school, from high school to college and from college into the business community.

There is also a danger of acquiring a neurotic frame of mind at other turning points in life. It does seem undeniable that all generations now have to face difficult situations living in a world characterized by rapid change compared to the pace of change in Morita's era. In particular, the technological revolution continues to accelerate the flow of information and to increase social complexity and also results in diversified, relativistic notions of value.

These changes undoubtedly provide more and more material abundance and convenience for human life. Unfortunately, however, the perception of that pathos of the human condition that is essential to living considerately in this world is apt to be ignored, creating a tendency to disregard the common human condition that fosters common sense and sensitivity. In other words, people lose the firm grounding that gives rise to the mutual understanding they need to acquire to live as mature human beings.

In view of this loss, values shared in common are obliterated, giving rise to a diffusion of nonsense.[26]

This kind of social condition places youths who are in a training period for acquiring the capabilities of self-reliance and social harmonizing, in the position of constantly facing anxiety-

[26] Nakamura, Y.: op. cit.

inducing situations, and this situation, in turn, lays the foundation for the development of neurosis. However, it is not true that neurosis is caused only by social conditions. The parent-child relationship in the home can also provoke neurosis as a concomitant factor.

The parental expectations that underlie the fine points of child training make it difficult for a child to attain a sense of self-reliance and harmony in living and to shift mentally in accord with changing social conditions. Much of this parental anticipation toward a child is communicated unconsciously from parent to child in the course of home life. This unspoken communication also extends to the tensions that develop when it is time for the child to depart from the enclosure of the *uchi* (home) into the outside community of the *seken* as a part of growing up, and it is such tensions that produce the frame of mind characteristic of inadaptability anxiety.

Morita finds that the hypochondriacal basic tone is one factor common to the various so-called neuroses observed in the early part of this century. He clarifies the pathological basis of the neuroses that develop in a psychogenic matrix as being the hypochondriacal basic tone and develops this construct into Morita *shinkeishitsu* theory. The hypochondriacal basic tone, which is the nucleus of his theory, is originally none other than the frame of mind that is adopted toward the basic adaptability of the human being, that is, the manifestation of the actions of *kizukau* and the *kizukau* mentality.

On the one hand, there is the *kizukau* stance toward self-reliance and self-development and, on the other, the actions of *kizukau* directed toward the protection of one's body and mind and toward the issue of winning acceptance in the *seken*, meaning the frame of mind of centripetal *shin-ki* (see Chapter 9), for preservation of oneself and for social harmony. This is the structural characteristic of the *kizukau* frame of mind, and it reverses its thrust in accordance with the specific situations that one faces. The hypochondriacal basic tone is the manifestation of this self-protective *kizukau*.

It is often said that a child grows up by observing his or her parents. The parents indicate to the child what posture to adopt to live properly in this world, reflecting even sociocultural fluctuations in their behavior. The child accepts that parental posture without awareness. Further, the parents expect the fine points of child training to guide the child toward attainment of practical habits.

This process does not consist of intellectual decision-making, being derived, instead, from the fundamental *kizukau* attitude of the parents to bring about the process, and it points out the course to take in the child's mind. This condition can be said to be the proper parent-child cultural matrix of the household.

This general household condition does not differ much from our case histories. It is characteristic, as shown in our case histories, that the *shinkeishitsu* persona is observed in many parents, particularly the father. The nature of that frame of mind, without specific reference to *shinkeishitsu* as such, is one of sensitivity, and it differs from a hysteric character in that the introspective and intellectual faculties are powerful. However, although shy, reserved and unsociable, this type of father is honest, does not neglect his duties and is tenacious in behavior.

If a person who has this character is a father, the child's impression is that the father is delicate-minded in regard to potency and, although loyal, is uninteresting as a source of sensory pleasure. However, because involvement with the child is basically loyal and honest, even if noninterferent, there are few cases in which a father of this kind is indifferent, leaves everything up to the mother and is not involved in the child's training in any manner. Even in a mother-dominant situation, particularly when the mother has total authority, there is no case in which the child feels that the father is altogether absent from the family relationship.

In many of our case histories, the patients became aware of their trend toward the *shinkeishitsu* character during early adolescence, and the principal influence on their character formation was the character of their parents (the father in most cases).

It is objectively evident that the existence of this character trend, whether or not expressed verbally, is such that the centripetal *shin-ki* milieu defined by the fine points of parental aims and goals in child training accelerates the same character trend in the child. The *seken* culture represented by the parents is adopted as the cultural form intrinsic to that family (the basic conceptual form of how to live properly in the *seken*), and adoption of this culture is communicated to the child through the particular milieu characteristic of that family.

Children first become aware of their character trend during early adolescence, as early as ten years of age, and many case histories indicate that no need was probably felt to pay close attention to one's character until that time. For this reason, the child accepted the parents' expectations and the household cultural milieu, adopting an obedient posture to fulfill those expectations.

The author can also draw this conclusion from the fact that, in many case histories, the children recollected that they were obedient and submissive.

Setting aside this point for the moment, we can note that, similar to the general trend, a *shinkeishitsu*-type child first becomes aware of his or her character during early adolescence and also feels that it is a disadvantage to facile adaptation (i.e., considered a defect). This observation indicates that socially, too, the opportunity for confronting new human relationships and life situations has increased in a life space that expands from a framework of ignorance. It is also a period of self-renewal, when a child begins to select values that are self-satisfactory.

As experience with many tense situations begins to occur, the stronger the desire for self-sufficiency becomes. This desire increases the impression of the household culture (proper subculture) stemming from the parents, in the process of contending with new and unfamiliar situations, and in the process of assimilating and absorbing this new experience, feelings of resistance and desires to endeavor to learn something new, due to the so-called culture lag, begin to surface.

These feelings of resistance and ambition give rise to fearful hesitation, which conflicts with the actions that are necessary for adapting mental and physical capabilities and one's character to new conditions. Centrifugal *ki*, namely, *sei-ki* (vitality), reverses to centripetal *ki*, namely, *shin-ki*. This feeling can flip over to motivate opposition toward the development of capabilities and toward the subculture to which an adolescent belongs, including the parents and other family members.

However, this rebellion and resistance toward the *uchi* (inside, homelike) environment arises initially from thwarted desires to merge facilely with a wider subculture that includes new conditions. This frustration increases the *kizukau* posture, that is, centripetal *shin-ki* directed toward one's quest for capability rather than resistance toward the *uchi* milieu.

In terms of actual social adaptability, an adolescent tries to move outward toward the *soto* society beyond the household but is unable to do so readily. Nevertheless, the adolescent cannot voluntarily continue to rely wholly on the *uchi* subculture and takes the *kizukau* posture of not being able to attain social adaptability at present, while pursuing an idealized self-image that is next to impossible to concretize. This situation gives rise to a condition of dilemma, of being held in check between the *uchi* and *soto* subcultures.[27]

---

[27] A. I have a timid character (inherited from my parents).

B. I do not know whether I can merge myself without resistance into new conditions like other people because of my character. (If I cannot merge, I blame it on my character and my parents.)

C. What can happen to me due to my character is that I will be hurt; therefore, the only thing I can do is confine myself within the *uchi*.

D. However, if I do so, I will betray my authentic self and my parents' expectations of me. At any rate, this dilemma is due to my weak character, and the only thing I can do is to correct this defect. In order to do so, I must leave my parents; but since I cannot do that completely on my own, my parents should help me so I can stand on my own two feet.

When an adolescent confronts this new living condition, awareness arises for the first time over anxious feelings concerning present capability and trends, and this awareness brings with it acknowledgment of feelings of hesitation and bewilderment.

This perspective dovetails with Fromm,[28] who holds that neurosis originates from the oedipus complex in terms of a child's reaction toward the pressures of irrational parental authority. Fromm construes this reaction to indicate that the child has failed to solve the conflicts that arise from this situation.

Although we concur with this conclusion in general, we have a different view of the mechanism involved. In our experience, many children do not consider involvement in parental training as something so heterogeneous that it can be called authoritative pressure. Even though there may be cases in which strict or overinterferent and overprotective parental training may take the form of severe scoldings or prohibitions and such controls as outright coercion, the children do not react by "fearing" the parents, as Fromm avers, and do not obey their parents only because it is unavoidable.

It is not altogether a fearful or compulsory power relationship but, rather, an affectionate and involuntary process of assimilation. Consequently, there is little tendency for a child to suppress will and spontaneity. However, the power to exhibit this tendency is apt to be suppressed by feelings of dependence on parents and on an introspective trend.

As a child grows older, opportunities for confrontation with new life situations increase, and the child departs gradually from parental protection. Independent decisions and actions are demanded, but the centripetal *shin-ki* frame of mind that arises from initial experiences direct the child's decisions and actions toward an introspective, cautious stance.

As a result, the child will newly direct his or her attention to his or her temperament, such as mental and physical capabilities and character. Before and after a tense situation, the consciousness of a child is such that his or her character is timid and sensitive. Further, there is a tendency to become conservative. Nonetheless, the child is aware of becoming conservative and rebels against that facet of self that is so afraid of losing and being hurt, in spite of the fact that the same self hates to be a loser and that competitive spirit is high.

However, the basic aim is to become capable of acting as *hito-nami* (an ordinary adult in *seken*), that is, someone who can merge into a new situation without resistance and who can manifest natural desires.

Nevertheless, even if this basic desire to become *hito-nami* in real life is concretized, other frustrations and conflicts will occur, with feelings of complete self-sufficiency unsatisfied. These desires than become inaccessible desires, the level of ego idealization is increased and real self-denigration follows. A sense of imperfection and a correlative consciousness of yearning for self-perfection will bob up and down.

A child in this condition is still not fully aware of the fact that he or she cannot sublate the *uchi*, in spite of the continuing desire to absorb the *soto* subculture consciously, because adherence to the ingrained *uchi* subculture is deep-seated. In actual situations, this is an attitude of constant yearning to overcome all kinds of obstacles and to be fully self-reliant, while experiencing inadaptability anxiety. Self-reliance is both fearful and desirable.

According to Morita, the authentic dignity of a human being lies simply in the expression of that activity that occurs naturally at the time one begins to exert an utmost effort to live successfully and is also this hope in itself. In concrete terms, this is the consciousness of . . . *tai* (want to); for example, I want to read, I want to associate with people. The opposite phenomenon, for example, is to regret that I was not able to read today or I was not able to associate

[28] Fromm, E: Individual and social origins of neurosis. *American Sociological Review* 9 (1944).

with people, which is oppositional to I want to do this or that, all of which are basically the same. This is authentic human dignity.

Full development of harmonized human life cannot occur if one cannot take independent action to deal with a situation, experience it and then later examine it introspectively. There can be no actual self-development if one only imagines a course of events in dealing with that situation, criticizing it or hesitating and taking no action. This only increases frustration and exacerbates tension.

A *shinkeishitsu*-type person will seek to avoid self-injury and become introspective to connote *sei-ki* (vitality) and will hesitate to fulfill expectations. Such a person will also be self-critical and resentful for readily adopting the centripetal frame of mind of *shin-ki.* Not a few instances of these feelings were observed in our case histories, and they indicated a resemblance to the *shinkeishitsu* persona of the parent. This also indicates that the image of the parent, particularly the father, has a strong influence on the character formation of a child, although the father seems weak, sincere but uninteresting, because this image appears to overlap with the child's self-image. A child rebels against this influence while being subject to it. A *kizukau* subculture condition in which a child cannot disengage from the parent or, of course, in which the child's self is created between parent and child, and centripetal *shin-ki*, that is, the frame of mind of dominating the hypochondriacal basic tone, is reinforced when some form of danger is encountered.

In conclusion, when the hypochondriacal basic tone is observed, as evidenced by obedience and resistance occurring between parent and child, it is desirable for that basic tone to develop not by a process of neurotic defenses but, rather, by having the frame of mind develop from obedience (involuntary) through resistance to final obedience (voluntary) as the process of opportunity that brings about structural reversal in favor of the manifestation of authentic human dignity.

The involvement of a child with the parents, until adolescence, is one of involuntary obedience and has the character of nonpersonality imitation within the family group. However, frustration and conflict occur readily from the onset of adolescence, and the child begins to rebel against the parents. This condition could be called the anxiety of taking wing. It can breed neurotic physical or experiential behavior patterns. However, capabilities for self-reliance and social harmonizing can be optimized if the child shifts to voluntary obedience and establishes a proper personal position in the cultural matrix at hand, accepting this position by willed self-decision. The *kizukau* frame of mind toward absorbing other subcultures and solidifying one's position can then be engendered gradually. Most young people can live without resort to any form of neurotic self-defense because they function by this kind of mental development.

13

Desire to Live and Fear of Death

It can readily be understood by reading Morita's writings that his aim was always to understand human nature, and the basis of this understanding was *seishi* (or *shōji*) *no mondai* (the issue of life and death). Morita thought of the mental structure of *shinkeishitsu* from the standpoint that the phenomena of life and death are in a relative relationship.

He first considered the hypochondriacal basic tone to be the primary cause for the onset of *shinkeishitsu* and came to place this concept at the crux of Morita theory. He had indicated, much earlier, that this basic tone is the manifestation of *seizon yoku* (the desire to exist), which is the true nature of human beings. However, for one reason or another, little explanation was given at that time concerning this *seizon yoku.*

He later replaced *seizon yoku* with the term *sei no yokubō* (the desire to live) and began to attach importance to the latter term as the central concept of Morita *shinkeishitsu* theory from the standpoint of the two mechanisms involved in its onset and cure. It may be that Morita did not revise his theory in principle but, rather, that his understanding of human nature had grown more profound.

What came to Morita's mind, when he first tried to understand human nature, was the notion of *shi no kyōfu* (the fear of death). Later, in clinical terms, he called this fear the "hypochondriacal basic tone." He considered *sei no yokubō* the phenomenon in relative relationship with *shi no kyōfu* and analogized it with the hypochondriacal basic tone.

Morita explains the relative relationship of *sei-shi* (life and death) as follows: "*Shi no kyōfu* becomes stronger whenever *sei no yokubō* becomes stronger and, conversely, *shi no kyōfu* is weakened whenever *sei no yokubō* is weakened. A high intensity of *shi no kyōfu* indicates that *sei no yokubō* is in vigorous condition; lack of *shi no kyōfu* shows that *sei no yokubō* has disappeared. Various problems of *seishi* or *shōji* (life and death) arise in accordance with the intensity of *sei no yokubō.* When one's self becomes replete with full recognition and acceptance of the infinite circumstances of *seishi,* this constitutes a perfect score of 100 on a figurative scale, and the problem of *seishi* is no longer problematical."

Later, Morita makes several remarks concerning *sei no yokubō,* the gist of which is as follows: What, in biology, we term the desire for the existence of the self, the desire to breed and reproduce, and the desire for preservation of the race, are all contained in this *sei no yokubō.* When this is expressed objectively, we use such terms as impulse, conduct or action.

If human beings are observed on a chronological scale, we see that the activity of living is not manifested completely in an infant . . . who will cry loudly when feeling discomfort in order to obtain protection from others, but will sleep calmly once the discomfort disappears. Even in the instance of a surgical operation, the infant will cry violently when cut, but will stop crying the instant the cutting is finished.

Although the mind of this infant could be compared to the *satori* state of mind in Zen, the two are similar only in that there is no attachment to material things. The actual content and utilization of these two states of mind are quite different.

Sei no yokubō is not thoroughly manifested in an infant. When the infant approaches the later childhood period, his life impulse increases; in comparison to an adult, the child is incessantly active while awake, much as in a manic state; his moods change easily, as in hysteria . . . his *sei no yokubō* is strong, but simple and crude. Consequently, his *shi no kyōfu* is also simple and transitory. When he reaches the age of 16 to 20 years-old, his desire for self-expression suddenly increases. This is the period in which *sei no yokubō* is most active. Consequently, *shi no kyōfu* is also strongest.

Conflicts of ideas occur between desire and fear, and he finally worries and suffers. *Shinkeishitsu* and hysteria occur most frequently during this period. The symptoms of *shinkeishitsu* arise from *shisō no mujun* (contradictoriness in thinking) between this desire and fear, and hysteria occurs in situations that give rise to sudden excitement.

At 30 to 40 years of age, the desire expands further and the ego is extended from *shō-ga* (the small self) to *tai-ga* (the large self).[1] For example, this man now ignores his own desire and fear out of love for his own child, and then proceeds to act out of so-called love for his neighbors and for human society. His mode of thought does not induce impulsive actions, like those of a child or self-centered youth, but is expressed in moderation.

At the age of 50 to 60 years-old, his body organs gradually start to show a retrograde metamorphosis, activity declines, and *sei no yokubō* gradually decreases in correspondence with this debilitation . . . which is a natural phenomenon that takes place in a living body. It should not be considered merely the result of experience and cultivation of the mind.

In other words, Morita expounds the idea that the relativistic manifestation of *sei no yokubō* in developmental psychology is a natural human phenomenon. He generalizes this idea further by stating that *sei no yokubō* is a pure human desire that is set in motion quite naturally but that it cannot be readily recognized amid the complications of everyday human life. However, if one places oneself in an isolated environment, remote from society, one will come to realize that this desire is present and that it is naturally set in motion from and by one's self. It is known as *sei no chikara* (strength of life).

Morita explains its content and direction of thrust as follows: "One should look at one's self, and have the desire to improve and develop oneself in the midst of the whole of creation." Further, "it is believed that all living creatures evolve and develop eternally and endlessly by action directed by the best of all methods, and with unremitting hour-by-hour effort involving both body and mind in line with one's respective status in life."

When it is viewed objectively, *sei no yokubō* is motivated most vigorously during the period of youth. Together with this, the desire to express oneself becomes strong. Nevertheless, friction and repulsion are experienced in confrontation with the various standards and restrictions imposed on self-expression by society, with the result that the hypochondriacal trait or *shi no kyōfu* is manifested easily and frequently.

Sociopathological phenomena and neurotic tendencies crop up readily during this period.

Morita has an appreciative understanding of the conflict and suffering that can occur in the minds of human beings, in line with their living conditions, and accepts these phenomena as natural reactions of the mind. He also takes the position that the true mental nature of human beings is for the self to act and overcome any such suffering. Morita also believes that a human being discovers, by himself or herself, the presence of *sei no yokubō*, which arises naturally, by following its motivation. He or she will, as a matter of course, reveal his or her true human character and be restored to his or her authentic self.

Morita uses the word *doryoku* (effort) to indicate the actions of human beings who strive to

[1] The original meaning of *taiga* is pāramātman in Sanskrit and is similar to supreme self. Namely, it is the condition of obtaining mind and body freedom by getting rid of persistence in oneself.

demonstrate their actual selves on the basis of *sei no yokubō* and considers its manifestation to be the *shizen no honsei* (natural character) of human beings.

However, the answer to the question of how vigorously this natural character, which does not appear often during the infantile period, will appear as an infant grows older cannot be inferred sufficiently from Morita's writings. The concept is probably natural for Morita, who takes the experienced position that it will appear gradually with development of the inner being as a psychological phenomenon that is a natural phenomenon of the living body. However, rather than believing this character to be acquired by experience, we believe that the principal point is as follows: Even if it is natural to consider the concept of Morita's *sei no yokubō*, which he advances as a natural phenomenon, to be the various biological desires that provoke evolution and development in ourselves as being the primary factors of human life, it is also inevitable that we consider this phenomenon to include another, higher level of psychological desire, such as "love for one's neighbors or for human society."

When we summarize Morita's *sei no yokubō*, we see it as the basic life desire that stimulates human beings to seek improvement, maintenance and development of the self in living. It is also the source of the collective activities that draw human beings together. In addition to instinctive desire, *sei no yokubō* contains a psychological component of a higher level. These two components are mutually harmonized. Both body and mind turn the self toward an infinite process of personal development through activities governed by the best method and by continuous effort. And this process is expressed as a manifestation of the whole of life among human beings.

Morita does, however, place importance on individual temperament, believing that human beings have an intrinsic temperament. The direction in which one moves and experiences the effect of *sei no yokubō* will depend entirely on one's intrinsic type of temperament (which is psychological). Morita seeks to classify *shinkeishitsu* or the "*shinkeishitsu* character" for exactly that reason and purpose.

Clarification of the psychological structure of *shinkeishitsu* was an urgent preoccupation for Morita until his *shinkeishitsu* theory was fully developed. His perception of the hypochondriacal basic tone as providing the momentum for the onset of *shinkeishitsu* was truly clear-sighted. It could be said to be a natural theoretical development.

The intuitive realization that temperamental tone or so-called true human character is actually the manifestation of the *sei no yokubō* in each human being cannot be readily acquired on the level at which pathological conditions are ordinarily studied. The discernment of this intrinsic human nature is not limited to the fixed temperament theory, called the "hypochondriacal basic tone," as Morita calls it, but, rather, is quite fluid. Morita's theory has a positive, constructive content and should be given high evaluation. His perception of *shinkeishitsu* as being an extension of normal human nature arises from his identification of *sei no yokubō*. A fundamental trust of human nature lies at the core of his theory.

14

Situational Elements as Pathogenic Factors of *Shinkeishitsu*

Morita considers *shinkeishitsu* to be a mental rather than a physical condition of hypersensitivity, as well as a manifestation of the entire personality rather than a matter of individual symptoms. Takeyama[1] later explains that "the conflict of *shinkeishitsu* is a personality reaction, not a biological reaction of the deep stratum. Essentially, conflict in the personality stratum at a high level is symptomatic of *shinkeishitsu*."

This explanation characterizes Morita *shinkeishitsu* as a situational reaction manifested in the personality by a person who has a pronounced hypochondriacal mental tendency. Ikeda[2] remarks on the *shinkeishitsu* structure as being the same in nature as an "impediment of intellectual attitude."

In Morita's view of human nature, human beings are engaged in constant activity, continually exerting effort and trying to develop and improve themselves because of *sei no yokubō*. Incessant mental activity tends to direct the self toward a more adaptive condition. However, when it is felt that this progress is obstructed by one's mental and physical condition, as a result of certain situational factors, personality conflict occurs. *Sei no yokubō* gradually shifts toward, and is strengthened in the direction of, the "hypochondriacal tendency" owing to the relativistic relationships that exist in the conscious mind.

The "inadaptability anxiety" defined by Kōra to mean the "anxiety of a feeling that one lacks adaptability because of one's own mental and physical condition" is also a state of mind that corresponds to this condition. Inadaptability anxiety will increase relative to the acceleration of the desire to possess the quality of adaptability.

An understanding of this personality reaction is of prime importance when we consider the process that triggers the onset of Morita *shinkeishitsu*. Morita's basic notion is that a personality characteristic relating to the *shinkeishitsu* condition, the so-called hypochondriacal basic tone, needs to be given the highest priority.

The process of the onset and development of the *shinkeishitsu* condition, with this personal characteristic as its base, takes place when a person's true human nature is not manifested naturally and when there is an absence of practical adaptability. How this process takes place can be generally understood from Morita's explanation. If, for example, a person rushes to jump on a train a scant moment before the train departs, there will be sensations of violent throbbing and palpitation of the heart and shortness of breath. These sensations will quickly subside and be forgotten. If, in a later situation, this person becomes aware of having the same sensations under similar circumstances, the latter situation will seem to be appreciably different, all the

---

[1] Takeyama, T.: Shinkeishitsu gakusetsu no tenbō (Views of *shinkeishitsu* theory) (in Japanese). *Japan Medical Journal* No. 1498 (1953).

[2] Ikeda, K.: Morita shinkeishitsu to sono ryōhō (Nervosity (Morita) and Morita therapy) (in Japanese). *Seishin Igaku* 1: 461–473 (1959).

more so if the sensations occur in reaction, say, to the news that someone close, a friend or family member, has suffered a heart attack.

Commonplace sensations ignored in the past now take on a sudden new meaning, provoking an intense anxiety reaction that cannot be ignored. The mental process of the person's attention slips out of the control of intention, and he begins, instead, to concentrate his attention on the sensations as such: the throbbing and palpitation of the heart and the shortness of breath occur, this time, because of his sudden anxiety reaction to the notion that he probably has a weak heart and is potentially prone to suffer a heart attack at any moment.

This reaction arises from a judgment based on his hypochondriacal tendency.

As a result, this person's receptiveness to such sensations becomes highly sensitized, and his tendency to impose a hypochondriacal interpretation of the events in his life is reinforced. This tendency acts to further intensify the sensations and to lower his practical functionability. His attention becomes more and more focused on the sensations.

This process is what Morita calls "psychic interaction," and it explains how awareness of being in the *shinkeishitsu* condition is intensified. Attention is centered exclusively on the sensations that provoke the anxiety reaction (with an increase in the inclination toward introversion) and on the mental condition experienced immediately before and after the sensations occur. The notion of progressive human life advancement is no longer borne in mind.

Morita calls this condition the "immediate object orientation of human consciousness." In this condition, the person's attention is fully preoccupied by the presumptive problem of possible heart failure; the natural fluidity of his attention comes to a halt. His incessant mental preoccupation with the condition of his heart, which is abnormally intense, brings the onset of fear and anxiety, and in that manner acts to reinforce his apprehension of potential heart failure as an autosuggestive effect. He thus becomes enmeshed and isolated in a vicious circle that has no end or exit because of what Morita calls the "antagonistic action of the mind," which intensifies the problem by means of strenuous mental efforts to deny that it exists.

Morita expresses the mental mechanisms that trigger the onset of the *shinkeishitsu* condition with this equation: Occurrence of *shinkeishitsu* = temperament × chance event × pathogenic factor.

His personal views on the etiological basis of *shinkeishitsu* will be discussed in this chapter by explaining the psychological mechanisms in terms of the pathogenic factor in which the symptoms of *shinkeishitsu* germinate, develop and become fixed.

Chance

The first element that plays the part of a causative factor in the onset of *shinkeishitsu* is what Morita calls "chance." According to Morita, chance is an accidental experience, perhaps a common, everyday event that has a direct, trigger-like impact that precipitates the onset of *shinkeishitsu.* Chance is usually called the precipitating factor. It can be an experience that occurs during the course of a person's ordinary day-to-day life. However, it is not analyzable in terms of relative strength or weakness, or in normative terms. Concrete examples of such chance events, in their role of precipitating factors, can be drawn from actual case histories.

1. Man, 25 years-old, company employee: phobic over possible loss of eyesight

One day, while filing away a pile of old newspaper clippings on the subjects of health and sanitation, this man's glance happened to fall on an article that dealt with glaucoma. Because the clippings he was filing had accumulated over a period of two to three years, producing quite a large pile, he was at that moment fatigued. After noting the item on glaucoma, he decided to lie down because his eyes felt extremely tired. He was gripped by the sudden sensations of palpitation and an apparent backflow of blood, caused by an increase in blood pressure that had overwhelmed him when he began to imagine that he might contract glaucoma and go blind. This sudden attack subsided after a short time, but he became captivated by the fear of glaucoma and loss of sight and began to experience chronic headaches, nausea and a feeling of photophobia.

2. Man, 22 years-old, student: pollakiuria, urophobia

Five years earlier, as a high-school sophomore, this man had experienced a need to urinate and had asked his teacher for permission to leave the classroom. He was reprimanded for asking. The need to urinate did not seem to be a problem at the time. However, three years later, when the man first sat down to take university entrance examinations, he felt a sudden need to urinate and became captivated by that sensation. Since that incident, he had experienced chronic pollakiuria and urophobia and could not attend classes.

3. Man, 39 years-old, seaman: phobic over alopecia

Some ten years previously, while having his hair cut, this man remembered a friend remark in jest that "your hair is falling out." Looking at his hair in the barbershop mirror, the man experienced sudden physical rigidity, his whole body became bathed in sweat and his face flushed. He became so agitated that he left the barbershop and went home before the haircut was finished. Since that incident, he had been captivated by the fear of going bald.

4. Woman, 44 years-old, housewife: cleptophobia

Some ten years previously, when visiting her older sister's home, this woman heard her sister jokingly remark: "I always feel that something is missing from the house after you visit me." The woman became captivated by this idea. She began to feel that salesclerks eyed her with suspicion whenever she went shopping. When the woman rode on a train, she suffered from a notion that other passengers would suspect her of being a thief if she even glanced at their belongings.

5. Woman, 31 years-old, housewife: psychosisphobia, mysophobia

The first attack had occurred about two years earlier. Immediately beforehand, the woman had experienced insomnia for two or three days. She believed, at the time, that she had read an article warning that the brain would function poorly if sleep were insufficient, and she became anxious about this possibility. Around the same time, she did not immediately understand something a friend had said and asked the friend to repeat the remark.

Afterward, she experienced a sudden fear that she was probably conversing with other people incoherently, without being aware of it. Since that time, she had become psychosisphobic and began to avoid conversation. During the time this symptom surfaced, her hands had touched feces when she was about to wash her child's soiled trousers. She began to wash her hands repeatedly. She felt that the towel that she had used to wipe her hands was also soiled, and she could not proceed with any subsequent activity until her presence of mind had been restored.

6. Woman, 32 years-old, housewife: fear of radiation poisoning

The onset of *shinkeishitsu* had occurred six years previously. After having had two abortions, this woman gave birth to her first child five years after marriage. Around the same time, she had been told that her husband had visited Hiroshima two weeks after the atomic bombing.

Because her husband still kept belongings dating from that time, the woman was seized by the fear that the entire household was contaminated by radioactivity.

7. Woman, 21 years-old, student (majoring in piano): fear of playing the piano in front of other people

This woman's fingers move freely, once she starts playing, but she feels that a long time passes before her fingers move in this manner, and her fingers tend to stiffen and become immobilized. This condition first arose three years previously. The woman had been taking piano lessons from the same instructor for some time but one day was mildly scolded. This experience was not unusual, however, and the rest of the day passed uneventfully. The following day, she felt that her fingers had stiffened and could not move because of concern that she would again be admonished. Her fear of playing in front of other people surfaced after this experience and had gradually intensified.

8. Woman, 26 years-old, shop clerk: fear of foul odor

This woman had experienced a fear of being disgusting to other people because of foul fecal odor. She also felt that other people treated her in that manner. The onset of *shinkeishitsu* had occurred four months previously. At one point, constipation and diarrhea had continued for four to five days. An internal medicine specialist had diagnosed her condition as colitis. The woman visited the hospital for some time as an outpatient. Once, during this time, the woman had soiled her underwear because of having diarrhea while riding a streetcar. She heard two men standing in front of her remark that "something smells bad." This remark was a great shock to her. Since then, she had developed the pertinent symptoms.

9. Man, 27 years-old, company employee: fear of one's own facial expression, anthropophobia

Two years previously, this man had been in love with a young woman, but she had married someone else. He had never expressed his feelings to her. Around the same time, after a friend's wedding reception, someone said softly to him: "You'll be the next to get married," while he was chatting with a group of friends. His face stiffened, and he was not able to respond with laughter.

Explanation of Chance Factors

Morita comments on the factor of chance as "something which commonly occurs to everybody, a commonplace situation in which an individual becomes obsessed by a feeling of illness due to some chance circumstance."

It is an experience by which the *shinkeishitsu* persona is directly motivated by the pathogenic mechanism that triggers the onset of the *shinkeishitsu* disorder, captivating the person in that condition.

Viewed from a general standpoint, it is a situation that could be experienced by anyone during the course of ordinary day-to-day life. The case histories we have cited above are no exception because they all involve commonplace events that are, in themselves, meaningless experiences.

In case 1, for example, the man's glance happened to fall on a news item on glaucoma while he was filling old newspaper clippings that had piled up over the past few years. At that moment, he was fatigued by this activity.

In case 2, the student had once felt a need to urinate during class and had been reprimanded by his teacher when he asked for permission to visit the restroom.

In case 3, the chance factor was a remark made in jest by a friend, and in case 4 a similar remark made by an older sister.

In case 5, the chance factor was an incidence of insomnia coupled with recollection of reading an article on the negative effects of lack of sleep; this case has elements in common with case 1.

In case 6, the woman had experienced anxiety over mental and physical distress similar to that in case 5, but this condition was triggered by a chance remark involving her husband.

In case 7, the piano student was mildly scolded by her teacher while playing the instrument; in case 8, the chance factor was the accidental soiling of the woman's underwear owing to an attack of diarrhea.

In case 9, the chance factor was a casual remark made by a friend, similar to the remarks made in cases 3 and 4.

People frequently experience all these situations: temporary mental and physical distress, small errors in interpersonal relationships, jokes and reprimands. The experiences have hardly any abnormal feature. The detonating force of the reactive condition is not set off by the objective strength or weakness of the incident or by its degree of importance as an objective phenomenon. If such were the case, the complementary or interactionary effects of a person's mental state and personality at the time would impel the person to decide whether or not the incident is to become a meaningful experience. The experience in itself is objectively meaningless. It is the sort of experience that a healthy person is aware of temporarily. However, a healthy person then moves on. A *shinkeishitsu* person fastens on the experience as something that is disadvantageous to his or her entire life, and this mental adhesion to the incident develops into a constant attitude of captivation. It acts to motivate the pathogenic mechanism that triggers the onset of the *shinkeishitsu* disorder.

According to Morita, these accidental experiences that he calls chance have no meaning, even if they do have a comprehensible relation, in pathogenic terms, to the onset of *shinkeishitsu.* Morita explains this point in the following way, in refutation of the Freudian point of view:

"Those of the psychoanalytic persuasion consider Morita therapy to be crude if causation is not scrutinized when, for example, obsession is caused by the fright experienced in reaction to the sound of a pair of scissors that has been accidentally dropped. If I do this by myself, it is more scientific because I actually see all of the phenomena and I write about the actual condition. In contrast with this, the position of the psychoanalytic school is that this approach readily becomes philosophical because an attempt is made to discuss the essence of the phenomena.

"The psychoanalytic interpretation may be that the fright experienced in reaction to the sound of the scissors is due to some sort of sexual shock rooted in the past, but I believe the dropping of the scissors is merely a matter of chance motivation. The true cause of the problem is the individual's temperament."[3]

The position of the psychoanalytic school may be that the meaning of being frightened by the sound and the dynamic mechanism of the cause of the *shinkeishitsu* disorder both lie in the subconscious mind. Morita, by contrast, considers the incident to be a chance experience and attaches no special meaning to it. It is the temperamental character of a person that infuses the incident with a special meaning. Given this temperamental character as an essential precondition, the question of why it functions in a motivational manner at one time but not at another is not clearly understood. However, it is possible to speculate that the exact mental state of a person, at a specific moment in the person's actual situation, is the key that triggers the hypochondriacal judgment.[4] This is due to its complementary effect on the temperamental character of the person.

In case 1, for example, the man had a keen interest in health and sanitation, particularly in connection with glaucoma; his mother had, at one time, been treated by an ophthalmologist. It was found, however, that she did not have glaucoma. There was no problem with her eyesight and no danger of losing her vision. However, the possibility of glaucoma lodged itself strongly in the man's memory. He had recently befriended an old man who had poor eyesight and felt an affectionate sympathy for the friend's condition. His mental state at the time is taken into account, along with the considerable weariness occasioned by filing the pile of old newspaper clippings. In that momentary mental condition, the chance experience of seeing an item on glaucoma sufficed to trigger his hypochondriacal reaction.

The same kind of situation is present in case 2. This man had twice failed the university examination. With the third test approaching, he was in the mental state of feeling driven into a corner. Under the circumstances, his feeling of perplexity, his uncertainty over what to do if he

---

[3] Morita previously makes reference to this factor of "chance" in association with the case of a 25-year-old, unmarried man in his thesis "On the Pathogenesis of the Obsessive-Compulsive Neurosis" (1934). This case of obsession had occurred five years earlier. One day before the patient's enrollment in the army, he was frightened by the sound made when his mother accidentally dropped a pair of scissors on a *kotatsu* (foot warmer) while he was resting in bed with a cold. This sound became the chance factor of his feeling a sudden chill and mental distress, since that time, whenever he saw a pair of scissors, resulting in a chronic fear of scissors.

The man went into the army after this incident. During that time, his symptoms improved. He was discharged three years later and returned to his family home. He did not find permanent employment outside the home but, instead, assisted in the family business. The man's obsession, during this time, was gradually aggravated. However, the focus of the man's fear expanded because he began to fear any object cut with scissors, for example, paper, cloth or leather. He felt both the chill and the mental distress on such occasions, experiencing extreme discomfort whenever he happened to look at any such material. In outline, the explanation given by Morita on the conditions that triggered the occurrence of the disorder is as follows: "What is pertinent in this case is that the obsession improved when he was in the army because he was absorbed in his military duties, but recurred after he returned to his home because he was idle and had time to again become absorbed in fear. The motivating factor of the obsession, in this instance, is that he was frightened and leaped to his feet when he heard the sudden loud noise of the scissors that had been dropped, precisely at a time when he was ill with a cold and had just fallen asleep. In such instances, most people would wake up wide-eyed, in reaction to the sound, and feel: 'What a frightful surprise!' But instead of directing their attention inward, toward the experience of being frightened, they would direct their attention outward, toward the source of the sound. By contrast, a person of the *shinkeishitsu* temperament is introspective and will concentrate attention on his or her own inner physical condition, rather than the outer objective reality, and will carry out a minute process of self-observation of the chill and mental distress aroused by the accidental sound. He will become obsessed with a subjective fear of experiencing such mental distress and will thus become controlled by the fear, in complete disregard of the original objective factor that gave rise to this fear. Consequently, his condition becomes detached from the incident which ignited the fear and he thus becomes captive to the feeling of fear in itself. This is the most important factor that ignites an obsession."

Morita also refers to the case of a 35-year-old man who suffered from obsession and explains the motivating factor of the obsession as follows: "When the patient was 15 years-old, he attended a lecture in school on the subject of the earth rotating on its axis and was struck by a fear so intense it made his 'hair stand on end' by imagining his body suddenly torn to shreds and scattered apart if he were ever shaken off the surface of the earth. He suffered constantly from this fear over a period of 20 years. He knew there was no possibility of his being shaken off the surface of the earth but clung to the fear so intensely that it continued to make his 'hair stand on end'."

This fear is similar to the fear of the scissors in the foregoing case, in which the man does not really fear scissors or the sound of dropped scissors but is, instead, afraid of reexperiencing his frightened feeling of having been "struck on the head" by the sound. Morita understood the nature of this situational motivating factor and of the fear that arises in reaction to any such chance events.

"Although the circumstances of the initial motivating factor of this fear are gradually forgotten, anything that recalls to the patient's mind the experience of being 'struck on the head' or 'making his hair stand on end' causes a recurrence of the fear. Therefore, even if it was only the sound of a pair of scissors at first, various forms of association arise, such as fear of any materials that are cut with scissors, or cutlery, shiny substances, needle cases, or hairdressings. Although these are complicated psychological conditions, they are set off by chance events. The school of psychoanalysis will probably attach importance to these chance factors and theorize about them in various ways. I do not place importance on the mental associations that spring up from these chance events as material worth consideration. I prefer to center my interest on the individual's feeling of being 'struck on the head' or of having his 'hair stand on end'." Morita considers these feelings to be emotional facts rooted in *sei no yokubō*, or in the fear of death, which human beings manifest in their living conditions.

[4] Ikeda, K.: See preceding text.

felt a need to urinate during the test period–and was not permitted to do so–became associated with that bitter experience in high school and thus triggered the anxiety that he had anticipated.

When an ordinary physiological or psychological experience, which can happen to anyone, becomes the incident that triggers the onset of *shinkeishitsu*, or the springboard for the condition to surface, we need to consider the complementary or interactionary effects of the person's mental state as well as his or her mental character, in other words, his or her hypochondriacal basic tone.

This springboard phenomenon is commonly referred to as the interaction between a preparatory condition and a fructifying factor. Kōra[5] suggests, with respect to the characteristic preparatory condition of a person, that the manner in which the person's temperamental tendency toward *shinkeishitsu* is related to his or her environment can readily trigger an anxious mental condition.

The factor of the chance experience that triggers the onset of *shinkeishitsu* is not directly detectable in some cases. The reason is that the triggering incident can be easily forgotten because even a completely commonplace incident can suffice to trigger the *shinkeishitsu* condition in many instances. Once a person has been captivated by the symptom of the *shinkeishitsu* reaction, his or her attention is directed exclusively toward the symptom, and not toward the mental condition that he or she was in at the time, as a result of what Morita calls the "peripheral nature of attention."[6]

Psychic Interaction and the Action of Autosuggestion

If the hypochondriacal basic tone is considered the primary cause of the onset of *shinkeishitsu*, the hypochondriacal tendency of a patient that has been triggered (motivated) by a certain chance incident and has then developed into *shinkeishitsu* also has a secondary mechanism–psychic interaction–that acts as a pathogenic factor.

Morita explains this mechanism as "a mental process in which attention is concentrated on a certain sensation; this sensation becomes hyper-sensitized; this condition of hyper-sensitivity fixates attention; the hyper-sensitized sensation and the fixation of attention mutually interact to increasingly intensify the sensitivity of the sensation."[7]

Thus, a man runs and jumps on a train a moment before it departs, heaving a sigh of relief (chance incident). He then suddenly becomes aware of breathing hard and feeling a throbbing of his heart (hypochondriacal experience). The sensations of breathing hard and heart throbbing intensify when he fixes his attention on a close observation of these sensations due to a hypochondriacal judgment that he probably has heart trouble. He then begins to experience the sensations even more acutely.

This anxious hypochondriacal tendency is further intensified when the man's attention is directed even more intently toward the sensations, which have been hypersensitized by an overanxious temperament. The interaction of the sensations and the attention paid to them causes these two phenomena to reinforce each other. The man maintains this hypersensitized state of sensation, so that it becomes a fixed state.

This factor of psychic interaction was cited, long ago, as a phenomenon of *circulus vitiosus* but was originally defined as a factor that was situated between psychic sensation and hypo-

---

[5] Kōra, T.: Shinkeishitsu no mondai (The problem of so-called neurasthenia) (in Japanese). *Psychiatria et Neurologia Japonica* 42(10):755–796 (1938).

[6] Morita, S.: See preceding text.

[7] Morita, S.: See preceding text.

chondriacal feeling. What Morita means by psychic interaction is somewhat different, because this term not only includes physical sensation but has a broader meaning as well, encompassing all the elements that contribute to the content of the *shinkeishitsu* symptom, that is, various feelings and mental concepts.

When the mechanism of this psychic interaction begins to function, a condition in which the "hypochondriacal humor" can be readily triggered has been set up, by the interaction between the man's mental condition and his personal character at that exact moment. A "hypochondriacal experience" occurs, by chance, when the man is in that interactive condition.

If we take case 9 as an example, we note that there was a young woman that the man had loved silently. She had married another man before he could venture to express his feelings to her. He was taken by surprise, in a single instant, completely losing his head when he was jokingly told by a friend that he would be the next one to get married.

This remark was made precisely at a time when the man was suffering over the matter of his timid character, and he was plunged into confusion. He laughed involuntarily but did not experience this reaction as genuine laughter; he felt that his face had twisted into an expression of grief. This feeling arose because the man was not able to conceal the weakness that he was assiduously trying to conceal and because he had formed the "hypochondriacal judgment" that he could probably not keep pace with other people in the future because of his weakness.

"Hypochondriacy," in essence, is the basic humor that maintains and improves human existence in the sense of "being concerned about things." The direction of its orientation is toward one's mental and physical condition and toward one's ability to cope with human relationships and social activities.

The flow of this humor called hypochondriacy contains the factor of an accelerative psychic interaction.[8] A hypochondriacal judgment in regard to certain sensory, emotional or conceptual phenomena as being abnormal, or indicative of an abnormal mental condition, is formed by the process of psychic interaction, which itself is accelerated by the hypochondriacal humor. This process intensifies the condition of "captivity" that arises from the *shinkeishitsu* trait.

The nature of this condition is such that it constitutes a state of subjective falseness.[9] When a person attains this condition, the consciousness of his or her field of attention is increased or a relative decrease in consciousness of the environment takes place[10] in such a way that anticipatory fear and anxiety can readily occur, strengthening the condition of captivity.

One factor that comes into play in this process is the action of autosuggestion. Because the suggestibility of the *shinkeishitsu* persona is intensified in this condition, anxiety can be anticipated. The person is easily affected by his or her senses, emotions or concepts, all of which are hypersensitized by the factor of psychic interaction, when the person is in the condition of the "hypochondriacal tend"; this hypersensitization sets off the continuous action of autosuggestion. The person hardens a hypochondriacal judgment into a virtual certainty and seals himself or herself into a subjective stance. As a result, the fluid action of the mind in its constant interaction with the environment comes to a halt. The person's attention is pinned tightly to hypersensitized symptoms unrelated to his or her intent. Anyone who is captivated by such hypersensitized symptoms is not aware of the process up to that point, simply succumbing unwittingly to feeling ill at ease all the time.

---

[8] Ikeda, K.: See preceding text.

[9] Kōra, T.: See preceding text.

[10] Kawai, H.: Shinkeishitsushō ni taisuru Morita ryōhō no seishin byōrigakuteki kenkyū hoi (A supplementary psychopathological study of Morita therapy for *shinkeishitsu* disorder) (in Japanese). *Tōkyō Jikeikai Ika Daigaku Zasshi* 74: 1214–1230 (1959).

Shisō no Mujun (contradictoriness in thinking) and the Antagonistic Action of the Mind

A detailed explanation of these two terms has been given in Chapter 5. Our focus here will be confined to their roles as psychodynamic phenomena in the pathogenic mechanism that reinforces the *toraware* (captivity) of *shinkeishitsu.*

A closed-circuit relationship, which is endless, is formed by psychic interaction. This relationship is further promoted by the hypochondriacal judgment connected with the antagonistic action of the mind, inducing a problematical condition between the mind and hypersensitive or heterogeneous feelings about objects.

Accordingly, in a person who suffers from this shackled condition, a mechanism that actuates *shisō no mujun* (contradictoriness in thinking) to protect oneself is engendered.[11]

All this stems from aspirations toward an idealized self-realization on a lofty level of "what one should be" or from the antagonistic desire of a strong, reality-negating mental condition that dictates "what one should not be." In case 9, for example, a closed-circuit mental condition in which there is no outlet has been formed in response to a conviction that one's facial expression is ugly owing to an oversensitized sense of warping, stiffening and twitching of facial muscles as well as to the hypochondriacal judgment that this disfiguring condition makes it impossible for oneself to live normally together with other people.

The man is shackled in this closed-circuit mental condition. Even if he escapes from the shackled condition, his desire for self-realization on a lofty level, dictated by a powerful mentality that is not daunted by any obstacle, and the antagonistic desire to repel forcefully his weak, timid, actual self are both activated.

In that manner, the *shisō no mujun* defined by Morita denotes the contradictory activity of simultaneously thinking about "what one might be" or "should be" and of "what one actually is." It is particularly true of the *shinkeishitsu* persona, whose hypochondriacal humor has been strengthened by chance incident, that self-evaluation of the true self is of a low level. Such a person aspires to an ideal self-image on a high plane called "what one should be." This aspiration sets into play the phenomenon of readily denying the fact of "what one actually is."

Case 9 demonstrates that a person who strongly yearns to maintain a stable condition in which the mind is never perturbed, under any circumstance, will become more and more attached to the sensitized object (so that he or she will not become aware of the fact that his or her desire is an impossibility). At the same time, the person will come to suffer more and more from this contradictoriness in thinking.

The reason is that the human mind is incapable of maintaining a fixed condition. It will normally indicate a great change at one time or a small change at another, in accordance with any specific situation. The natural human mind cannot remain immobilized.

A large disparity arises between the lofty idealizing self, with its desire for "what one should be" and the true self of "what one actually is." This persona suffers in the mental trap of a vicious circle that has no end or exit. What further complicates the suffering of the *shinkeishitsu* persona is thinking that the ideal level of self that desires "what one should be" is not too lofty and impossible for realization but that it is, rather, a condition clearly achievable by any healthy human being.

By judging the issue in that manner, the person's evaluation of his or her true self is low, and the tendency to consider himself or herself inferior continues to increase. As a result, the thrust of the person's hypochondriacal humor is even more directed toward his or her psychosomatic states on a secondary level. This process reinforces the person's belief in the lowered function of the oversensitized or heterogeneous object of his or her fear and anxiety. The person's mind becomes completely preoccupied with escaping from this hypofunctional or heterogeneous condition; that is, the mechanism of the "antagonistic action of the mind," which we will discuss next, is more exacerbated, and this result further reinforces the endless vicious circle and further complicates the *shinkeishitsu* suffering.

A condition Ikeda[12] calls the "absolute self-contradiction of being in the intellect for its own sake" is generated by this mental attitude. A person in this condition can no longer feel merely uneasy about the anxiety that is inherent in the condition. The person does not wish to feel uneasy about fear and anxiety, which can be anticipated, trying, instead, to resist the experience of such feelings. In this condition, an attempt is made to resolve the illogical, emotional prob-

---

[11] Schema of development of symptoms according to pathogenesis on the basis of psychic interaction, antagonistic action of the mind and action of autosuggestion.

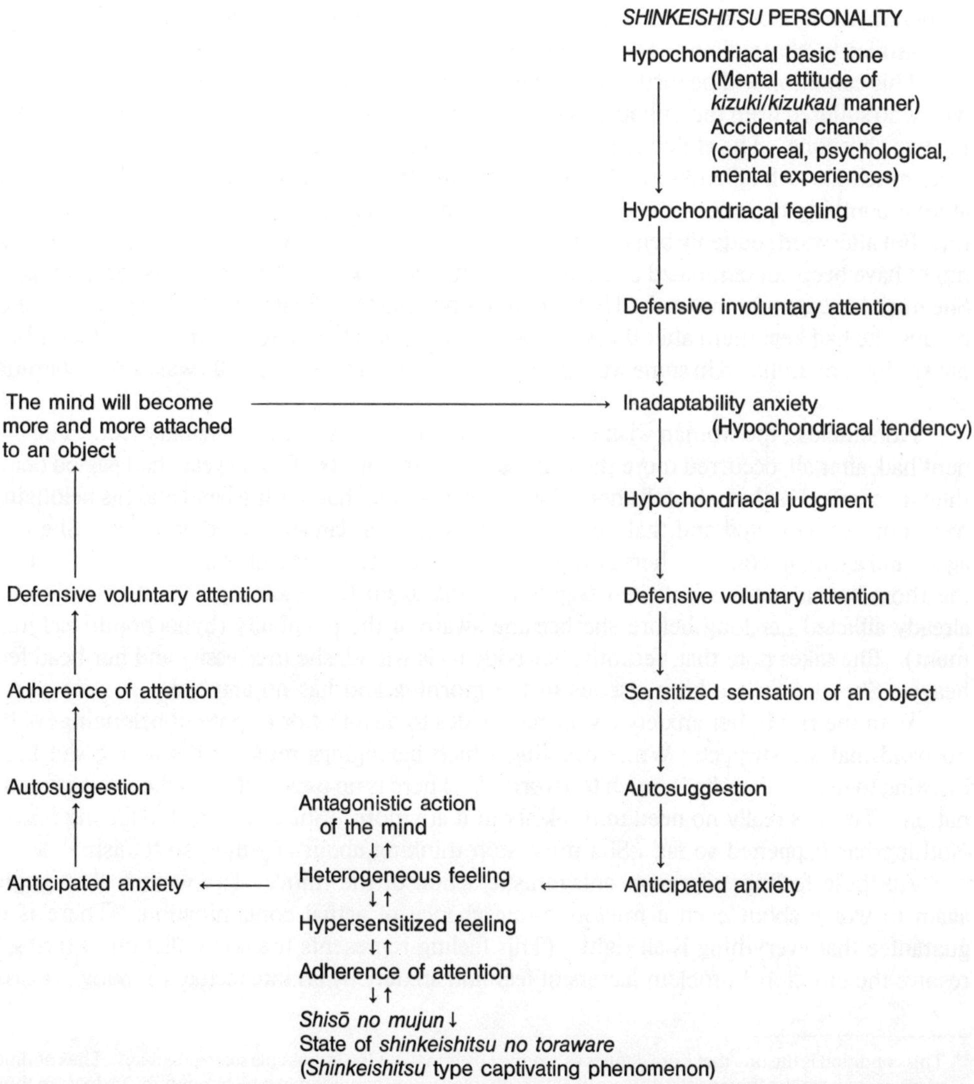

[12] Ikeda, K.: See preceding text.

lem factors called fear and anxiety by an intellectual (rational) process of "thinking." However, this approach does not work; it culminates in driving the person into a mental blind alley.

The intellectual resistance created by thinking that "I should not be like this" stems from what Morita defines as the "antagonistic action of the mind." It is a phenomenon in which the intellect strives to negate and reject fear and anxiety experienced in response to any physical or mental phenomenon considered disadvantageous or heterogeneous not only in regard to certain oversensitized objects of concern but also in regard to one's fundamental fitness for living.

A person in this condition struggles to control his or her emotions by an intellectual attempt to repel the self that experiences fear and anxiety in response to oversensitized objects, for example, by intellectual insistence that "fear and anxiety must not be experienced," "I must stop worrying" or "I must not allow myself to be aware of what I feel."

However, because mental tension and restlessness occur naturally in this condition, with worry and anxiety incessantly anticipated, a complex and powerful state of conflict is engendered, because all attempts to resist and repel fear and anxiety end in abject failure.[13] This phenomenon accelerates psychic interaction to a level that is endless in duration and to a level that is also similar to contradictoriness in thinking.

This condition will be further described in reference to case 6 as an example. The housewife who suffered from radiophobia gave birth to her first child five years after marriage, following two abortions. The childbirth was a happy event, but the infant was handled with extreme care, much like a fragile object. During that time, the woman's husband told her about the atomic bombing episode. She did not feel much of anything about these comments at that time but afterward suddenly began to think that there was considerable danger that her husband might have been contaminated by radiation, even two weeks after the bomb had been dropped. She must have ignorantly touched her husband's belongings at that time, and many times since, because he had kept them after the wedding. Quite apart from that matter, he must have been physically contaminated in some way, meaning that their entire household was also contaminated.

Nonetheless, the woman wishes to dismiss the matter as one of imaginary fear. The incident had, after all, occurred more than 12 years earlier, and six of those years had passed before they married. Further, she tells herself, it is also possible that her husband and his belongings were not contaminated and that he is completely free of dangerous radioactivity. She tries, again and again, to convince herself (rational resistance) that her fear is unfounded by reiterating those considerations but then begins to think again that radioactive contamination had already afflicted her long before she became aware of the possibility (hypochondriacal judgment). She takes note that, recently, her body feels wilted, she tires easily and her head feels heavy. She also feels a bit nauseous in the morning and has no appetite.

With the rise in her anxiety level, she decides to disinfect or dispose of belongings of her husband that are suspect. While deciding which belongings must be discarded, she keeps insisting to herself that she is much too worried. There is no possibility of radioactive contamination. There is really no need to think about it anymore. She needs to stop feeling uneasy. Nothing has happened so far. She must stop thinking about anything so foolish.

All these feelings represent antagonistic action of the mind. The woman then begins again to worry about even a million-to-one chance of actual contamination. There is no guarantee that everything is all right. (This feeling represents the contradiction of trying to resolve the emotional problem factors of fear and anxiety by an intellectual thinking process.)

---

[13] This condition is the one that Kōra defines as "conflict over making the impossible seem possible." The condition of *arugamama* in the therapeutic process of Morita therapy is one condition in which "contradictoriness in thinking" and "antagonistic action of the mind" are overcome.

It is clear, in this case, that the woman is captivated by an obsessive radiophobia. Both "contradictoriness in thinking" and "antagonistic action of the mind" act in a complementary manner to create the woman's hypochondriacal state of mind and to reinforce the mechanism of incessant psychic interaction.

Consciousness and Attention Activities: Voluntary and Involuntary Attention

Morita considers one factor of the *shinkeishitsu* symptom to be a phenomenon of a subjectively fabricated nature (Kōra[14]), which occurs when a *shinkeishitsu* person has concentrated his or her attention autosuggestively on sensations, emotions or conceptions that are disadvantageous, or at least unpleasant, to his or her existence and when the patient clings more and more to this subjectively fabricated material. The process of this mental structuring, with its powerful subjectivity, will be described here from the perspective of attention activity.

According to Morita, the process of human mental activity is directed toward adaptation for self-preservation, naturally. From that standpoint, a so-called threshold of consciousness is produced, in manifesting adaptive human function by conscious effort or strain. Numerous conscious efforts or severe strain accompanies the activity of new learning, for example, and for this reason the threshold of consciousness is also high.

By contrast, consciousness directed toward the activity decreases as time goes by and as learning progresses; consciousness and attention are then directed toward the object of study in a centrifugal manner. For example, when a person learns to hit a ball with a bat, consciousness is first concentrated on the ball (while proficiency in batting is learned), rather than on the motions of the hands and whole body.

All attention, in the case of the person we have described, was directed to concentrate on his hard breathing and his violent heartbeat, experienced when he jumped aboard a train just a moment before the doors closed. His consciousness was not directed toward his condition before or after this brief incident. It was, instead, directed toward his sudden fear of heart failure. This phenomenon is what Morita calls the "peripherality" or "immediate object orientation" of human consciousness and attention. Contradictoriness in thinking occurs readily when these factors of human mental phenomena are not kept in consideration.

Morita classifies attention activity into voluntary, active attention and involuntary, passive attention. He discusses the former from a temporal-spatial point of view. In summary, his line of thought is as follows:

When attention activity is observed from a spatial vantage point, it can be described as a "field" of attention or consciousness, in the sense of "field of view." For example, fix your attention on one point or small object. If your attention is fully concentrated on that point, and if your mental state is generally tense, consciousness is most clear in its close focus on that single point of attention. However, this clarity will decrease if you shift attention toward the surroundings. Finally, a limit is reached beyond which your consciousness cannot be broadened.

If you increase efforts to concentrate attention on the initial fixed point (so-called secondary attention), or if your attention is already fixed on that point, with tension absent and relaxation evident, the condition becomes one in which you are conscious only of that point and do not become conscious of the surroundings. Fluctuations of attention in this conscious condition may occur owing to a rhythm in the intensity of the attention devoted to that fixed point of

[14] Kōra, T.: Morita therapy. In *Essays in Commemoration of Takehisa Kōra's Appointment as Professor Emeritus*, 1964. (Printed in Japanese)

consciousness, but you will finally lose awareness of that concentration of attention, and it will become involuntary and passive in character.

This condition could be called one in which consciousness has reached its finite limit and has lost any objective awareness of its function. For example, a person slips into a condition of loss of self-consciousness due to a certain vivid impression. Not becoming aware of fear in a condition of conscious fear, or not aware of courage when acting with determination, is a case in point.

During attention activity, passive fixation of attention takes place in close correlation with the effect of autosuggestion. If one is in a condition of passive, involuntary acceptance, usually when anxious or distressed in response to an unpleasant concept or in response to conceptual/sensory phenomena experienced as stimuli, a concentration of attention on those mental phenomena will arise. In the case of the *shinkeishitsu* persona, this process of attention fixation is reinforced by one's underlying hypochondriacal humor.

Consciousness toward the surroundings of an attention point will decrease relative to any increase of conscious activity in the field of attention,[15] and consciousness of wide-ranging changes in one's environment will become impossible. As a result, freedom of action will be sacrificed. There is a tendency to examine only inner objects of consciousness, and such objects are increasingly given the status of facts, which is the process that forms the subjectively fabricated structure of the *shinkeishitsu* symptom.

Once conscious activity becomes fixed in the passive, involuntary condition, it becomes more difficult to escape from that condition. The harder the mechanism of antagonistic action of the mind acts on this condition, the stronger the involuntary fixation becomes.

For example, a person engrossed in reading suddenly becomes aware of the sound of an air conditioner. If the person tries to resist listening to this sound by consciously insisting "I will not listen to it" or "I will not let it concern me," the sound becomes obstructive and disturbs his or her reading. The more the person consciously resists listening to it, the more it will disturb him or her, despite the person's intense efforts to ignore it, and finally his or her entire consciousness becomes concentrated on it. The sound becomes a loud noise that threatens the person's reading rather than a soft hum associated with control of room temperature. The sound was, of course, present in the room before the person became aware of it–it was objectively, not subjectively, present.

While the person's conscious activity was concentrated on reading, in a condition of involuntary attention, this sound was in the surroundings of his or her field of consciousness but not sensed in awareness. When the person's attention was shifted from reading to listening attentively to this one sound, he or she thus became aware of its presence in the room and began to resist it as something disruptive. As the person further increased his or her level of attention devoted to the sound, it finally became a disturbing noise.

This phenomenon is the principle of manipulation used to overcome the mechanisms of "contradictoriness in thinking" and "antagonistic action of the mind" in Morita therapy. The basis of this principle, when the example cited previously is referred to, is that the natural condition of the mental activity of a healthy person is such that his or her attention will be focused naturally on the content of the book that he or she is reading, and the person continues to read while hearing the sound of the air conditioner (but not shifting his or her attention to it). Eventually, if the person's attention continues to be devoted to reading, the activity of reading will become repositioned in the center of his or her field of consciousness. The sound will shift to peripheral awareness and will not be consciously heard. In that manner, the reader complies obediently with this natural mental process in a mental state of *arugamama.*

---

[15] Kawai, H.: See preceding text.

The *Toraware* State of Mind

Kawai[16] understands the symptom of *shinkeishitsu* as being a self-defense reaction directed against inadaptability anxiety and explains selection of concrete symptoms by referring to a mechanism of internal projection. Kōra[17] attempts to explain the mental attitude (*toraware* attitude) of the *shinkeishitsu* persona by using a method of understanding that he calls the defense reaction. To Kōra, an essential form of adaptability anxiety can occur in anyone. In a healthy person, this anxiety is life-positive in that it incites actual adaptability. It is not something confined to a certain object, and it is not fixed. Human life is finite, and human beings lack omniscience. Consequently, situations arise in which anxiety will inevitably occur, even when things seem stable and settled. Anxiety cannot be extinguished as long as the anxious human being is alive. For this reason, human beings can learn to cope with unknown, limited situations in a frame of mind called adaptability anxiety.

In this frame of mind, attention is not confined to one fixed object. However, the *shinkeishitsu* persona displays an attitude of directing anxiety toward a fixed object by means of various pathogenic mechanisms. This phenomenon can be considered a kind of defense mechanism.

Kōra thinks that the captivation of the *shinkeishitsu* persona by a certain fixed object is due to the effect of the so-called mechanism of the principle of energy conservation, which can be considered a conservation of mental energy. He calls this effect an apparent simplification of the defense mechanism.[18]

He interprets this phenomenon not in the sense of the Freudian formation of symbols but, more generally, as the formation of *toraware* by limiting attention to a fixed object that stands forth as the symbol of a more pervasive condition of adaptability anxiety. This *shinkeishitsu* simplification of the self-defense mechanism seemingly acts efficaciously, in line with the energy conservation principle. Such objects are limited in mental activity to the mechanisms of "contradictoriness in thinking" and "antagonistic action of the mind."

According to Kōra, these two mechanisms accelerate the process of limitation of an object (with the *toraware* formed in reaction to a certain fixed object) in exactly that manner. However, these mechanisms accelerate the *toraware* viewpoint in a magnified, absolutized cognitive manner to form one characteristic of the attitude adopted by the *shinkeishitsu* persona. This process consists of functionally universalizing the symptom throughout the entire persona with a limitation of the symptom. The anthropophobic man, in our case study, believes that he could live much as a healthy person does if only he did not blush. However, he is paralyzed into inactivity because, in fact, he does blush. (This fact is not related to frequency or intensity.) He universalizes this fact to take in his entire body and forms an absolutist conviction that he is not a healthy person because of this single phenomenon of blushing.

This universalizing tendency indicates a development toward further reinforcement of attention attachment by the sheer concentration of energy directed toward this one limited object (blushing). The condition of *shinkeishitsu no toraware* is, however, different from conditional images, such as overconcern for one's body[19], and from the condition of Stekel's

---

[16] Kawai, H.: See preceding text.

[17] Kōra, T.: Shinkeishitsu shōjō hassei no kiten to Morita ryōhō no tokushitsu (The mechanism of *shinkeishitsu* incidence and the characteristics of Morita therapy) (in Japanese). *Kūshū Shinkei Seishinshi* 20(2): 115–119 (1974).

[18] Kōra, T.: See preceding text.

[19] Laughlin, H.: *The Neuroses in Clinical Practice.* W. B. Saunders, London (1956).

nosophobic, hysterical, paranoid and obsessional neurotic hypochondriasis (Nervöse Angstzustände und ihre Behandlung, 1924. See footnote 20). Even if excessive attachment is indicated by the condition of one's mind and body, it is not a mental structure of simple concern about illness and health, of experiencing fear and anxiety or of having an obsessive notion that is entirely heterogenic to oneself, much less one having a psychotic structure, such as a hypochondriacal delusion.

Rather, *shinkeishitsu no toraware* is a strong concentration of attention on a fixed object and an autosuggestive hypochondriacal judgment. At the same time, it is a condition of suffering from a conflict that a person cannot repulse, even if he or she tries to. It could be said to be a condition in which a person has strong anxiety focused on a fixed object but is frightened by his or her condition, which is anxious, quite apart from the object for its own sake. The major source of anxiety for the *shinkeishitsu* persona does not lie in the objective nature of any object but, rather, is one's self in a state of anxiety. The strongly subjective mental structure of the *shinkeishitsu* persona is, we might say, motivated by a dual structural psychology composed of the asthenic hypochondriacal humor and the sthenic *sei no yokubō* (desire to live), as Kōra believes.

The phenomenological features of *shinkeishitsu no toraware* differ considerably from the attachment phenomenon exhibited by ordinary hypochondriacs in the strong functional application of such impressions as asthenia, hypersensitivity and depressiveness. Ladee[20] has written on the subject of the aggressiveness observed in hypochondriacs, but it is believed that this phenomenon is basically different from the *shinkeishitsu* condition. Jahrreis[21] mentions, in regard to the development of the hypochondriacal notion from information he derived from his cases, that a certain depressive condition, or at least a mildly depressive tendency, observed in the emotional life of hypochondriacs produces a hypochondriacal notion, or is needed to sustain it, and that if this hypochondriacal notion embodies an acutely emotional content, it becomes an exaggerated tendency. If the emotional content of the hypochondriacal notion is low, it becomes more of a delusive trend.

Jahrreis's observations are of great interest. It is unfortunate that it is not possible to comprehend fully, from his writings, the differences or similarities of the mildly depressive condition or the tendency toward hypochondriacal humor by comparison with Morita.

Jahrreis also explains introspective emotional egotism in hypochondriacs as a generally isolated, precautionary trend intended for self-defense and self-preservation. Doubtless, the *shinkeishitsu* persona pays careful attention to self-defense and self-preservation and, as a result, exhibits a pronouncedly self-centered trend. However, a more sthenic tendency is also evident, because such a person desires improvement and development of the self to attain the level of ordinary people or to attain an even higher level (the perfectionistic, idealistic trend).[22] Even if this desire is manifested as an introspective emotional egotism, any depressive or pessimistic feeling does not interfere with its primary importance.

The *shinkeishitsu no toraware* persona has a certain similarity to a "strong capacity for imagery as an introvertive activity"[23] in that it manifests a strong introvertive tendency, but the self is not fixated in a completely rigid condition, in spite of strong subjectivity; the immediate object of *toraware* is an error that stems from the insatiable challenge of emotional facts by the intellect, as is frequently expressed by the statement that "I understand the problem logically,

---

[20] Ladee, G. A.: *Hypochondriacal Syndromes.* Elsevier, Amsterdam (1966).

[21] Jahrreis, W.: Das Hypochondrische Denken. *Archiv für Psychiatrie und Nervenkrankheiten* 92: 686–823 (1930).

[22] Kondō, A.: Morita's theory of nervosity compared with the psychoanalytic theories of Freud and Horney on neurosis (in Japanese). *Tōkyō Jikeikai Ika Daigaku Zasshi* 73: 2077–2123 (1958).

[23] Schipkowensky, N.: Wesen der Hypochondrie. *Zeitschrift für die Gesamte Neurologie und Psychiatrie* 174: 1–65 (1942).

but I am still captivated by it." This error is apparently caused by the dualism that exists in human beings in the form of "oneself as subject" and "oneself as object" within the context of the underlying condition of the hypochondriacal basic tone.

Part IV

Problems in the Therapeutic Process

15

Description of the Therapeutic Process

Practice of Morita Therapy

Morita states that a prerequisite for practicing Morita therapy is to determine whether such therapy is indicated by ascertaining a patient's diagnosis. Morita therapy is a specific therapy for Morita *shinkeishitsu* owing to its pathological view of the symptoms, with an appropriate therapeutic method being based on this view and with a mutually regulative relationship existing between these two elements.

As will be pointed out in Part V, there are several variations on the specific type and content of Morita therapy, although the essential therapeutic principle is universal and consistent. The different variations will be explained in this chapter along the lines of Morita's thinking in relation to hospitalization therapy, which was the original form[1] of Morita therapy.

Principle of Morita Therapy

According to Morita, the ultimate goal of Morita therapy is educating and training a patient to deal effectively with the hypochondriacal basic tone. This goal signifies the importance that the personality of a *shinkeishitsu* patient has in the therapeutic process. The means used to achieve this goal consist of absolute, isolated bed rest, work therapy and social-life training, which are structured in a systematic manner to form a therapeutic system. Underlying this therapeutic method is the pathological view of *shinkeishitsu* adopted by Morita, as was explained in Part III. This point of view can be summarized as follows:

Morita's attention was drawn to the fact that the psychological tone of the personality indicates the hypochondriacal tendency in *shinkeishitsu* with a specific peculiarity of a hyper-

---

[1] Apart from carrying out the original therapeutic method in its initial form according to Morita's description, there are a number of variations that depend on the various conditions of each patient. One variation is shortening the work period that follows the absolute, isolated bed rest stage in the instance of inpatients. The procedure of changing and increasing the quality and quantity of the patient's life in stages as prescribed in the original form is omitted; therapy dealing with the irregular life pattern characteristic of the fourth stage is started immediately, to shorten the time required for therapy on the whole. Another method, for outpatient treatment, is carried out in a similar manner, applying the inpatient methods of absolute, isolated bed rest and work therapy; that is, bed rest is carried out in the home, with the cooperation of family members, and work therapy is carried out by having the patient visit the hospital after the bed rest stage. This variation will be explained elsewhere in more detail, but in brief it is a method by which persuasion is applied, based on the principle of Morita therapy, for outpatient treatment.

sensitive temperament when it is ranked among the various categories of the seven abnormal personality types that he classifies; he calls this factor the hypochondriacal basic tone and makes it his central concept when explaining the process by which Morita *shinkeishitsu* is engendered. Expressed in another way, this hypochondriacal basic tone is a form of introvertive character trend. It is characteristic that the introspective trend is strong and that such patients have active intellects, although they are mentally hypersensitive, and for that reason Morita differentiates this condition from the hypersensitive condition that is typical of hysteria.

Morita notes that the hypochondriacal basic tone is essentially a manifestation of the desire to live, which is the nuclear characteristic of all human beings. In this respect, it is a core trait that all human beings possess. However, in the relative relationship between the two factors, the desire to live recedes into a *shinkeishitsu* patient's mental background and the hypochondriacal basic tone becomes concomitantly dominant, with a chance experience being the random factor that precipitates the onset of *shinkeishitsu.*

Morita considers this condition as being a type of degeneration that develops out of that precondition as the root cause of illness (*shinkeishitsu*) in his *shinkeishitsu* theory, which is based on psychogenic theory. More importance is placed on the factor of temperament than on the factor of the environment, but the condition is a defensive reaction of the personality that can be understood as a functional conflict[2] of intelligence within the ego. The element that reinforces the posture of defense and the conflict of intelligence within the ego is the so-called antagonistic action in Morita theory. Simultaneously, the mechanism of the mental interaction effect is activated, and the *shinkeishitsu* person falls into a vicious circle of ceaseless contradictoriness in thinking, as if falling into an antlion-like trap called *toraware*, which decreases effective mental function. This is the gist of Morita's *shinkeishitsu* theory.

In principle, the ego struggles to eliminate anxiety from the factor of adaptability linked to the desire to live, that is, the anxious concern to improve and develop oneself. This concern is both rational and explicit; in most cases, it functions without self-reflection. However, when a condition that makes a person mentally hypersensitive is precipitated, the person becomes self-reflective and intellectualizing, and in that state the mechanism becomes conspicuous. The person attempts to resolve these anxieties (most of which are sensual and emotional factors) in life through adaptation by assuming an intellectualizing disposition, although there is no possibility of success (because the attempt has the inherent contradiction of struggling to resolve emotional problems with an application of mental logic), and the struggle only strengthens the internal contradiction, which leads to the onset of *shinkeishitsu.* The ego does not become aware of the contradiction. Attention is directed only to the object(s) of anxiety, and the acceleration of sensitivity occurs in conjunction with a weakening of the control over both mental and physical condition.

Morita therapy holds that this intellectualizing process and its effects must first be interrupted to break the closed circuit of contradictoriness in thinking. The incessant recycling of the mental interaction is brought to a halt with absolute, isolated bed rest and subsequent work therapy techniques. Anxiety is endured as it exists, and the habit of improving and developing oneself in accordance with one's authentic human desire to live is instilled for the purpose of cultivating goals and training the personality.

---

[2] Ikeda, K.: Morita shinkeishitsu to Morita ryōhō (Nervosity (Morita) and Morita therapy) (in Japanese). *Seishin Igaku* 7:461–473 (1959).

Precautions and Procedures for Conducting Morita Therapy

Before instituting Morita therapy, the therapist must explain the following points to a patient so that the patient understands the instructions because they are integral to the proper performance of such therapy.

The therapist provides a general explanation of the essential components of Morita *shinkeishitsu* and points out that psychotherapy of the Morita form is most suitable for the patient because his or her disorder is Morita *shinkeishitsu*, which has developed psychologically as a result of a mentally hypersensitive character trend.

In most cases, this therapy can be carried out only with close cooperation between the therapist and the patient, each in his or her respective role. For example, the patient has thought only about escaping from the symptom and has exerted almost all his or her energy to try to eliminate the suffering. At this juncture, however, the patient must entrust the therapist to apply effective therapy. The patient should expend his or her energy on realistic, life-enhancing methods to perfect, as much as is possible, the content of his or her life, which cannot be entrusted to other persons. In the therapeutic situation, the patient must consider therapy as being an experiment carried out to improve his or her activity. Together with the therapeutic instruction given later, the role of the patient is to begin life activity in this new direction and to cooperate in the therapeutic procedure.

Explanation given to a patient during the performance of Morita therapy includes the following components:

• Basic explanation of absolute, isolated bed rest

Other than going to the lavatory, washing one's face and eating meals (setting and clearing the table are carried out by the person in charge), a patient rests in bed at all times.

All such activities as needless conversation, receiving visitors, reading, listening to the radio, watching television and smoking are prohibited.

The period of absolute, isolated bed rest lasts about 7 days; the therapist will inform the patient one day before this period ends that he or she is free to get out of bed.

There is no restriction on thinking during this period. The patient may think about anything he or she desires. The patient should think as much as he or she can and suffer as much as he or she can endure. During this period, the patient may sleep whenever he or she desires. The patient may start thinking again as soon as he or she awakes. This condition must be endured as it is, even if the patient begins to experience doubts about the therapeutic method as a result of acute anxiety and suffering. Everything must be left to the course of nature as the patient's mind directs, without opposition, while he or she lies quietly in bed.

• Precautions given after the second stage of therapy

Although there are seasonal differences the patient will generally be instructed to go to bed around 10:00 p.m. and to wake up around 6:00 a.m.

The patient may go outdoors after the second stage of therapy. However, the patient should do so only for unavoidable reasons, such as shopping for necessities, visiting a barbershop and going to a public bathhouse. Taking a walk for relaxation and going to a coffee shop or a movie theater are prohibited activities.

Watching television, playing board games, such as *go* or *shōgi*, and playing cards or musical instruments, such as the piano, are permitted activities after the third stage of therapy, but even these pastimes are restricted to short rest periods after lunch or dinner.

Receiving visitors is a permissible activity only after the fourth stage of therapy.

The patient should recognize at all times that he or she is undergoing therapy and thus must act responsibly and prudently.

General Explanation for Practice of Morita Therapy

After explaining the instructions to the patient, the therapist initiates therapy in the following sequence: absolute, isolated bed rest; light work therapy; heavier mental and physical work therapy; and, last, life activities training therapy.

The basic explanation given in the following sections is centered around Morita's description.

First Stage: Absolute, Isolated Bed Rest

The patient is placed in a private room. Direct illumination and stimulation from outside elements, such as scenery, sounds and voices, are restricted as much as is possible to provide a truly isolated condition. The patient must be completely isolated, with visitors, conversation, reading and smoking prohibited and with bed rest imposed at all times except for use of the lavatory, washing the face or eating at mealtimes. Progress during the bed rest stage proceeds typically with an increase in appetite during the first day as a result of isolation from the troublesome stimuli encountered before therapy was instituted. The patient is in a state of mental and physical rest. This stage ordinarily lasts four to seven days. (A general psychopathological description of a patient's experiences during this stage is given later.)

Second Stage: Light Work Therapy

In general, this stage also consists of isolation. Similar to the first stage, conversation, visitors and games are initially prohibited. The patient goes to bed between 9:30 and 10:00 p.m. and wakes up at 6:00 a.m. The period of bed rest is restricted to about eight hours. The patient is instructed to go outdoors during the daytime for exposure to outside air and direct sunlight; the patient is not permitted to lie down on his or her side or to take a nap in the room, even if he or she experiences physical fatigue or simply feels tired. The patient must write in a diary the events of the day because the entries will provide helpful information for understanding his or her mental and physical condition. Unpleasant physical sensations or obsessive states are managed with the spirit of *arugamama* endurance and in a quiet manner. The purpose of this stage is to have the patient endure the suffering and to experience tedium to spur him or her to voluntary activity, that is, to engender the desire for exercise and work. The therapist never imposes instillative or transitory work. This stage lasts four to seven days. Conversation is gradually permitted from around the fourth day, although fraternization with "outsiders" is still prohibited. However, the therapist does promote the patient to engage in some activity throughout the day outside his or her room.

Third Stage: Heavier Mental and Physical Work Therapy

Means for spurring spontaneous activities of the mind and body are chiefly introduced during the preceding stage, but during this stage, the therapist promotes endurance and perseverance in work, helps the patient gain self-confidence and engenders courage by helping the patient feel pleasure from being successful in work activities. The patient is directed toward laborious chores as much as is possible and in accordance with physical condition; examples of such chores are digging holes, chopping firewood, working in a field and taking care of plants. Reading is gradually permitted. Going out is also permitted but only for shopping for necessities, taking a walk without a specific objective or meeting friends or family members. Such amusements as board games are still not permitted. The patient is restricted to working and reading alone. The third stage lasts about seven days.

Fourth Stage: Life Activities Training Therapy

This stage involves training the patient to adapt to changes in the outside world and to prepare for living outside the therapeutic environment. Communication with the patient's family, reading and going out to attend to business matters are permitted activities during this stage.

Patient Experience During the Four Stages of Morita Therapy

First Stage: Absolute, Isolated Bed Rest

Morita calls this stage a period of suffering and tedium and, at the same time, "a period of separation from social communication." Strictly speaking, this separation continues until the second stage and, as a rule, social communication is prohibited until the fourth stage, although limited communication is permissible during the third stage. In Morita therapy, one's mind confronts itself in a condition of complete isolation from social contact until the fourth stage. At the same time, during the first stage, the self-image confronts its gregarious nature, as represented by its *seken.*[3]

It is believed that self-discernment is accelerated by this stage. A patient's consciousness and its transition during this stage are generally as follows:

On the first day, tension is experienced owing to expectations and anxieties toward the new life condition that the patient will experience from this point within a context as yet unknown. Even then, however, the patient will gradually feel at ease and, in many cases, can sleep comfortably in a quiet condition, freed from the troublesome irritations experienced previously.

On the second day, the patient becomes aware of anxious mental associations and varied imaginative notions and pain of one kind or another. This awareness may revolve around personal concerns, the cause of the disorder and what lies ahead in the future, although there are individual differences in this regard.

Morita's explanation of this condition is that "if the patient slips into imagination, he should not try to distract his attention or try to forget or destroy such imaginative activity, but rather try to exercise imagination self-assertively, and if he cannot endure the associated pain, he should still try to confront it by gritting his teeth or clenching his fists, and simply wait to see how it finally turns out, as in the instance of a toothache or a stomachache. He must not leave his bed and go outside the room or complain about his suffering to someone else."

Morita further explains this condition by refering to the Zen precept that an attempt to destroy unpleasant mental associations is akin to "the desire to erase one wave with another wave, which only results in generating a myriad waves one after another." One's mind is in resistance to itself and, consequently, will become even more jumbled. Likewise, if something

---

[3] Fujita, C.: Nihon ni okeru shūdan seishin ryōhō—Morita ryōhōteki tachiba kara no kentō (Group psychotherapy in Japan—Review from Morita therapy) (in Japanese). *Seishin Ikagku* 10(7):525–529 (1968).

frightening whose true character is unknown appears in a patient's mental vision and he or she tries the utmost to avoid looking at it, the mind will become more and more attached to it, and the patient cannot forget it; however, if the patient ventures to be bold and examines the frightening vision head-on, it will turn out to be something of no concern.

If the patient tries to escape from pain, he or she will plunge deeper and deeper into anxiety, but if the patient confronts it directly, face to face, acknowledging the pain as pain, it will be an action on the order of the military tactic of burning the proverbial bridges behind him; the pain will soon be alleviated and eventually vanish, and the patient will have the feeling of coming into contact with a refreshing flash of hope. This flash of hope does not represent the elimination of pain, indicating, instead, that pain will soon be alleviated if the patient plunges into it aggressively. For example, in midwinter swimming, one hesitates to jump in at first, thinking the water will be so cold that the intestines will be jolted into the diaphragm or that breathing will be paralyzed by shock the instant one leaps into the cold water. As a result, one becomes even more agitated and frightened of jumping in. However, if one, instead, resolutely dives in, it is immediately realized that swimming is possible without difficulty. Later, when coming out of the water, one will feel that the chill in the air is even more intense than the chill in the water.

A *shinkeishitsu* patient will feel twice as much suffering owing to fearful anticipation of pain and anxiety. Further, this fear will seem to intensify threefold as a result of the patient's additional attempts to defy his or her fear of suffering.

In this stage, then, a patient is made to experience directly, by mental experimentation, various changes in the progression of his or her condition, and this mental experimentation becomes the basis for accelerating the relief of the *shinkeishitsu* symptom. This treatment procedure is basically different from an intellectual, persuasive approach alone; verbal communication is not necessary because this stage is one in which self-realization lies beyond verbal concepts.

In experiencing this stage of pain, a patient moves rapidly through the process that relieves the symptom because the pain is acute, and it is sometimes possible for a patient to complete this stage within two to three hours. In many cases, however, the resultant condition becomes conspicuous and can be clearly observed only on the fourth or fifth day. Patients who move slowly through this process tend to resort to some means of mental distraction, such as smoking, frequent visits to the lavatory or gazing at outdoor scenery through a window, diverting attention from the pain. However, when a patient acquires the requisite experience of facing the pain and coming to terms with it, actually overcoming it, he or she will begin to feel at ease (usually on about the third or fourth day) and can then look back at the pain of the previous day. Even if the patient tries to summon up and experience the same pain once again, he or she cannot induce it willfully and systematically and will be in a condition in which he or she can in no way compel the self to suffer.

Idle notions that occur with the passage of time will be experienced as being disconnected from oneself and can be confronted objectively, by inserting a psychological gap between them.

Around the fourth or fifth day, a feeling of tedium supersedes such idle notions. The patient wants to get up early and do something, or to speak to someone—anyone. (This phase is the tedium = stimulus-starved stage.) Various elements of which the patient was initially aware, such as anxiety, difficulty in concentration, a feeling of heaviness in the head and sleeplessness, have almost completely disappeared. In most cases, after completing this first stage, a patient experiences mental and physical repose, as well as decreases in irritability, physical disharmony and fatigue. In some cases, however, a feeling of decreased mental and physical activity, resulting from the absolute, isolated bed rest condition, persists.

Second Stage: Light Work Therapy

The ground rule for a patient during this stage is continued isolation from all social communication, in principle. Social association, conversation and going out elsewhere are prohibited activities. The patient goes to bed around 9:00 or 10:00 p.m. and awakes at 5:00 or 6:00 a.m. During the daytime, the patient is instructed to go outdoors for exposure to outside air and direct sunlight but is not permitted to lie down, even if he or she feels physically fatigued. The patient is requested to enter the events of the day in the diary before retiring.

On the first day, a patient's activities are limited, and he or she is not permitted to perform heavy work that requires muscular exertion or to take random walks. In the yard, the patient may sit and gather weeds or dry leaves on the lawn as his or her mind directs or simply observe the activities of ants. The object of this phase is to suggest voluntary activities to the patient to engage his or her mind and body by artificially imposing certain restrictions on activity. With the patient restricted in this manner, he or she naturally feels bored and does not feel content if not engaging in activity. Consequently, spontaneous activities of the mind and body are engendered. In view of this, only passive restrictions are imposed, with specific work not being assigned.

This stage is not instillative but, rather, spontaneous. It has the same intent as stimulating voluntary activities in a young child by the educational method created and espoused by Maria Montessori (1870–1952).[4] A patient becomes interested in work during the afternoon of the first day of the second stage and actually yearns to do something.

For example, if a patient pulls a cluster of weeds to clean the lawn, he or she will feel a craving to look around for other weeds and dry leaves to make the entire lawn immaculately clean. As a result, the patient will become interested in sweeping and collecting dry leaves in the yard and burning them and will also sweep the yard and keep the gardening tools in good order. This *ki-kubari* (attentiveness) to trying to improve this condition as much as is possible is called the "wholehearted desire to experience feelings." This craving will not surface, nor will interest in work arise, if the proper psychological groundwork has not been laid down in advance to bring the patient to this new plateau.

Morita says that this interest in activity and yearning to perform work can arise only if one always keeps busy. If, for example, any such work activity is prescheduled and the patient is instructed to clean the yard by pulling weeds or sweeping dry leaves, a mood of troublesome hardship will develop and the patient will not be in the proper mood to engage in self-motivated activities.

Getting things done one after another is, by human nature, difficult. Frequently, one does something without being aware of it right from the beginning. The work is done by getting in the mood without realizing that one has actually started to work. Therefore, during the second stage, there is a need to select an activity that is isolated from a patient's actual life, that is, something that seems meaningless and unrelated to practical matters or to productive activity. The main objective is to induce spontaneous activity in a *shinkeishitsu* patient's mind and body and to urge the patient further and further in that direction. Because a patient's vital power is restored to normal by the second or third day, the first-day restriction on work is relaxed, and

---

[4] Maria Montessori's book, *Il Metado della Pedagogia Scientifica Applicato all'Educazione Infantia nella Case dei Bambini* (Scientific Education Method Applied to Infant Education in Children's Homes) was translated into Japanese in 1914; when Morita read an essay titled, "The Essence of Montessori's Educational Method," written by Kiyomaru Kohno, a Montessori student and advocate who had a great interest in infant education, Morita appeared to be favorably impressed.

the patient is permitted to perform almost any sort of work that captures his or her interest. However, strenuous manual labor is still prohibited.

Gradually, conversation with other patients and light reading will be permitted, but communication with the outside world is still prohibited. Even if a patient becomes interested in reading, he or she is not permitted to read while confined to the room; reading is a permissible activity only during spare time between work periods. Reading matter is restricted to history, natural science and biography; special efforts to understand and memorize are prohibited, with only light scanning of reading material a permissible activity.

A *shinkeishitsu* patient customarily suffers because the meaning of what he or she reads is not retained in his or her mind; the patient's faculty of memory cannot be concentrated owing to the incessant anticipation of fear that occupies his or her consciousness, and because the patient is controlled by this anticipation of fear, his or her attention is dispersed. The movement of the patient's mind is not directed to what he or she is reading, being directed, instead, to his or her mental condition as such.

During this stage, then, a patient may read lightly if he or she desires and may stop reading if interest is lost, similar to what the patient does during voluntary work activity. No specific reading plan is needed because the patient may read while standing in the shade of a tree, for instance. Around the fifth day of this stage, interest in physical and mental work will accelerate gradually, much as when an infant begins to find pleasure in manifesting his or her vitality by taking some sort of action. The patient begins to undertake more laborious work, finding satisfaction in hard work out of a motivation for concern for good health. This phase is the end of the second stage. Around this time, a patient's facial expression, attitude and manner of speech become charged with vitality, as if he or she were a new person compared to his or her condition before entering therapy.

Third Stage: Heavier Mental and Physical Work Therapy

Continuing from the second stage, the quality and quantity of work begin to become gradually higher. A patient becomes absorbed in some kind of work throughout the day. This work may include wiping windows, cleaning floors, making objects out of wood or taking care of the lawn. Tasks that have clearly recognizable results are preferable.

The scope of permissible reading material is expanded. A patient may now read publications pertaining to his or her special interest or school textbooks during work breaks. However, the permissible content is still similar to that of the preceding stage.[5]

Going out is a permissible activity, although such activity is still confined to shopping for necessities or conducting simple business matters. Walks for pure relaxation or idle talk with friends is not a permissible activity at this stage. Sports and games, such as catchball, volleyball or pingpong, *go*, *shōgi* or card-playing, are still not permissible activities. A patient is permitted only to work or read by himself or herself. Further, even if a patient's activities are still restricted by his or her obsessions, such as a fear of going out or a fear of moving vehicles, the patient is instructed to go shopping or to run errands, if necessary by using public transport facilities, such as buses or commuter trains. However, it should be fully understood that the objective of such activity is to take care of errands. Going out or riding in vehicles is permissible only as a means to that end.

As a rule, reactions toward treatment take several different forms around the end of this period, that is, approaching the fourth week after the start of therapy. Although the *shinkei-*

[5] Full-scale reading is permitted from the beginning of the fourth stage. Morita initially started to broaden the quality and quantity of reading matter from the third stage, but several years later postponed this step to the fourth stage.

shitsu symptom may continue to be manifest during the early part of the third period, even in patients in whom therapy has resulted in considerable improvement, it will have abated markedly or disappeared almost completely, and daily life in the therapeutic environment is such that a patient becomes engrossed in work assertively and independently. A patient employs great effort to comply with the therapist's instructions, even if he or she still has doubts because there has been no dramatic change in the symptom, or alternates between joy and sorrow consistent with alterations in the severity of the symptom.

Even if a patient's performance in life activities has improved so much that he or she does not differ from a healthy person when viewed objectively, the patient still subjectively evaluates his or her condition as inferior to the condition of other people. The patient believes that his or her condition has gradually been improving but continues to have an apprehensive anxiety that it may take a turn for the worse in the future.

In most cases in which the progress of the therapeutic process is not fully satisfactory, daily work activities end in attempts to alleviate the symptom. There can be a tendency to isolate oneself from "real work" to consider how working can relieve the symptom or what kind of work is most appropriate for that symptom.[6] In certain cases, a patient frequently enters feelings of disgust in the diary, claiming that the assigned work alone is useless because it is completely unrelated to alleviation of the symptom.

Until the third stage, the purpose of the therapeutic process is to prepare a patient for the chance to transcend the self by self-examination and self-interrogation while he or she engages in a struggle with the self as an individual isolated from social communication (gregariousness). The time of the transition from the third to the fourth stage is an especially important period for both a patient and the therapist. This transition has the following characteristics:

- The therapeutic process is progressing well, with simultaneous, if only gradual, relief of the subjective symptom.
- The symptom remains at about the same level of intensity, but the patient has become self-assertive in his or her daily life attitude.
- The patient is ready to confront directly a condition that is much like that of actual daily life as soon as is possible. An example is a patient who has a symptom of an obsessive nature, such as fear of going out (including fear of moving vehicles), anthropophobia, agoraphobia or claustrophobia. (In most such cases, the suffering is relieved temporarily because the patient is isolated from stimuli that readily provoke fear; that is, he or she is isolated from the outside environment by hospitalization.) The time at which a patient feels every day during the third stage that he or she is busy because of the large number of tasks the patient sees before him or her, one after another, is a turning point for proceeding to the next stage.

Fourth Stage: Life Activities Training Therapy

Morita calls this stage the "complex actual life stage."[7] It is the stage of preparation directly connected with the patient's actual living conditions in the outside world. The therapeutic goal of the third stage is to have the patient acquire voluntary experience in discovering the authentic

---

[6] The therapist reads a patient's diary every day and comments on the patient's respective experiences or directs the patient's attention to practical applications but does not tell the patient that his or her condition will improve or that his or her interest in daily living will arise if he or she follows the therapist's instruction. The therapist only gives a patient instruction on limitations of work or other subjects of immediate importance. It is necessary to have the patient understand this beforehand. The reason is that the will to acquire voluntary experience is weakened if a patient anticipates or obtains suggestions from the therapist as to the efficacy of work therapy.

[7] Morita, S.: Shinkeishitsu no hontai oyobi ryōhō (The substance of *shinkeishitsu* and its therapy). Tohōdō, Tokyo (1928). In *Morita Shōma Zenshū*, Vol. II (edited by T. Kōra et al.). Hakuyōsha, Tokyo (1974). (Printed in Japanese)

self while enduring suffering caused by the symptom. For this purpose, the daily living condition is regulated so that social communication is restricted or prohibited; relaxation, amusement and passing time uselessly are prohibited activities.

Endurance training, discovery of latent spontaneity, awareness of the struggle against symptoms and acquisition of self-confidence are emphasized.

However, all these restrictions are removed in the fourth stage because it is one of preparation for returning to actual living conditions by means of training for adaptation to the conditions in the outside world. The quality and quantity of reading matter and opportunities to go out are broadened, communication with family members and friends is permitted and efforts are directed toward life objectives that a patient is aiming for. The patient may vary bedtime or even stay up all night if he or she desires. Engaging in various types of exercise, participating in sports, going to movies, attending lectures, playing board games and taking walks are permissible activities during leisure hours.

The chief objective is to get a patient to participate in everything spontaneously as the need arises and, further, to make the patient feel, in this manner, that he or she can do whatever he or she wants to do. The therapist thus helps engender a self-presence that includes self-confidence by dispelling the prejudicial self-inferiority complex that the patient has so far had.

The condition of a patient's consciousness during this stage can vary, but common to all patients is a growing awareness of change in themselves. A patient who was previously so intensely concerned about his or her symptom now feels like a new person. A patient experiences happiness from having something within that makes a smile appear naturally, and the patient feels that something akin to self-confidence is welling up.

However, this feeling is still unstable and generally changes from time to time. At certain times, a patient feels fully confident that he or she has been completely cured but at other times has the opposite feeling of losing self-confidence and falls into despair. The patient evaluates himself or herself as being in good or poor condition.

Nonetheless, the pendulum swings of these extreme and alternating experiences of joy and sorrow gradually become weaker. This development takes place shortly after the first week of the fourth stage. A patient begins to evaluate his or her changing status in a manner characterized by level-headedness and a self-critical attitude, although this changing attitude depends on the acquisition of a psychological distance with respect to oneself. Although the symptom still exists, it does not unduly distress the patient even when it comes to the forefront of awareness. Suffering is no longer as intense as it had previously been. Tasks that the patient felt he or she could not accomplish in the past can now be accomplished, to such an extent that the patient is not even aware that he or she has begun to disregard the symptom.

This phenomenon does not represent a conscious change of a conspicuous improvement. The patient in no way is able to determine whether he or she has been cured, but he or she takes a stance of tackling actual living conditions to the best of his or her abilities. An optimistic attitude of having become extremely opened outward –"Now I am absolutely all right and completely cured"– is not, of course, a true discernment of oneself, and the therapeutic process is still incomplete.[8]

[8] Diagram of *shinkeishitsu*'s process of pathogenesis and process of cure.

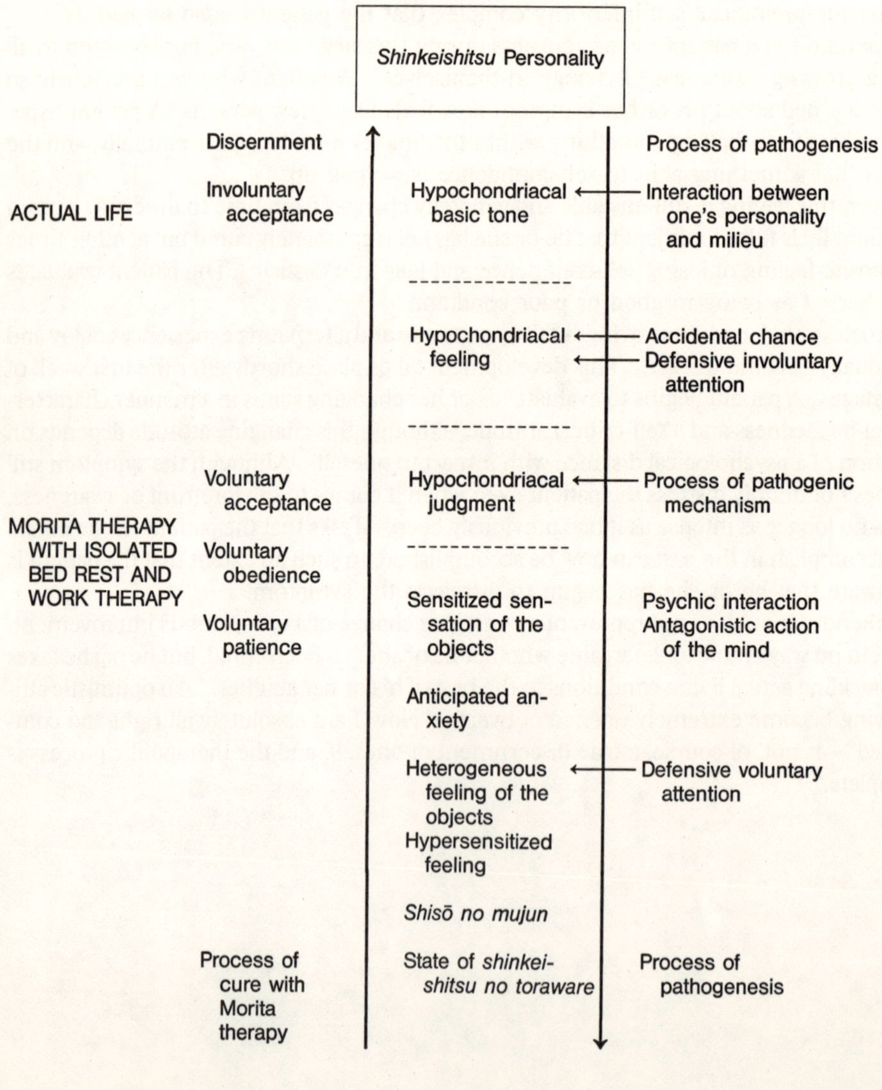

Summary and Explanation of the Therapy Process

The author has now examined the sequential steps in Morita therapy, which are summarized in the following paragraphs.

In Morita therapy, physical rest or recovery from chronic fatigue is induced by absolute, isolated bed rest. At the same time, a feeling of tedium is induced by cutting off a vicious mental circle and thereby reducing suffering. Next, natural therapy (see Part VI) to induce spontaneous activity in physical and mental functioning by means of work therapy is instilled, promoted and properly guided for body-mind training by work therapy. This training process progresses gradually from single to multiple tasks and from easy to difficult levels, in the sequence of (1) isolation from social communication; (2) light physical labor; (3) heavier physical and mental labor; and (4) ending isolation from social communication with life activities training similar to the requirements of actual daily living.

According to Morita, various kinds of chemotherapy and suggestive methods were carried out in the past but were useful only for temporary relief of symptoms. Patients readily placed confidence in these therapies, but satisfactory results could not be obtained. Such patients therefore tried even harder to obtain relief from the symptoms, and almost all of them ended in a condition of ineffectiveness, making the symptoms even more complicated than before, precipitating themselves into a more extreme condition of *toraware.* These treatment procedures disregarded the essence of Morita *shinkeishitsu.*

In view of this observation, Morita discarded the former therapeutic approach for the management of this neurosis and developed a newer form of therapy. This therapy was not designed to make patients forget about therapy for the time being to isolate their actions from the concept of *toraware.* A patient's dependence on therapy means an attachment to his or her disorder. Therapy must, instead, start by changing a patient's attitude of dependence on therapy to an attitude directed toward actual life realization. Complicated mental activities are accelerated by work therapy, and functional activities as a body-mind unit are cultivated. By this process, a patient gradually becomes aware that harmonized life activities are naturally possible.

Therapeutic Benefits of Absolute, Isolated Bed Rest

The benefits of this phase of therapy, in Morita's words, can be summarized as follows:

1. Isolation by cutting off social communication
2. Alleviation of mental and physical fatigue
3. Usefulness of the preceding two benefits for the differential diagnosis through observation of the existing mental state
4. Experience of suffering to a degree sufficient to lead to its subsequent relief
5. Induction of a feeling of tedium
6. Creation of a foundation for voluntary training with these processes

These processes are explained in greater depth in the sections that follow.

• Morita therapy attempts to accelerate the overall process of change by placing a patient in a special environment, isolated from society, to disrupt the patient's erroneous concepts of therapy and illness and to deprive the patient of contact with stimuli from the outside world so as to eliminate the condition of mental conflict that had existed before therapy was begun. In Morita's words, this environment induces cultivation of *junna kokoro* (authentic mentality). The patient is isolated from social communication and accepts the therapist only by confronting himself or herself as an individual, in a state of mind that discards all contrivance because there is no alternative except to rely entirely on the therapist. This attitude is related to self-acceptance. The patient can, then, cooperate as much as is possible and can allow everything else to take its own course. This is the reason that Morita considers this stage as the starting point for building the foundations for spontaneity training.

• A patient is instructed to remain in a state of absolute, isolated bed rest so that mental and physical fatigue can be relieved. Suffering is relieved and eliminated by a natural process of feeling once troublesome external stimuli have been eliminated, and the patient rests quietly exactly as he or she is.

According to Morita, from the standpoint of the psychosomatic theory of identity,[9] the life functions of human beings are harmonized by the rhythm of various life phenomena. Mental phenomena are life functions and are no exception to this rule. Interference in the harmony of life functions will arise if this rhythm is disturbed. Although *shinkeishitsu* patients do not initially have an organic disorder, the rhythm of mental phenomena will become further disturbed by a mistaken form of recuperation because of doubts about the cause of the trouble or fear of probable character trouble or psychosis, owing to suffering from subjective symptoms that cause disharmony and a lack of integrated life functions in many patients. The objective for such patients is recuperation through rest, but when they resort to trial and error actions in their search for various therapeutic remedies while still in an anxious state of mind, instead of true rest, they will experience greater fatigue. True rest is achieved through absolute bed rest carried out in social isolation, with stimuli from the outside world eliminated. The environment that is thus created adjusts the disturbed rhythm and promotes a harmonizing of mental and physical functions in preparation for the work therapy that will follow. From this standpoint, absolute, isolated bed rest becomes a means for obtaining an opportunity to motivate a patient's natural healing power.

• On the first day of bed rest, many patients rest and sleep better than they had expected because they feel reassured that they have been released from throublesome external stimuli that had previously persisted. This feeling arises out of a hope for success with the treatment that has begun, even if there is still anxiety over the uncertainty of an unknown therapeutic experience. On the second day, however, anxious associations of thoughts will again arise because of various mental anxieties and obsessions that lead to renewed suffering. However, patients undergoing Morita *shinkeishitsu* therapy try to bear this suffering as much as they can so that they may comply with the necessary isolated bed rest. On the one hand, some patients experience the isolated bed rest condition without complaints of anxiety or suffering, and other patients experience a feeling of tedium after only two or three days or as long as five or six days. (Differentiation from schizophrenia, melancholia and borderline cases is pertinent here.)

On the other hand, some patients lose their composure and are not able to adhere to the absolute, isolated bed rest condition. Such patients frequently get out of bed and look out the window, read, walk around the room, leave the room and talk unnecessarily with other patients or go to the restroom frequently. They have complaints that seem indicative of Morita *shinkeishitsu* during initial interviews, but the difference in their attitude during treatment is considerably clarified by the bed rest stage. Such patients have other forms of neurosis, for example, schizophrenia, melancholia, abnormal character reaction (e.g., asthenic character or weak-willed character) or hysteria.

---

[9] Morita, S.: op. cit.

Such patients, especially those with symptoms of an obsession, often cause difficulty from the standpoint of differentiation. For example, in some cases, such actions as washing the hands and confirming cleanliness are particularly frequent, resembling Morita *shinkeishitsu* superficially. However, the ego action is weak, conflicts are few and the actions are repeated impulsively.

Case in point: Man, 38 years-old, obsession, compulsive actions

When anything this patient is anxious about, such as a gas cock or an electric cord, comes to his mind, he repeats the act of confirming the lack of danger several times impulsively, until he is satisfied that there is no danger. Further, he does not confine such compulsive actions to himself. He persistently requests the cooperation of other persons. On his first day of absolute, isolated bed rest, he became anxious about whether he had forgotten to shut off the gas cock of the water heater that he had turned on to wash his face, and he left the room innumerable times to confirm that the gas cock had been turned off, regardless of the time of day. When he was cautioned not to leave the room, he persistently called out to ask other patients to make sure that the gas cock had been turned off. He pointed out emphatically that he becomes restless when he thinks about the accident that could occur if he forgot to close the gas cock by any chance, and he was unable to rest because he persistently requested the cooperation of other patients. This example represents a character reaction of a weak-willed person, and the patient's compulsion was managed successfully with pharmacotherapy.

• The experience of *hanmon soku gedatsu* means to shift from suffering by a complete change to enlightenment or to abandon suffering and become spiritually enlightened. Together with the stage of tedium, which is explained next, the experience of suffering is so important that Morita also calls the period of absolute, isolated bed rest the stage of suffering.

Although other means have been used in an attempt to alleviate symptoms, they have not been successful. In fact, such approaches induce a complex mental state of aggravation against a patient's express will, and the patient gradually becomes more and more anxious about being in a state of anxiety. Although such patients are partially aware that self-defensive efforts to eliminate suffering and anxiety by force of will bring only temporary consolation, not only do they not attempt to stop such efforts but they fall into a condition of repeating the efforts more and more intensely. Much of their natural energy for self-development and self-improvement is consequently squandered on actions intended to resolve their anxieties. When their motions of daily living are completely brought to a halt by absolute, isolated bed rest, the suffering, for which there is no outlet, reaches an extreme. In many cases, this phenomenon takes place around the third day. The patient's consciousness will open into a new phase when it is driven into an ultimate condition in which there is no possible means of escape. This condition is a new experience similar to liberation and precedes the feeling of tedium, which occurs next.

Because a patient cannot take any evasive or buffer-like stance of mind that relieves anxiety, the anxiety will be temporarily aggravated. However, the complex conflicts that arise within the patient as he or she becomes anxious about anxiety will gradually shift to simple conflict because there is no other means at hand than to face the anxiety directly.

Defensive measures taken against external stimuli will be reduced by cutting off actual, complicated and direct stimuli, but the patient's conceptual image of neurosis will then increase in relative proportion, and intellectual, defensive activity in opposition to this state of mind will also increase. However, because this condition is now separated from actual life activities, and because the intellectual measures are only conceptual, defensive effects will cease, and suffering will reach an extreme due to the impasse imposed by isolated bed rest.

Strong emotional tension will gradually subside, similar to a sea of mountainous waves becoming calm. This feeling can be considered akin to feeling liberated, as though a heavy load has been removed after extreme suffering has been endured, and the patient moves into a mental state in which some hope, although slight, bubbles up from the bottom of the heart. Morita expresses this attitude as *hanmon soku gedatsu*, believing that it has an association with the Buddhist term *hanmon soku bodai.* In other words, this attitude is a method of "not cutting off anxiety" but, rather, of "leaping into anxiety as it is." This attitude is also one of determination, called *omoikiri* (self-resignation) or *ketsudan* (decisiveness), that is, confronting reality face to face in the anxious present exactly as it is and accepting this condition without discretion.

• The next change that takes place in a patient's consciousness is a seeping feeling of tedium. This feeling engenders a desire to awake early and do something. According to Morita, one's mental and physical functions become relaxed unawares when one is placed for a long period in a condition in which there is no stimulus to arouse a feeling of boredom. Also even when a stimulus is strong, it will not be felt too strongly if it is continued for a long period because one becomes accustomed to it and is no longer aware of it. Thus, one's life functions take fluid actions naturally, in accordance with any situation. One's mental and physical functions always act toward adaptation. When one withstands the condition of absolute, isolated bed rest in which one is isolated from social communication and overcomes this situation, the stance of the hypochondriacal mind, which has held a dominant position until now, undergoes a complete change to a stance in which the condition that Morita calls *sei no yokubō* (the desire to live) becomes dominant, and the flow of the mind becomes directed toward the outside world. Morita expresses this concept as follows:

"Generally speaking, a healthy mind cannot pass time without thinking about anything or doing nothing" (see Chapter 4).

". . . When you place yourself in a solitary situation isolated from society, you will only then understand the desire which is motivated naturally. This is *sei no chikara* (the strength of life)." A Morita *shinkeishitsu* patient does not become aware of the presence of this *sei no chikara*, which he or she naturally possesses, because he or she does not have the time to spare from constant preoccupation with a buffer-like stance of self-defense."[10]

A Therapeutic Meanings of Work Activities

Morita characterizes the role of work in his special therapy with a basic mode of thought, as follows.

There can be no sense of life if motion or work activity is absent from human life. This condition is much the same as if a human being is deprived of food. Similar to the appetite for food, each human being has an inherent appetite for motion and work activity. Such activities are performed essentially by harmonizing mental and physical functions. This harmonization is linked with materializing the desire for self-development, improvement or innovation. If, for example, one's physical work is restricted or one is deprived of the opportunity to perform it, one will suffer from a disharmony of mental and physical activities.

Morita recommends work activities for patients undergoing *shinkeishitsu* therapy based on that standpoint.

• In the special therapy for Morita *shinkeishitsu*, the concept of therapy is not expressed to a patient from the first to the fourth stage. Emphasis is placed on becoming free of any such

[10] Morita, S.: Shinkei suijaku oyobi kyōhaku kannen no konjihō (A complete cure treatment for neurasthenia and obsession). In *Morita Shōma Zenshū*, Vol. II. Hakuyōsha, Tokyo (1974). (Printed in Japanese)

conceptual attachment. Therapeutic work activities are designed to provide work that enhances a patient's practice at living.

• In much the same manner as stimulating an increase in appetite, measures were taken by Morita to induce in his patients a state of ennui and tedium, as has already been mentioned, to create a desire for work activities. This approach effectively elicits the desire for spontaneous activity that all human beings possess. Morita believed that previous modes of work therapy for mental diversion and training were unsatisfactory because selection of specific work activities and development of a work schedule had been carried out mechanically. Human beings generally suffer and feel resistant when work is assigned heteronomously, as a result of emotional antagonism. This result is similar to the resentment that occurs when an array of rich food is placed thoughtlessly and indiscriminately in front of a person who has little desire to eat.

• Interest in work can arise only through the actual performance of the work. Engaging in an activity is the best method for acquiring interest in that activity. It is generally recognized that great interest in work may not arise at first in view of individual tastes and preferences, but that interest will arise during the performance of the work, and in due time the work will become tasteful.

Interest will be engendered by acting, devising and learning. For example, an 18-year-old man who had mysophobia also had a fear of small birds. When the man went into the third stage of therapy, which necessitated more strenuous work activity, he decided to build a bird cage at the suggestion of another patient. After consulting the therapist, these two patients made a simple sketch and had the framework of the cage made by an iron foundry. The foundation for the cage was made in a few days, the framework was affixed to it, all preparations were completed by wrapping wire netting around the frame and then the perch, nesting box and feeding stand were installed. The finished cage was roomy enough for two adults. The work role that each patient had was determined by drawing lots. The 18-year-old patient became the person in charge of feeding. It was obvious that he disliked this assignment, but he still had the final decision. One week soon passed. The patient wrote the following comments in his diary: "As the days passed, I did not hate the birds, which were so dirty, as much as I had before. Not only that, one day when I approached the cage to feed the birds as usual, I became aware that they had gathered at the feeding stand and door as though they knew I was coming. I was surprised, since this was entirely unexpected and, at the same time, I was deeply moved. Since then I have begun to feel a deep affection for the birds."

• The dignity and decency of work are disregarded in Morita therapy. Any valuation of work is ignored, and any work that attracts one's eyes or that one become aware of is then carried out. Attempts are made to improve any aspect of work of which one becomes aware, such as dealing with objects that are scattered around, not set in order or dirty: dry leaves may be scattered about, weeds are growing in the middle of the lawn or some area is too dusty to be used as it is. Just as a child feels pleasure in the manifestation of his or her functionality through vigorous action, work motivates an intention toward devising means to make something even better and, further, makes one discover an ability for handling labor with no regard for any dignity or value of the work activity, and this experience is eventually interlinked with self-confidence. This experience gives rise to an interest in any kind of work as such, with the dignity and decency of whatever kind of work it is disregarded. The patient begins to work independently and, unexpectedly, becomes aware of no longer being held in captivation, instead being fervently absorbed in working.

• Morita recommends work that can be done outdoors rather than work that can be done only indoors. At first, such work is simple, requiring little labor. Everything is left up to the mood of a patient, such as weeding the yard, gathering leaves and branches, observing the activities of ants and butterflies or looking at plants and flowers. The patient is instructed to stay outdoors for half of a day or a whole day and is permitted only to take a rest in a chair if he or she becomes tired. Walks, games and conversation are prohibited activities. The therapist, who directs this activity, does not give concrete instructions or strong recommendations or commands to the patient. It is only necessary for the patient to carry out the work independently by having him set an example for himself.

On rainy days, there is other work concerned with daily life indoors, such as cleaning floors or hallways, wiping windows, polishing doorknobs, scrubbing toilets, cleaning the communal bath and shower stalls and peeling potatoes. It is requisite for the therapist always to consider what kind of work is suitable for a particular time and situation to prevent work activity from becoming too mechanical and affording no opportunity for devising, maneuvering and adaptation. Also, as a rule, it is necessary for the therapist to be aware of the efficiency of work performed throughout the day and to be alert for the onset of a feeling of fatigue. Work is begun as light labor because, in general, efficiency is not too good in the morning. Because efficiency improves after one to two hours of working, heavier work can then be assigned and, although slight fatigue may be experienced after lunch, efficiency will improve afterward when the patient again becomes active. Efficiency will decrease again at around 3:00 or 4:00 p.m. The therapist needs to make a patient become aware that work efficiency changes with the passing of time and needs to have work conform to that natural rhythm or pattern.

Another general rule is that work should be carried out independently; in many cases, this rule is a basic tenet of Morita therapy, and working together with other patients is an exception. According to Morita, this approach is used to avoid the negative effect of making a patient feel anxious by needlessly stirring up a spirit of rivalry, overzealousness in activity or a pessimistic notion that a patient's work ability is inferior to that of other patients.[11] However, this rule is simply a general guideline, and there are cases in which cooperative work is carried out for the purpose of stimulating mutual assistance or improving common efficiency.

• After physical work has progressed, mental work is gradually added, but even at this point, Morita places the major emphasis on physical work, and precautions are taken not to lean too much toward the mental aspect of work.[12]

Morita cites as mental work such initial activities as simply observing ants or plants and flowers. Mental activities that are appropriate at a later stage include sketching, calligraphy, writing diary entries, essays and poems, versifying, reading, listening to music, playing musical instruments and creating handicrafts. Diary writing is begun at an early stage and will be discussed in more detail later.

Along with keeping a diary, reading is one of the activities on which Morita places great emphasis. Generally, diversion of attention and relaxation are the chief objectives of reading for use in therapy, but Morita stresses its utility from the standpoint of mental work as being similar to physical labor. The fundamental rule is to permit reading after physical work has begun to progress rhythmically. Morita explains that if physical work is considered a staple food, mental work is subsidiary nourishment. In other words, performance of work and experience at working are considered the principal aspects, while the intellectual or sentimental factors of mental work can be construed as secondary aspects.

Reading during the course of therapy begins with a book laid open in the shade of a tree during spare moments of outdoor work, to be read in a light frame of mind. Reading at a desk indoors is prohibited. Beginning with reading by this method is effective for patients with Morita *shinkeishitsu*, who often complain of lexiphobia (fear of reading) due to poor compre-

---

[11] Morita, S.: Shinkeishitsu no hontai oyobi ryōhō (The substance of *shinkeishitsu* and its therapy); ibid.

[12] Morita, S.: Seishin ryōhō kōgi (Lectures on psychotherapy). In *Morita Shōma Zenshū*, Vol. I. Hakuyōsha, Tokyo (1974). (Printed in Japanese)

hension or memory because of dispersal of attention or of not knowing what they are reading because their mind is not clear. The method of reading is to open a book to any page at random and read cursorily, just scanning without an attempt to force understanding or to memorize anything. A patient can stop reading after half of a page if he or she is not in a mood for reading. Also, if a patient has a desire to start reading again, he or she may do so. This casual approach to reading is an effective method for overcoming anticipated anxiety toward reading. When a patient with lexiphobia takes a book in hand, his or her mind is not always concentrating on the present moment, and the patient's attention can be further distracted from reading because he or she infers his or her feelings or thinks about what could occur afterward. Even if the patient does read, he or she will only become impatient, and what has been read will not be retained. Consequently, the approach to reading in Morita therapy is intended to alleviate a patient's sense of valuation, fulfilled desire or anticipatory sentiments in regard to the act of reading. All recreational reading matter is prohibited, as is reading matter of a truly literary or ideological nature. Only simple, practical, descriptive, scientific topics selected from the fields of zoology, botany, astronomy, geography, psychology, history and biography are permissible for reading. Poems are convenient as reading matter because fragments can be read without starting at the beginning, and because their rhythmical structure may well strike a sense of measured flow in being read.

Morita stresses that this reading procedure must be carried out with an attitude similar to that which is applied to physical work. In brief, various speculations that can arise from reading must be completely discouraged because they can disturb the act of reading; such contrivances as concentration of attention must be sublated, and a patient needs only to read to the extent that he or she can. If a patient can read even a little bit of something, he or she can accept this activity as being an activity having importance and continue to repeat it. This training method in which a patient reads with a submissive mental attitude devoid of deliberate artifice is the goal of mental activity encouraged by the act of reading.

- Keeping a diary is also a form of mental activity. A diary is essentially a record of a personal nature. To a patient, a diary is a meaningful record of daily or other topics and personal activities, associations with other persons, personal impressions or comments on weather conditions that have meaning to the patient. For this reason, a diary is an item of private property and, in principle, is not supposed to be exposed to the eyes of other people. However, the number of cases in which the objective is an anticipation that other people will read the record is not small. Although there may or may not be a positive intention, the fact that a diary does not remain in the hands of the person to whom it belongs, having been given social status instead, seems inevitable in all parts of the world. This phenomenon seems to be especially characteristic of Japan. It is evident not only in the history of literature but also in sociocultural or political history. Diaries of excellent literary caliber are still read by people of much later eras.

The high valuation that the Japanese have conferred on diaries stems from the fact that they have been a staple item in Japanese culture for a long period; each Japanese citizen views a diary as being a worthwhile contribution to human life, and it can easily take on an intimate character.

The diary method used in Morita therapy is akin to this point of view. Morita recommends that a diary be kept by a patient starting during the second stage of therapy, and he uses it as one form of access to the inner condition of the patient or his or her life situation.[13] However, a diary also has an important role in improving mutual understanding between the therapist and a patient and in making the patient acquire the ability to view his or her experiences objectively.

---

[13] Morita, S.; ibid.

A diary in Morita therapy is not only a record of private, daily experience but also a record of a patient's awareness of the therapist as a reader of the diary as an important source of information relating to therapy. Using a diary, a patient thus can converse with the therapist by means of the written word, without feeling much resistance as compared to the resistance that arises in direct conversation. A diary therefore acts as a vehicle for mutual emotional openness. The therapist usually informs a patient of the following essential points for writing entries in a diary:

1. As a rule, no restriction is placed on content. The patient can write anything, but it must be centered chiefly on the experiences gained by the patient's activities each day.
2. The time spent on writing entries must be 30 minutes or less per day.
3. The entries should be limited to one page of a 179 × 252mm notebook per day.
4. The writing must be legible enough to be read easily.

The method of instruction for writing diary entries is explained by the following example (underlines in the text and comments within parentheses have been added by the therapist):

Case in point: Man, 20-year-old student, fear of direct eye contact and confrontation

I get out of bed. This is the first day. After washing my face, I came face to face with two female patients. *Greet them with my eyes averted. Become agitated,* probably because it is the first time I have met other people after being released from complete isolation. (It felt good to greet them even if your eyes were averted and you became agitated. Do this again in the future.) No one was in the sitting room when I entered it, although I thought someone else was there. *My heart beat rapidly because I was so agitated. I thought this is not good because I would not be able to mix with others.* (Remain in that same frame of mind. Everyone experiences a similar mental condition when not accustomed to doing something new. Try to gain more experience in contact with other people.) . . .

I went out into the yard. New shoots have begun to appear on summer plants. I extended my hands in an attempt to pull them out. I realized that my frame of mind began to feel normal while doing this weeding work. *I can converse rather easily when I meet people if I turn my eyes away.* (The matter of turning your eyes away or not will be set aside for the time being. Rather than that, focus clearly on the fact that you were able to converse.) . . .

After supper, two or three people were talking in the living room. *As I thought I would try to participate, I introduced myself while trying to form a suitable facial expression by desperate efforts.* (You introduced yourself because you wished to participate. Doing this in itself is sufficient. Avoid any artifice.) . . .

This is the third day. *I believe I was probably a somewhat self-centered person.* I thought only about my own gaze and facial expression, and did not think very much about other people. No, it was not that I did not think about people but that my thinking was superficial and *I did not try to truly understand them.* I had therefore overlooked something important and of value. (Becoming aware of this indicates great progress.) . . .

Today, Mr. S. was discharged from the hospital. He seemed very happy surrounded by his family. I also wished to congratulate him from the bottom of my heart. I will be next. I was somewhat uneasy about how the farewell party will turn out, but still, I thought it is so sad to say farewell. When I began to think about whether I will be able to give as good a speech as Mr. S. did, *I began to feel some apprehension about whether I will be able to express my opinions like other people* at the seminar when I return to university life. (Such mental perturbation is quite natural.) . . .

This condition of living will end in another five days. Time flies very fast. Today there were four men to talk to, without any women present. *Conversation, after all, will be livelier if many women are present and life will have more savor.* (This is an aspect of a natural mind. Resistance will not arise while you accept this feeling as it is, and you will not suffer over this matter. However, there are some anthropophobic persons who suffer because they believe such a feeling is demoralizing and unclean. This is quite the same as the suffering you experience when you become aware of your eyes.) . . .

The television stand was completed today. I exerted great effort to finish it because I felt responsible as the one who had decided to design it, assemble materials and build it. Mr. K. saw that I was doing my best and I was very happy because he did his best to help me. (You must cultivate this as a valuable experience.) . . .

Today was a truly splendid day. I was deeply moved because everyone, including Mr. O. and Mr. K., sang for me at my farewell party. In contrast to this, when the time came I was not able to sufficiently communicate what I had been thinking about from the previous evening. I had the feeling that I spoke falteringly and incoherently. I regretted this very much, but I was glad to find out that human beings are not altogether worthless. When I return to student life again, *I will do my best one way or another by making the most of this experience.* From now on, I will not run away no matter what may happen, and I vowed to myself that I will say whatever needs to be said. (Whether this determination will be fulfilled or not will depend on how you put this into practice in your daily life.)

The preceding paragraphs are excerpts from a diary kept by a patient who had been hospitalized for 29 days; only a very small part of it has been quoted here. However, guidance by diary communication was carried out along these lines. This patient was asked to submit his diary to the therapist every day or every other day. The therapist read the diary at times other than during interviews (or, in some cases, during an interview) and carried out communication with the patient on that basis.

If it was possible, the therapist added simple explanatory comments in the diary in red ink, underlined the parts that he considered as being most important to the patient and, after the interview, had the patient give considerable thought to the comments and underlined passages. Changes of mind in accordance with each situation were indicated as being one factor in guidance and explanation. Concrete explanation or a strong stress on the therapist's mode of thought or efforts of persuasion were avoided, as we will explain later.

If there are words or contexts that are difficult to comprehend or if the writing style is too verbose, the therapist will ask the patient to make the diary more readable in such instances. In most cases, however, comments are confined to the initially generalized precautions, and the therapist looks forward to the patient becoming aware of this on his or her own and taking corrective action. A patient who writes in the diary by putting himself or herself in the position of the other party (reader) will become aware that this approach represents practical training for exercising care during social association with other persons in everyday life. The main points for concern are to have social manners that are not unpleasant to other people, to communicate one's ideas and intentions accurately and to elicit the opinion of another person smoothly. This concern can be understood as representing cultivation of a consideration for other persons' opinions.

Diary guidance of this nature provides one type of reference material that a patient and the therapist can acknowledge in longitudinal terms and, transversely, in the progression of changes in the mental attitude of the patient during the therapeutic process. Moreover, it can become a sort of guidepost for the future life of the patient. A large number of patients begin to keep a diary as a new habit and continue to keep for a long time, even after therapy has been completed. The diary becomes a form of spiritual nourishment for the person who writes it.

16

Instructions and Explanations Provided in Morita Therapy

We have so far provided a description, as a matter of form, of the therapeutic method in connection with absolute, isolated bed rest and work that is used in the practice of Morita therapy. We will now discuss the features of verbal association used in the therapeutic relationship between a patient and the therapist.

We may have given the impression that emphasis is placed on nonverbal rather than verbal communication in the therapist-patient relationship. The reason is that absolute, isolated bed rest and work therapy are the essence of the therapeutic format. Verbal communication in the face-to-face therapist-patient relationship was not a subject for consideration to much an extent, and even when this subject was considered, it was in the context of *fumon* (disregard) or in the context of persuasion, dealt with perfunctorily without in-depth discussion as characteristic of the therapist's authoritative attitude (see Part VIII). To expand our discussion of verbal and nonverbal treatment techniques, *fumon* and acceptance will be explained at length in the next chapter. In this chapter, the nature of verbal communication between a patient and the therapist vis-à-vis persuasion will be discussed.

In most cases, verbal involvement between the therapist and a patient is apparently interpreted as persuasion. However, because the essence of Morita therapy may be distorted by this notion, we must correct any such misunderstanding.

In summarizing Morita's views and intentions, we need to stress that he emphasizes the actual state of a patient's mind (based on the facts of human nature). A patient is not aware of this emphasis because his or her mind is in the *toraware* state of captivation. Morita places supreme emphasis on the experience of a patient. Changes of mind occur by emphasizing the kind of living condition that arises from a patient's mind, in terms of time, place and human relationships. Persuasion may be used only to supplement this experiential approach.[1]

Accordingly, verbal communication in Morita therapy is composed of explanation and instruction rather than outright persuasion.

In general, persuasion is defined as bringing a patient into compliance by a process of rational exposition used to convince the patient to adopt a new attitude toward life. It is a process intended to give the patient a logical understanding of his or her predicament and its resolution. Creating awareness in a patient and having the patient understand his or her problem is inherent in the instructions and explanations provided in Morita therapy, but logical understanding does not have a direct role. Convincing a patient by means of outright persuasion is intentionally avoided.

The persuasion method proposed by Dubois is representative of this method of psychotherapy. This method of convincing by concrete logic is used as a means to replace a patient's

---

[1] Morita, S.: Seishin ryōhō kōgi (Lectures on psychotherapy). In *Morita Shōma Zenshū*, Vol. I. Hakuyōsha, Tokyo (1974). (Printed in Japanese)

pathological concept with realistic judgment and understanding. A patient is encouraged, for example, to "increase self-confidence," "live in the present," "remove the mental fear of suffering from illness" or "pay no heed to suffering from illness and acquire the attitude of overlooking hypersensitive feelings," so that he or she can prepare for ongoing living.

This method may be effective with a healthy person who has mental adaptability, but it is not likely to have any practical effect on a patient who is captivated by *toraware*. In fact, it is possible that aggressive use of persuasion may exacerbate the condition of captivation. Such patients characteristically use this method without success, by repeatedly telling themselves to do this or that to alleviate their suffering, but this method only aggravates the symptoms. Self-persuasion is an immensely complex process, and to some extent a patient is aware of this fact.

We will now provide examples of how instructions and explanations are communicated to a patient in Morita therapy.

Verbal communication between a patient and the therapist centers around the patient's experiences throughout the therapeutic process. This communication is carried out not only directly, during interviews, but also indirectly, by means of a patient's diary and at other opportune times during the hospitalization period.

For example, when a patient experiences severe anxiety because of palpitation and an oppressive sensation in the chest and feels that he or she may die at any moment of heart failure, the patient may temporarily experience relief if he or she is told that medical tests reveal no cardiac abnormality. However, in many cases, such a comforting statement is insufficient. Even if such patients try to reassure themselves over and over again that there is no possibility of sudden heart failure because even they think that there is nothing wrong with their hearts, they have found from prior experience that their anxiety is still not relieved. Their past experience is that the more they try to deny such fear, the more they suffer from it.

Nevertheless, such patients still try to persuade themselves repeatedly, whenever gripped by fear, that there is nothing to fear because there is nothing abnormal about them. No matter how concretely the therapist tries, by means of rational persuasion, to remove the fear of a patient who is in that condition, the effort is mostly in vain.

It is natural that fear and anxiety will arise in any patient who experiences palpitation and an oppressive sensation in the chest. Such patients may try to avoid having these sensations, but the more they try to escape, the stronger the palpitation and oppressive sensation in the chest will become. The therapist may counsel a patient not to try to evade and escape the anxiety and fear but, rather, to accept these feelings as they are and wait with forbearance until the fear and anxiety have abated. Such patients have, in fact, noted that anxiety and fear have disappeared any number of times in the past.

Morita, instead, advises such patients to take an attitude of carefully observing the phenomenon from beginning to end and to accept its occurrence with self-assertiveness.[2] After enduring the characteristic paroxysm in that manner, such patients must continue to proceed with their ordinary life activities with self-assertiveness. The therapist instructs a patient at opportune times to accept any such experience calmly as part of a life pattern that rejects evasion and escape. By facing the experience as it is, the patient is led to consider the complicated neurotic anxiety that he or she misinterprets as a fear instead of a simple, real anxiety. This method is not one of rational persuasion because it has the effect of bringing a patient to an awareness of an actual change of the mind exactly as it is.

Patients with mysophobia who repeatedly scrub their hands whenever they have touched something "soiled," taking into consideration the number of times they must wash their hands

---

[2] Morita remarks that "the patient must let the symptom occur, observe its essence, and experience his fear self-assertively." The object of this method is to put an end to a patient's fearful anticipation of experiencing fear.

before all the threatening bacteria can be completely removed, finally suffer because this scrubbing activity goes on endlessly and they are unable to stop it until they are thoroughly satisfied. This is a complicated conflict that is not simply one of washing away unsanitary substances but, rather, one of trying to interpret a phobia in terms other than fear. Such patients are not aware of any contradiction in persuading themselves by reasoning what the limit of hand washing should be vis-à-vis their unsanitary feeling. The therapist sometimes provides the following explanation to such a patient. If his or her toilet were completely sterilized, would he or she be able to eat or drink something out of it? Considering the toilet sterile because it has been completely sterilized is logical, but the patient will still not be able to eat or drink out of it without resistance even if he or she has been logically convinced. The unsanitary associations of a toilet constantly overshadow pure logic, as a fact of the action of the mind. The unsanitary feeling that such patients experience toward their hands is, in all respects, emotional, and they cannot be persuaded even by logical reasoning, that their hands are clean after they have been thoroughly sterilized. They are not aware of this emotional factor.

As another example, suppose a person is convinced that, theoretically, traveling by plane is completely safe. Even so, the feeling of anxiety when the moment comes to board the plane is a different matter. Although people generally experience the same factor of anxiety toward danger, they board a plane with the awareness that it is simple anxiety as such. The practical factor of flying is given priority by habit, and anxiety recedes. Anxiety and apprehension are not simple enough to be eliminated by reasoning, especially in the instance of a complicated neurotic conflict. The factor of anxiety is subject to the growth of practical activity, and it may finally disappear owing to ongoing shifts of mentality. The therapist must explain this to a patient by verbal communication at an appropriate time so that the patient can accept it by means of his or her subsequent experience.

A similar approach is frequently carried out during interviews with outpatients.

For example, the therapist will ask a patient to listen carefully. "Can you hear anything?" The patient may reply that he or she can hear a particular noise, such as that of a ventilator. The therapist then tells the patient to disregard that sound. The patient follows that instruction but replies, "I can't do it, because the more I try to do it, the more I hear it." The therapist simply affirms this fact and moves on to the next subject. After continuing the interview for some time, he asks casually, "Do you still hear the noise you heard a while ago?" The patient will reply, "I don't hear it now."

This is only a trivial example of what the patient experiences all the time, but to him or her the noise is not something subject to intentional manipulation of his or her feelings, irrespective of whether it is pleasant or unpleasant. This therapeutic approach is more effective than simple, logical persuasion for having the patient realize that he or she will eventually become unaware of the noise, that it will disappear naturally in his or her awareness as he or she moves on to another activity. It will be impossible to disregard the noise during the time the patient tries to ignore it intentionally because it interferes with his or her life activities as a type of feeling that is disturbing and unpleasant due to a certain neurotic condition. However, by drawing the patient's attention to the noise, the therapist gives the patient a chance to realize that unpleasant, anxious feelings can change or disappear before he or she is aware of it because the patient carries out activities arising from his or her desires one after another while leaving the disturbing factor alone as it is.

Going through this experience is effective for controlling the mechanism of contradictoriness in thinking, which is one of the pathogenic factors of Morita *shinkeishitsu*, and also for diluting any deliberate, misguided attempts to eliminate fear or anxiety willfully.

For example, if a compulsive act, such as neurotic confirmation, is repeated over and over again, it is not confirmation any more, before one is aware of that fact, even if it is confirmation based on some kind of imperfection when it begins. It finally becomes an impulsive activity for eliminating anxiety, which has become a synonym for confirmation. A patient feels that he or she cannot bear not to confirm it, but the patient is not aware that the effect of the activity is something quite different from confirmation as such and that it is, in fact, an attempt to escape from the anxiety that would arise if that activity were discontinued. As a result, the patient's entire life lacks unity and the patient is thrown into confusion. Instead of the activity of the patient's consciousness being such that it surveys the whole situation, his or her attention is riveted on the one facet of confirmation. Consequently, the patient believes that he or she is someone who is more nervous or more fearful than other people, and this hypersensitivity (what Morita calls the hypochondriacal basic tone toward normal awareness is further aggravated by any willful attempt to be unconcerned about it.

This hypersensitivity is also conspicuous in the mentality (see Chapter 9) of patients with anthropophobia. The bodies and facial expressions of such patients become rigid from the high level of tension that arises when they have to face other people, and such patients suffer because they cannot converse easily with other persons. Because anticipated fear of facing other people is increased, they fry to avoid the company of other persons. They become disgusted with their weak will and timidity, and they suffer in the grip of a dilemma that they cannot resolve. Such patients long strongly for a state of mind in which they will not, like other people, experience such tension, but this wish makes them even more conscious of that extreme degree of tension.

The therapist provides the following explanation for a patient who has any such complaint.

Shifts in state of mind occur constantly in response to changes in the conditions that one faces. However, such shifts are not within one's awareness at all times, and even more so when one is absorbed in conversation with other pepole. In associating with another person, there are occasions when one needs to be more alert than usual, depending on the identity of the other person(s) and the particular environment. At any such time, when one may, by chance, direct one's attention to one's state of mind, one will become newly aware that one feels especially tense. State of mind goes through constant, delicate shifts, becoming severely strained or quite relaxed, depending on differences in the persons one meets or the circumstances one confronts in the meeting.

This is quite similar to feeling cold or warm with shifts in temperature and humidity. If a patient wants to feel warm when it is, in fact, cold, can he or she feel warm by mere exercise of willpower? The therapist will sometimes ask: "If you wish to learn how to swim but cannot do it because you are afraid of the water, what can you do if you wish to overcome your fear of the water by one means or another?" In many instances, the answer to this question is that the only way is to get into the water. If you are afraid of the water, you must become accustomed to being in it. Interest in learning how to swim will increase, and fear will decrease, if you get in and learn to swim a little.

The therapist can then say: "Isn't this the same as the condition of anthropophobia?" However, even if a patient can understand this question objectively, when it concerns the patient, he or she will not become subjectively aware of it or will think that he or she alone is an exception.

There are other cases in which patients are frequently instructed to make a firm decision by separating their feelings from their actions and doing something if they think it is better to do it or even if they are unable to decide whether to do it. Likewise, a decision should be made to do something with tension and feeling left alone as they are if a patient thinks the action is necessary.

In general, the feelings and actions of people in daily life are not necessarily compatible. For example, housework or studies, or associating with other persons, cannot always be handled self-assertively in a pleasant mood. It is also necessary to explain to a patient that there are many instances when actions are taken even when one is not "in the mood" or when one feels extremely anxious and excessively tense.

There are other cases in which patients are frequently instructed to make a firm decision by separating their feelings from their actions and doing something if they think it is better to do it or even if they are unable to decide whether to do it. Likewise, a decision should be made to do something with tension and feeling left alone as they are if a patient thinks the action is necessary.

In summary, the instructions and explanations provided in Morita therapy are communicated by placing emphasis on illuminating natural changes in a patient's state of mind and making him or her aware of that factor. If we adopt Morita's view that the hypochondriacal basic tone and *sei no yokubō* have the same root cause, the mental phenomena of *ki wo kubaru* (be concerned about) and *ki wo tsukau* (be watchful) are expressions of the natural action of the mind (force and direction) in seeking a place for realization of self-development, self-improvement and self-assertion and, at the same time, in maintaining one's safety under such circumstances. Consequently, the essence of anxiety and fear in a *shinkeishitsu* patient should be understood as originating from overconcern or *ki-zukai* (worry; see Chapters 2 and 9) in the process of life adaptation or self-realization and also from the factor of a safety valve for self-preservation. In that definition, mental shifts take place within an *onozu-kara-naru* (natural or spontaneous) mentality in response to whatever conditions we confront, and this phenomenon cannot be manipulated intentionally, irrespective of our wishes. It is thus clear that the instruction and explanation provided in Morita therapy are not simply of a logical or speculative nature because Morita therapy is "basically a natural therapy,"[3] as indicated by Morita's statement[4] that "the activities of man's mind and body are natural phenomena. It is not possible to control them artificially."

---

[3] Morita, S.: Shinkeishitsu oyobi shinkeisuijaku no ryōhō (The therapy for *shinkeishitsu* and neurasthenia). In *Morita Shōma Zenshū*, Vol. I. Hakuyōsha, Tokyo (1974). (Printed in Japanese)

[4] Morita, S.: ibid.

17

The Therapist-Patient Relationship in Morita Therapy: *Fumon* and Acceptance

When psychotherapy is carried out by means of empathetic contact, the human relationship between the therapist and a patient becomes an important subject for consideration. The reason is that the treatment process differs in accordance with the manner of involvement of the therapist, and this variable has a great influence on the effect of treatment.

Moreover, the relationship between the therapist and a patient differs from ordinary human relationships because it is not merely a friendly association; it also incorporates the fundamental qualifications for conducting psychotherapy, such as the personal character, professional technique and private sympathy of the therapist.

Further, the nature of the therapist-patient relationship and the interpretation of the treatment process differ from a psychotherapeutic standpoint. In some kinds of psychotherapy, this relationship is considered particularly important, whereas in other modalities, it is not.

Analytical therapy, for instance, belongs in the former category. In this therapeutic modality, the therapist-patient relationship is an important variable because it is a prerequisite of the psychotherapeutic contract, with the therapist acting as the listener in a process of free association. A patient's emotional history can be grasped from understanding the various defensive and transferential phenomena developed by way of the patient's resistance to the therapist. The entire treatment process lies in having the patient discern this behavioral pattern by correlation with the existing symptoms.

By contrast, Morita therapy does not attach any importance to the form or structure of this relationship and does not give it much consideration. Whether or not there is such an intention, a therapist-patient relationship exists in Morita therapy insofar as this therapy is a type of psychotherapy, and that relationship doubtless has an important role in the treatment process. However, almost no information is available concerning the therapist-patient relationship in Morita therapy.[1] The reason is that the chief treatment process in Morita therapy is centered on the actual life activities of a patient; the therapist-patient relationship is secondary and serves only as a setting in which the patient's activities may be stimulated.

The meaning of the therapist-patient relationship in regard to the therapeutic process has been mostly veiled. In reality, however, the meaning of a patient's life experience can be understood only by actively pursuing the patient's human relationship with the therapist.

To understand Morita therapy, the meaning of the patient's human relationship with the therapist needs to be considered even if it seems weak on the surface.

---

[1] Morita occasionally comments on the consciousness of the therapist engaged in psychotherapy or the importance of the role it plays, but it appears that he did not specifically study the therapist-patient relationship as a formal subject. A. Kondō was the first investigator to discuss the matter assertively from the standpoint of Morita therapy.

The therapist comes into contact with a patient in analytical therapy with the characteristic *kikite* (listener) attitude. What attitude, then, should the Morita therapist adopt in association with the patient?

In addressing that question, Kondō[2] explains that "understanding" is the most important variable in the therapist-patient relationship. This understanding comes from the therapist's personal experience of suffering from *shinkeishitsu.* The therapist can empathize with the patient's feelings as a result of his or her self-illumination through educational analysis obtained in self-applied analytical therapy.

There is a great difference in terms of depth, breadth and truth between this self-illumination and the understanding obtained by technical considerations. The "accepting" attitude that the therapist adopts as the basic condition for conducting psychotherapy is inherent in the unfalsified, unconscious psychotherapeutic attitude. Kondō explains that the therapist-patient relationship becomes self-evident if Morita therapy is carried out with that premise accepted as a natural fact that need not be questioned. He also explains that the understanding of a person with such experience is that the pathological basis of *shinkeishitsu*, in Morita therapy, is that of a normal condition rather than a form of mental illness. Combined with the attitude of acceptance, that experience makes it possible for a patient to proceed toward self-acceptance. Actual acceptance takes place only with acquisition of the experience called life practice, and this experience develops further into self-realization. Kondo's explanation is quite lucid, and it is probably most helpful to understand the therapist-patient relationship in this way. However, can this relationship be considered with an even more positive attitude?

If the therapist is the "listener," that is, the dialogue partner, in analytical therapy, it can be said that the therapist in Morita therapy has the attitude of "cutting off a dialogue role." This basic attitude lies beyond any differentiation of verbal or active approaches.

Kondō discusses the general therapist-patient relationship on the premise that many therapists who carry out Morita therapy have experienced *shinkeishitsu* themselves. However, having had this experience does not make the role of the therapist universal. Even if it is a fact, it should be assumed that the relationship between the therapist and a patient in Morita therapy can be discussed as having that special characteristic of individual experience. Empathy and understanding can emerge if the pathological nature of a patient's suffering has an understandable correlation. If such is the case, it is not necessary for the therapist to have experienced *shinkeishitsu.* The reason is that a person who has experienced the condition is not necessarily someone who understands it well. This issue should be discussed with the professional qualifications of a psychotherapist as a basis and should be considered as being separate from the role of the therapist in working with a patient.

Role of *Fumon*[3] in the Therapist-Patient Relationship

When the phrase "cutting off a dialogue role" is expressed in another way, it is called *fumon.* This term denotes the technical role that the therapist assumes to have a patient sublate his or her symptoms, and it is the most characteristic therapist-patient relationship in Morita therapy.

The term *fumon* signifies that a silence called *ma* (pause) appears by cutting off a dialogue. Dictionary definitions[4] of *ma* (pause) include *aida* (space), *ai* (between), *sukima* (opening), *itoma* (leisure), *hyōshi no utsuri-kawari* (change in rhythm), *koroai* (suitable time), *shio* (tide),

[2] Kondō, A.: Therapist-patient relationship in psychotherapy—On Horney's school and Morita therapy (in Japanese). *The Japanese Journal of Psycho-analysis* 7(6) (1961).

kikai (opportunity) and *sonoba no yōsu* (situational context). It is a word that expresses the connective aspect of change from one phase to another. This connection has both spatial and temporal qualities, and it comprises both static and dynamic properties. *Ma* is present within the phenomena of change.

Ma[5] in psychotherapy stands for the relationship between the therapist and a patient, and this relationship has several important characteristics. One characteristic can be considered the therapeutic distance[6] that exists between the two persons. The therapist who adopts an analytical stance creates a problem from the standpoint of having this distance constitute a neutral role. The meaning of *ma* differs in accordance with the reason that a neutral role must be taken. For the Freudian therapist, this distance is needed to prevent, as much as is possible, any emotional engagement with a patient. For the Ferenczian therapist, an attitude opposite to that of avoiding engagement is taken. This attitude is no longer neutral and probably exceeds the boundaries of neutrality considerably. However, distance is naturally established in mutual relationships between human beings. The analytical therapist long ago adopted the method of relationship in which the distance is neither too far nor too close.

A proper distance[7] is maintained in accordance with the situation. Some patients try to form an intimate connection with the therapist, at times rejecting this distant attitude, ignoring it and then trying to get free of it. A cure is in progress if a patient's attitude becomes the same as that of the therapist.

In Morita therapy, an attitude of becoming close to, but not overly familiar with, a patient[8] is generally requisite. The necessity of a proper distance is also included, but it does not mean that *ma*, in this instance, requires the therapist to maintain a neutral position. This *ma* has meaning not only from the standpoint of interpersonal relationships. It is quite the same inside oneself; it is possible to control oneself by maintaining a proper distance.

As a rule, maintaining a psychological distance[9] means that the strength of impression of the emotional factor decreases, as distance increases, from an emotional standpoint. A condition of seeing the self is understood as indicating a condition in which a distance has been established and cool, intellectual decision making is possible.

---

[3] Linguistically, *fumon* means "ignore," but in this instance the word means a silence based on the essence of linguistic relationships and on continuity of human involvement premised on dialogue. It does not mean only that communication by speech has been disrupted. It is an opportunity to open up the self and to grow by means of a momentary silence in the mutual relationships that take place between human beings, and to let the essence of life suddenly come forth in a manner similar to the effect of a pause in a theme played out in a musical rhythm. Max Picard says, in the preface of his book *Die Welt des Schwegens*, that "silence does not simply mean that human beings stop talking. Silence is something more than simply the interruption of speech." And at the end, he says: ". . . . the completion and meaning of silence for human beings is that of using speech only in places other than a place of worship. However, in worship, the silence of human beings receives its meaning and affords completion of the self by meeting a godlike silence." Picard cites Kierkegaard's remark that "the condition of the present world, on the whole, is sick; if I were a physician and was asked what to do about it, I would probably say 'create silence.'"

[4] Shinmura, I. (Ed.): *Kōjien*, Iwanami Shoten, Tokyo (1967).

[5] Fujita, C.: Discussion on a problem of temporal conditions in Morita therapy (*in Japanese*). *Shinkeishitsu* 7(1) (1967); On the meanings of *fumon* (disregard of symptoms) in Morita therapy; practice and theory of psychotherapy (in Japanese). *Shinkeishitsu* (retitled) 1(1) (1967).

[6] Doi, T.: *Seishin Ryōhō to Seishin Bunseki* (Psychotherapy and Psychoanalysis). Kaneko Shobō, Tokyo (1961). (Printed in Japanese)

[7] Kasahara, Y.: Seishin ryōhō ippan no chiyu kiten no ichi kōsatsu (Onto-analytic investigation on psychotherapy) (in Japanese). *Seishin Igaku* 9(4):273 (1967).

[8] There is no doubt that this attitude is based on what Freud calls *ärtzliche Diskretion*, but since the therapist resides together with the patient for a long period, it is difficult to keep a private life concealed from the patient. Even if no kind of personal contact during therapy can be construed as being not entirely private in nature, the professional consideration of communication with the patient is not lacking, and it is natural that a mutually intimate feeling arises and that the patient has feelings of respect and friendliness toward the therapist as a physician, teacher and father figure, brother figure or partner. The relationship does not truly conform to Lawrence Kubie's admonition to be analytically incognito or to maintain complete neutrality.

[9] Fujioka, Y.: An essay on pictures of personality by Rorschach's test (in Japanese). *Jinbun Gakuhō* 20(82) (1962).

Thus, *ma* expresses the way in which the human mind is opened intellectually and emotionally. Considering the past relationship in psychotherapy relative to temporal changes, such as *koroai* (suitable time), *ori* (occasion) and *shio* (tide), also has great importance.

In general, there should be communication between the therapist and a patient in psychotherapy. Naturally, speech is the medium for this communication. When therapy is carried out with speech as the principal connective, there are cases in which communication is present as well as cases in which there is none. Speech is not always the chief connective. In both instances, *ma* plays an important part in the process of communicating.

In Morita therapy, a special human relationship situation called *fumon* is necessary. The attitudes of *towanu* (not asked) and *toi-tadasanu* (not elicited) are infused into the patient. The therapist cuts off the attitude of *kikite* (listener) and, instead, adopts the attitude of *suteoku* (let it be as it is). It appears that disruption of communication has occurred, owing to both of these attitudes from a phenomenological standpoint. The mutual therapist-patient relationship has become one of *ma* confronting *ma*, which cuts off both time and space connectives. This situation appears to be hollow, empty, and it may be supposed that something meaningful will not be produced for either the patient of the therapist.

Then why is that disruption by *ma* so requisite in Morita therapy? If the therapist seeks a location to carry out this technique of *fumon* during the treatment process, the most suitable location is that of absolute, isolated bed rest because it is a condition in which questions are enclosed in suspended brackets, so to speak, and because there is no alternative to expression of one's authentic self in a cutoff condition that forbids speech or action. Physiologically, this condition is a kind of sensory deprivation; sociologically, it is isolation from the group. However, shutting off communication by speech by substituting *ma* does not mean that there is no communication. Communication is carried out in a different dimension, and preparations are made to return to communication by speech later.

A patient who has become a captive of his or her symptoms and who has continued to complain now has an *ori* (occasion) when complaints of uneasiness and pain are cut off, during this time of absolute, isolated bed rest. This condition represents an important *kikai* (opportunity) and also becomes *utsuri-kawaru ori* (an occasion for change) to lead the patient to the next therapeutic level. In this sense, absolute, isolated bed rest, which has a relationship with *ma* from a temporal standpoint, becomes a condition in which the self must face itself and thus a chance for self-interrogation. Perceiving *ma* as a method of preventing communication by speech, acting as a substitute of "silent communication," offers the opportunity to recover communication with oneself. Even if it appears that any human relationship between the therapist and the patient has been cut off, communication in the form of *sonoba no yōsu* (the situational context) is maintained.

Fumon is a consistent factor of the therapist-patient relationship throughout the process of Morita therapy, except during the period of absolute, isolated bed rest. *Fumon* includes work periods or outpatient therapy. This condition differs from absolute, isolated bed rest because communication by speech increases, and *fumon* becomes even more characteristic. *Fumon* is an attitude of completely "cutting off the therapist as a listener to the patient's complaints." Also, the evaluation of immediate daily life does not focus on subjective content, such as pain, uncertainty, distrust and difficulty felt during the process of activity, but, rather, is limited to activities that are goal-directed. Any subjective evaluation connected with a patient's symptoms is sealed within suspended brackets as *fumon.*

From a patient's standpoint, the activity of complaining is disrupted, and if communication by speech concerning the patient's complaints, except on matters of daily life activities as such, is not permitted, one is limited to self-expression within a restricted situation, similar to the situation in the absolute, isolated bed rest condition. Due to this situation, *ma* (in its meaning of "change in condition") is put into play as the turning point a patient takes toward the cure process.

The therapist-patient relationship in Morita therapy is not considered only a background process but, rather, as a treatment process that emerges more and more on the surface. The meaningfulness of the relationship lies in the phenomenon of shutting out communication, that is, *fumon.* There is a situation called *ori* (occasion) that changes (called *ma*) from a space-time standpoint in the process of human living, and the role of the therapist in Morita therapy is to adopt this *ma* in the form of *fumon* during the treatment process. This mode of involvement is the form of a consistent therapist-patient relationship.

18

Situational, Spatial and Temporal Aspects of Morita Therapy

As has been mentioned previously, the basic format of Morita therapy consists of absolute, isolated bed rest followed by work therapy. The purpose of this format is to accelerate the anxiety peak of a patient and, at the same time, to activate the adaptive abilities of the natural mind and body of the patient from within to allow the patient the opportunity for shifting his or her attitude toward self-development. Because Morita had a unique therapeutic situation for putting this format into practice, its features will now be explained.

Therapeutic Situation

As a rule, Morita therapy is carried out in a hospital setting. The conditions of the therapeutic situation, particularly space and time considerations for conducting therapy effectively, have not been examined in depth in the past, having been described only as characteristic features of such therapy.

However, the therapeutic situation must not be overlooked. Aizawa[1] makes this observation and describes the therapeutic situation in detail. Space and time considerations have important roles in accelerating the process of Morita therapy.

Morita set up the therapeutic model and policy by trial and error experience and devised the homelike therapeutic format.[2] To counteract a poor environment, which contributes to the mental alterations that result in symptom fixation in the *shinkeishitsu* persona, any chance factors or opportunities that can give rise to neurosis (induced by such elements as precautionary activities as the causal mechanism of *shisō-no-mujun*) must be overcome.

Morita also decided that the therapeutic objective is a patient's acquisition of a mental attitude that allows him or her to accept his or her mental structure and functions. For this purpose, it is necessary, first of all, to bring a patient into an environment that has a homelike atmosphere. In such a receptive environment, a patient discerns the origin of his or her symptom and discovers how he or she needs to behave in the future on the basis of direct experience. This is accomplished by means of the patient's human relationship with the therapist.

In the basic therapeutic process, before there is any intellectual activity effected by verbal communication, Morita established, as fundamental principles, absolute, isolated bed rest,

---

[1] Aizawa, O.: Morita ryōhō no jissai—chiryōteki kankyō (The practice of morita therapy and therapeutic situation). In *Gendai no Morita Ryōhō* (Present-day Morita Therapy), edited by T. Kōra and K. Ōhara. Hakuyōsha, Tokyo (1977). (Printed in Japanese)

[2] Nomura, A.: Morita Shōma: Sono hito to gyōseki to sono go (The human figure and his personal achievements and later publications) (in Japanese); ibid.

which shuts off contact with the outside world, and a working relationship with a patient through the latter's performance of nonverbal work assignments.

A patient is brought into a homelike environment[3] and conducts his or her life activities by concentrating on the most effective way(s) to spend each day. During this time, the therapist, as a rule, handles the patient by the method of *fumon* (disregard of the patient's symptom; see Chapter 17). The value of the patient's work is not considered. The sole objective is accomplishment of work assignments, but in a gradual manner suitable guidance is given to improve work quality and productivity. At the same time, the attitude of *toraware* is gradually changed. This natural change in the attitude of *fumon* and acceptance by the therapist may appear to be contradictory at first glance, but it does become the characteristic feature of the human relationship between the therapist and a patient and is one of the major turning points in therapy.

Guidance is given so that the therapist quickly senses any sign of change in a patient's attitude, so that the patient can observe his or her symptom independently in the *arugamama* condition.

The therapist can conduct therapy smoothly in each case because such patients, as a group, are mostly similar in the sense that they are well suited to undergo and benefit from Morita therapy.[4] In addition, the groups are composed of a small number of patients. A patient group does not receive supervision of daily life activities within the framework of a hospital environment. Rather, each patient spends each day by himself or herself, under self-supervision, almost autonomously. Further, the time spent in therapy needs to be meaningful to each patient. Needless to say, living with patients in this special environment is an important role for the staff.

Space and Time Considerations

On the basis of personal experience, Morita devised a hospital program of therapy for Morita *shinkeishitsu* patients; he used his home as a clinic, actually living with his patients.

This approach has been used consistently by Morita's successors, who have constructed

---

[3] Kondō, A.: Therapist-patient relationship in psychotherapy,–on Horney's school and Morita therapy (in Japanese). *The Japanese Journal of Psycho-analysis* 7(6):8–13 (1961). Kondō describes the psychological importance of being accepted into a homelike environment as follows:

- A special resistance is not experienced because the facility is so similar to a patient's home environment. Friendliness toward the patient is shown openly.
- A patient is conscious of the fact that he or she is a patient; however, a patient is not treated as a patient but, rather, as a healthy person.
- It is difficult for a patient to request that he or she be given special treatment, as in a hospital, and also difficult to evade the treatment procedure.

[4] Kōra, T.: Morita therapy. In *Essays in Commemoration of Takehisa Kōra's Appointment as Professor Emeritus*, 1964 (Printed in Japanese). In this essay, Kōra describes the *shinkeishitsu* persona as follows:

- The Morita *shinkeishitsu* persona has relatively strong willpower and a determination, as a patient, to recover and restore himself to a healthy human being by successfully overcoming his or her problem.
- If a patient has a competent therapist, the *shinkeishitsu* persona will acquire the capability of self-examination and be able to comment on the patient's inner condition.
- The development of the psychological process of *shinkeishitsu* can be indicated by an ordinary psychological schematic, and every aspect of it can be elucidated by psychological inference.
- The *shinkeishitsu* persona has a hypochondriacal trait and is initiated by some factor that acts as a trigger in personal experience. This mental impediment is further exacerbated by mental interaction and, as a result, becomes fixed as a neurosis.
- The symptom of *shinkeishitsu* can be produced by the subjective nature of a patient.
- The *shinkeishitsu* persona is probably nonsocial but not antisocial.
- The *shinkeishitsu* persona does not exhibit intellectual retardation or any factor characteristic of an emotional flatness.

their own clinics on the basis of Morita's guidelines. Since that time, the many clinics that have been constructed for this purpose have been functionally identical. However, the current trend is to have the clinic and the therapist's home physically separated. Nevertheless, Morita therapists have continued to function in their respective capacity in the therapeutic environment.

Instead of having the atmosphere of a confined hospital environment, the clinic is spacious and homelike. Fewer than 20 patients are accommodated at any given time because of administrative rules that govern operation of private clinics. In general, ten patients are accommodated, mostly in private rooms. Bed-rest rooms are usually separated, but in all cases a private room of some type is provided. Ten square meters of floor space is considered adequate for a private room (or bed room). In most clinics, the bath, toilet and wash basin are communal. The bed-rest rooms are constructed to satisfy the need for quiet isolation. Consequently, the windows have coverings that shut out direct sunlight and noise from the outside to eliminate irritating external stimuli as much as is possible.

In addition to the facilities customarily available in any general clinic, such as an examination room, pharmacy, consultation room, staff room and waiting room, the space in which Morita therapy is carried out also includes a kitchen, living room, drawing room and workroom. Outdoor facilities vary from clinic to clinic, but even small Morita therapy clinics have vegetable gardens and flower gardens large enough for cultivation.

A patient begins the treatment procedure in a nonverbal spatial environment. The important point is that the period of hospitalization is fairly limited in Morita therapy. (Morita limited this period to approximately 40 days, but it currently lasts about 60 days.) A patient undergoes treatment under this time constraint with the assistance of the therapist with the goal of acquiring adaptability to actual life situations.

Private and group consultations are provided, even though a specific appointment time for each patient, as is characteristic of many other treatment modalities, is not given.[5] In other words, the time limit imposed on hospitalization represents the total treatment period available to each patient. The question is how, within that time limit, each patient puts the guidelines of Morita therapy into practice.

The time and space conditions that characterize a Morita therapy clinic have been developed to provide the following:

- A life-style that can be accepted in the home
- An environment for life that has a direct connection with the treatment program
- A natural connection among a patient, other patients and the therapy staff

Let us examine each of these items in turn.

- *A life-style that can be accepted in the home*

Morita states that his hospitalization therapy is essentially home therapy, so the environmental condition is that of a homelike atmosphere rather than a hospital setting. The clinic is set up in a manner similar to an ordinary private home, and a patient lives there as a member of his or her family. In other words, the patient is accepted into a setting that resembles his or her familiar home environment.

In this treatment environment, the therapist must first prepare a patient to realize that the *shinkeishitsu* persona is inclined to slip into the blind alley of the *shinkeishitsu* symptom called *toraware* by thinking in circles. A patient in this oversensitive condition must learn to put a stop to such mental contrivance voluntarily.

Further, the therapist must bring a patient to a mental state of self-adaptability to actual life situations while he or she is still suffering from this mental condition. For that purpose, the

---

[5] Doi, T.: *Seishin Ryōhō to Seishin Bunseki* (Psychotherapy and Psychoanalysis). Kaneko Shobō, Tokyo (1980). (Printed in Japanese)

therapist must utilize the homelike hospital environment to provide acceptance for the patient and his or her symptom.

Patients undergoing Morita therapy suffer from anxiety and inner conflicts and from an inferiority complex as subnormal social misfits. Such patients are accepted into a homelike therapeutic situation that confers a keen awareness of mental relief and the anticipation of being treated as healthy persons.

The oversensitive, defensive posture characteristic of such patients is gradually relaxed by the acceptance of that homelike setting, and their strong subjective view of their inner condition will then decrease to its original intensity. Such patients come to perceive that their existence, their mental and physical life conditions, are abnormal, but they also begin to consider these conditions as being "foreign matter," becoming aware that they are not abnormal according to any comprehensive definition of the word.

This change in a patient's subjective perception becomes the springboard that allows the patient to understand the cause of his or her symptom and then to discover how he or she can behave to overcome it in the future. The patient begins to form, through his or her experiences, the conviction that he or she can associate successfully with other persons, and live as other people do, in his or her daily life by sublating intellectual considerations and impediments. A patient's experience of acceptance in the therapeutic situation, by the staff, is the first step in Morita therapy.

An important concern for a patient during this initial phase of the program is his or her association with the staff, chiefly the therapist in charge, and with other patients. Each patient learns to associate with a plurality of people in the two-sided situation of living with oneself and also living with each member of the group.

Therapist-Patient Relationship

First of all, the therapist's human relationship with the patient must be considered and explained. As in other commonly used psychotherapeutic modalities, it is quite natural that the therapist-patient relationship has an important role. However, in Morita therapy, this relationship is not the directly decisive factor that effects the therapeutic turning point in therapy.

Verbal communication and nonverbal measures in Morita therapy accelerate the process of absolute, isolated bed rest and the work program in line with the principles of therapy.

As has been mentioned, the human relationship between the therapist and a patient takes the form of *fumon* (see Chapter 17). The most conspicuous manifestation of *fumon* becomes evident during the first stage of therapy (absolute, isolated bed rest). Even after this stage has ended, the therapist does not, as a rule, treat a patient's complaint as a direct therapeutic object.[6] Any attempt to make a patient understand his or her condition intelligently, by providing a direct interpretation and explanation of the condition, will reactivate the locus of mental discre-

[6] With regard to the symptom of an individual Morita *shinkeishitsu* persona in Morita therapy, as a rule, the therapist first investigates specific peculiarities during the initial consultation and in the life history of the patient. The patient's relationships with other family members are also examined and clarified to pinpoint the cause of the symptom. If it is ascertained that the patient does, in fact, suffer from Morita *shinkeishitsu*, on the basis of that examination, the patient's problem is not treated as uniquely individual during the therapeutic process but, rather, is reduced to a psychological factor common to human beings as such. (If the patient wishes to live a better human life, a natural human reaction of being conscious of that wish is consistently experienced.) The therapist adopts the professional attitude of *fumon* toward the patient's complaint. Therapy is focused on how the patient accepts and resolves problems by means of authentic human responses to life situations within the framework of Morita therapy.

tion, or thought control, that the patient has exercised in the past and will drive the patient back into the blind alley of *toraware.* It is important to avoid deliberately attempting to alleviate a patient's symptom or attempting to change his or her mental set through the mechanism of thought control at this stage of therapy.

The goal of the therapist is to determine how a patient carries out daily life activities in the face of his or her complaint. However, the patient's complaint is not completely ignored. The condition in which the symptom is readily sensed by a patient in daily life, or the manner in which it differs from an ordinary, healthy personal reaction, psychologically or physically, is scrutinized from time to time on a case by case basis, in a spirit of objective investigation and examination (see Chapter 16).

The essence of the therapist-patient relationship is that the therapist neither completely disregards the complaint that arises from a patient's symptom nor, conversely, completely condones the complaint, instead taking a flexible, middle-of-the-road attitude, with *fumon* as the basic guideline. A patient learns to evaluate the achievements of the work that he or she has done in daily life. At the same time, the patient is invested with the *ma* capability of objectively observing his or her mental and physical reactions independently (see Chapter 17).

A patient then becomes aware that he or she can become self-assertive toward his or her work. *Ma* provides the patient with the means to realize his or her *mokuteki hon'i* (original intention to serve his or her own purpose). There is no strong repulsion or resistance felt by a patient in this *fumon*-based therapist-patient relationship. A confidential relationship is formed, and the patient's behavior shifts toward the objective anticipated by the therapist.

The final feature of the therapist-patient relationship that accelerates the therapeutic process can be considered, in philosophical terms, as a view of human existence adopted by the therapists who succeeded Morita. It is an attitude of trusting the constructive human temperament, the natural self-curative capability inherent in the *shinkeishitsu* persona, with encouragement provided by attempts to elicit this capability therapeutically.

The consistent attitude of the therapist (which may be likened to a characteristic atmosphere of Morita therapy) is one of accepting a patient naturally while moving through the *fumon* process. The patient is naturally infused with this atmosphere. The conviction that the patient can win acceptance as a person in society begins to form without him or her being aware of it. The same atmosphere shifts the patient's vision to other patients who are living with him or her under the same conditions. The patient begins to realize that other persons whom he or she believed to be heterogeneous and unrelated to him or her are much the same as he or she is. The patient suddenly begins to experience friendly feelings and senses that the speech and behavior of other persons are mirrors in which he or she can scrutinize himself or herself.

A patient carries out his or her life separately in this manner. A patient realizes that each person lives cooperatively by playing his or her part and, further, the patient becomes more conscious, day after day, of the situation of being naturally accepted and of spending the greater part of each day together with the staff centered around the therapist.

The staff has a double relational role of "family member" as well as therapeutic agent, combining an attitude of emotional participation with one of emotional neutrality. The anxious defenses of a patient are gradually disarmed by mutual observation and participation with other patients. Mutual sympathy and impartiality arise. The patient begins to reexamine himself or herself and his or her symptom with a new perspective.

As Kondō[7] mentions, "the patient is treated, each and every day, as if he is a member of a family comprised of doctor, nurse and other staff members, as one collective entity moving

---

[7] Kondō, K.: Tanki seishin ryōhō to Morita ryōhō (Short-term psychotherapy and Morita therapy) (in Japanese). *Shinkeishitsu* 6(2):47–61 (1966).

along with him throughout the therapy period. The patient is not treated as a 'special exception' but included and integrated into the therapy relationship as a full member of that 'family'."

The staff consists of the therapist as the central figure and a nurse, psychiatric social worker, clinical psychologist and cook. An additional staff member assumes a somewhat mother-like role. This staff member encourages a patient to engage in daily life activities among the staff members and acts as an assistant to the therapist to enhance the effectiveness of therapy. She assists in the therapeutic process and, at the same time, plays the part of surrogate mother.

To a patient, this staff member is someone who helps him or her sincerely, so that his or her daily life has a relationship neither too close nor too far from the therapeutic process. She makes a patient become aware of–and teaches at opportune times–information and manners that the patient needs to incorporate in daily life, acting as a reliable consultant and supporter.

Morita therapy is homelike therapy because of the inclusion among the staff members of such a mother figure. A mother figure was present when Morita began his hospitalization therapy, and it is probable that a close cooperative relationship existed between Morita and this mother figure because she was his wife, who played the part of cotherapist.

Morita explains this matter briefly, stating that "the assistance of the wife is important because the therapy is home therapy, and she acts as an assistant in therapy in the role of chief nurse." This statement provides evidence of Morita's therapeutic experience, which was more personal than is usually the case because at first he used his home as a clinic for conducting therapy. However, the number of clinics in which a cotherapist plays the part of a mother figure is currently not small.

A mother-like cotherapist is an important component of the environment in which Morita therapy is carried out, and such a staff member lends a homelike atmosphere to this setting. It is not essential for a cotherapist to be the therapist's wife, even though Morita's cotherapist was his wife. Any woman of appropriate character and skills, as major requirements, can fill this role.

There is still heated debate as to whether the conditions of a homelike environment and the presence of a surrogate mother are essential components of the underlying concepts of Morita therapy. As is true of the original form of therapy carried out by Morita, most present-day variations on Morita therapy tend to be based on the individual techniques of each therapist. In other words, Morita therapy is truly a "home-made" treatment modality.

This observation raises several questions, as Aizawa[8] points out, and it also is the basis for claims that there are limitations to the means by which Morita therapy can be carried out. Nonetheless, there are many real problems[9] in conducting Morita therapy in a general hospital setting. It is difficult to anticipate genuine success with Morita therapy unless a specialized team of staff members can be organized or unless a similar cooperative system can be provided.

Considering this matter again, the receptive, homelike atmosphere of a Morita therapy clinic has been shown to be essential for achieving the therapeutic objective. However, as will be discussed in Chapter 19, the effectiveness of a Morita therapy clinic will not be correctly understood if it is overemphasized.

---

[8] In the above publications, S. Aizawa points out that the environment of a Morita therapy clinic is advantageous precisely because it provides a receptive, homelike atmosphere that enhances the process of such therapy. On the other hand, such an environment has the following disadvantages:

- The influence of the therapist and his home can be too overpowering.
- The weaknesses of the therapist may be too readily revealed, and it may be difficult to maintain a proper interpersonal distance between the therapist and a patient during therapy.
- It may be difficult to keep the clinic in operation because the number of patients is small.

The first and last disadvantages impose the decisive limits on a home therapy schematic.

[9] Uchimura, H.: *Toraware* (neurotic preoccupation) and the therapeutic situation in Morita psychotherapy (in Japanese). *Seishin Igaku* 12(9) (1970).

The environment in which Morita therapy is carried out has not only a receptive, homelike atmosphere but also an atmosphere that promotes socializing to help strengthen self-confidence and to accelerate self-acceptance in a complementary, hand-in-hand manner.

An important feature of the therapeutic situation is that it prevents direct communication with the outside world for about one-third of the therapy period. Patients gradually learn, not by verbal communication but by simple association, that they must come to depend on their own strength and not evade the situations of ordinary day-to-day life. They learn this approach to living in a special setting in which they cannot avert their vision from the self that has been too dependent and evasive in the past.

This so-called process of self-acceptance brings a patient to understand gradually what it is that he or she has actually wanted to accomplish, and the patient will then move on to become involved in the real world on his or her initiative. The therapeutic environment provides the double structure of a homelike condition as well as the group setting that is needed to accelerate the social functioning of such patients, with the ultimate goal of therapy always being to open outward toward society.

• *An environment for life that has a direct connection with the treatment program*

One of the conditions for carrying out Morita therapy effectively is, as was mentioned previously, a homelike atmosphere. A patient proceeds with his or her daily life activities according to the plan developed using Morita therapy, but when the patient's activities coincide with the therapeutic process in a close interrelationship, the structural function of Morita therapy progresses effectively.

A patient will experience the absolute, isolated bed rest condition as well as work therapy (see Chapter 15), but throughout some periods of bed rest and during work, the patient will have human relationships with the staff and other patients while being cut off from the outside world. The objective for the patient in this regard is to think out how his or her time should be spent, within the context of the schedule set for each therapy period.

A patient must work for a specified time in this environment, according to the instructions given by the therapist, and must take the actions that are necessary for achieving the objectives of the work that has been assigned. Such actions are exclusively practical and materialistic; the patient experiences the activity of performing work self-assertively if he or she considers the work beneficial. (Some patients hesitate and think about this and that in carrying out these actions whereas other patients take no action because they spend their time trying to determine whether the work is of value. Such patients pass the time entrapped in the *toraware* condition of the symptom, and the therapist must instruct them to recall their original wish to enter therapy.)

A patient needs daily practice in the series of decisions that accompany such activities, their continuation, developmental stages and completion. The extent to which daily practice is instilled in a patient by voluntary decision-making is important.[10] The attitude of becoming self-assertively involved in such activities while still suffering from the symptom and while feeling defensive is not easily formed by a patient, but the defensive attitude is gradually relaxed,

---

[10] For instance, activities important in day-to-day life include those relating to the essential human needs of food, clothing and shelter. Food-related activities can be examined as one example. Patients who have completed the third stage of therapy autonomously discuss and decide the work role that each one of them will assume and carry out in a commitment to mutual cooperation. In concrete terms, the patients purchase foodstuffs, prepare menus, cook and set the table in consultation with the therapy staff. Meals are prepared and served on the basis of whether each and every work role assignment is or is not carried out satisfactorily. Morita comments that cooking rice is the most important task. Once the cooking process begins, it must be completed. The cook has to see it through to the end, even in spite of anxiety or loathing. The cook prepares the food not only for himself or herself but also in direct connection with the lives of the other patients with whom he or she lives. Cooking represents a type of training for self-realization of the importance of carrying out a work role satisfactorily.

and the patient can then scrutinize and self-evaluate the relatively serene reality of the situation in which he or she is placed throughout therapy.

This shift in attitude usually is evident in the entries made in a patient's diary, in interviews with the therapist or the patient's conversations in group meetings. Evidence of this shift in attitude also is apparent in a patient's daily conversation, in the manner in which the patient selects subjects for discussion, in the manner in which he or she meets people and in other forms of self-expression.

These changes appear gradually, as though thin layers of onionskin were being peeled, or at decisive times, such as *καιρος* (Greek), meaning sudden conversions of "turning points." This change in attitude and in an increasing degree of volition leads to the manifestation of *jijitsu hon'i*. Each hour of each day has new meaning, and each hour encourages the conscious orientation of a patient.

The therapist quickly senses such changes and communicates to the patient a proper evaluation, by comments made in the diary or during interviews. In many cases, a patient's self-evaluation is lower than that made by the therapist, but the therapist does not comment on this disparity directly. Instruction is limited to pointing out that a patient's comments are not confined to his or her consciousness, extending and making up an evaluation of his or her entire self. Or, again, the therapist only advises the patient regarding his or her life behavior concretely in the homelike therapeutic environment.

Morita therapy encourages a patient to acquire adaptability to actual living conditions in the outside world, accelerating the patient's understanding of his or her symptom and thus speeding up the curative process in a manner that the patient can accept. The therapist will at times strictly observe the *fumon* position toward a patient's complaint but at other times will instruct the patient to observe himself or herself and his or her environment dispassionately. At the same time, the therapist commonly takes the attitude of accepting the patient as someone who has the capability of a healthy person of adapting to actual living conditions as a member of society. This attitude displayed by the therapist can be said to be both paternal and maternal. It is also both mood-neutral and mood-participatory. This attitude is one characteristic function of the environment that is directly connective with the therapeutic process in Morita thrapy.

• *A natural connection among a patient, other patients and the therapy staff*

A patient lives in a therapeutic environment that has the features that have already been discussed. In general, however, a patient lives in a situation that prevents communication with the outside world, one in which he or she lives independently. Communication with society outside the clinic and association with other patients within the clinic are restricted. In fact, communication is restricted almost entirely to mealtimes until the third stage of therapy. (Even when this restriction is removed, conversation with other patients concerning one's complaint is prohibited.)

While suffering from his or her symptom, a patient carries out his or her life activities together with the staff. This situation might seem to represent a state of constant isolation, but a patient is not alienated from the staff or from other patients. A patient is initially concerned about whether he or she can live a normal life under a condition of personal separation but then begins to realize that he or she is fully accepted by those around him or her. The patient also realizes that he or she has gradually come to trust and accept the therapist. The patient, then, will foresee that, in this situation, he or she can live a life similar to those of other people.

Further, the patient recognizes that he or she would like to actualize authentic human desires more assertively, appearing in public, and wishes to have other persons perceive this attitude in him or her. This mental shift is a sign that a natural and pliant state of mind must be revived. The patient begins to consider, in response to reality, what it is that he or she truly wants to actualize. The patient begins to realize that he or she did too much to safeguard himself or herself from various sources of irritation, even if reluctantly, and, moreover, has tried with the utmost strength to escape any situation that might carry the risk of emotional injury.

When a patient reaches this point, the patient begins to realize that he or she has suffered because of thinking he or she had to live in complete self-isolation. The patient is not, in fact, isolated and now perceives that he or she can face and overcome the symptom that has caused inner torture. When the patient looks at and listens to other patients, he or she has a realization of living a life similar to their lives, but the patient also persists in thinking that he or she is partially different from them, so the patient cannot seem to adapt himself or herself to actual living conditions as well as healthy people do.

Nevertheless, the patient begins to entertain a faint hope that he or she could be like those patients, or even that this will now be inevitable. The part played by the staff members, particularly the cotherapist, who assumes the surrogate mother role, gives considerable assistance to this change in a patient's mentality. This mental shift occurs during the fourth stage of therapy for many patients.

In this stage, whether or not a patient is strongly aware of it, he or she begins to experience the positive feeling that he or she is fully accepted by the therapist as a whole person. However, the therapist does not communicate this acceptance openly, and the patient's complaint is kept in the state of *fumon* as his or her social association with other patients begins. The patient's awareness (or being accepted by the therapist, whose presence is equated with *seken*[11]) shifts to the hope that he or she can be accepted by all people as being a healthy person.

In particular, participation in group discussions (see Chapter 19) about life in the clinic and about group work assignments makes a patient become conscious of being opened up to life in the outside world. The environment in which Morita therapy is carried out has the double aspect of being homelike and also equivalent to the social setting of the *seken.*

This process of change in a patient's awareness is closely related to the following factors. First of all, it is a process that naturally induces and actualizes the desire of a patient to participate and experience self-actualization in the *seken.* A patient first experiences a therapeutic environment similar to actual living conditions but with the inclusion of the *fumon* factor, which excludes dependency on other persons and cuts off social communication. This experience occurs in a receptive, homelike environment that enfolds the patient, who has had a characteristic attitude of evading his or her *seken*, even if reluctantly.

In the physical environment of Morita therapy, a patient must participate as an individual. The environment has functions to elicit a spirit of group participation even before a patient becomes aware of it, in the process of going through individual treatment by means of his or her relationship with the therapist.

---

[11] A circumscribed world that serves as a personal sphere or reference and that delimits the range of one's activities.

Part V

Morita Therapy: Scope of Application and Practice

19

Special Forms of Morita Therapy

Morita therapy is applicable only to psychogenic disorders (i.e., neuroses) for which psychotherapy is effective. However, this treatment modality is effective only in the management of a specific group of neuroses that have the psychopathological structure that Morita calls *shinkeishitsu.*

Patients with symptoms of *shinkeishitsu* who visit a hospital for consulation and treatment do not consist only of those who have the basic form of *shinkeishitsu* or the psychological mechanism for manifestation of the symptoms. If the neurosis for which Morita therapy is most suitable is considered to be the pure form, there are also impure types[1] that deviate somewhat from this pure form.

Morita therapy is generally carried out in a hospital setting, as has been explained in detail in Part IV. However, all of the patients who wish to undergo Morita therapy cannot be accommodated in available hospital space, so relatively few patients actually receive treatment on an inpatient basis. Other drawbacks of this therapy are its cost, which is prohibitive in some cases, and the length of the hospital stay that is required. Last, there is the structural aspect of basic character and psychological mechanism, or the extent to which a particular neurosis is inclined toward an impure type.

To overcome cost and time limitations, Morita sometimes resorted to outpatient therapy or to diary guidance by means of written correspondence. Diary guidance therapy is carried out on a case-by-case basis, but experience has shown that the strength of a patient's desire for a cure, his or her capability for introspection and ability to evaluate the neurosis and the patient's willpower in adhering to the treatment procedures are important considerations in predicting the outcome of these alternative forms of standard Morita therapy.

As Morita says, symptoms of *shinkeishitsu* are originally based on a normal mental state and are phenomena that can occur in anyone who has a hypochondriacal tendency (the tendency of a solicitous character of being concerned or paying attention, which everyone originally has). People who have this tendency become overly anxious due to some chance factor. For this reason, Morita therapy does not consist solely of inpatient treatment measures, being applicable as well on an outpatient basis through the use of life guidance for patients with *shinkeishitsu.* Compared with Morita's era, the scope of therapy has been expanded considerably to include group therapy in combination with drug therapy for the impure types of *shinkeishitsu.* Outpatient therapy, group therapy and pharmacotherapy as adjuncts to basic Morita therapy will be discussed in this chapter.

---

[1] Takeyama, T.: Shinkeishitsu no fujun kei ni kansuru kenkyū (Clinical study on impure types of *shinkeishitsu*) (in Japanese). In *Collection of Theses in Commemoration of Mourning for Professor Morita* (1938).

Outpatient Therapy

The psychiatric clinic of the Jikei University School of Medicine, with which the author was formerly affiliated, has carried out therapy and studies of *shinkeishitsu* for more than five decades since Morita's time. Morita's successor, Kōra, and other practitioners have carried his work forward to the present. A large number of patients with *shinkeishitsu* have undergone Morita therapy, and the number of patients receiving such therapy has grown markedly since 1950, when it became so well-known that the need for outpatient treatment grew swiftly. Before 1950, few patients were able to receive Morita therapy in hospitals because of its cost or a patient's work or school schedule. Also tending to limit the number of hospital admissions for Morita therapy was the failure of family members to understand a patient's suffering because he or she appeared to be in good health and was thus reluctant to undergo treatment because the condition was considered merely a product of his or her imagination.

To overcome these obstructions to the widespread acceptance and use of Morita therapy, Takeyama[2] wrote a short report that described treatment on an outpatient basis. A medical system based on the medical care insurance law was put into effect in Japan after World War II, but an appropriate standard of application for psychotherapy is not included in the system. This omission has had a deleterious effect on clinical paractice of Morita therapy, with its fundamental principle of hospital treatment. The need for hospitalization in Morita therapy does not differ from the more obvious need for hospitalization in the management of other health problems.

Thus, this special characteristic of Morita therapy was not taken into consideration by Japanese policymakers, so that many clinics used to conduct Morita therapy are not eligible for medical care insurance. Morita therapy is, in effect, considered to be an optional form of medical care, and thus almost all its costs must be paid by a patient. For this reason, it is difficult for patients other than those from wealthy families to receive inpatient treatment. Thus, the need for treatment on an outpatient basis increased.

To meet this need and to improve the effectiveness of outpatient treatment, researchers in the field developed new forms of Morita therapy for outpatients, which included the concurrent use of various tranquilizers that have recently seen widespread application. Outpatient treatment was restudied. A number of problems arose in carrying out Morita therapy for *shinkeishitsu* on an outpatient basis. These problems will be explained in relation to clinical experience.[3,4]

Considerations

Morita therapy for outpatients is not radically different from therapy for inpatients as long as it is based on Morita's theory of therapy. Some researchers[5] consider Morita therapy to consist

---

[2] Takeyama, T.: Shinkeishitsu no gairai ryōhō (Outpatient treatment of *shinkeishitsu*) (in Japanese). *Shinkeishitsu* 7:542 (1936).

[3] Fujita, C.: Morita ryōhō ni tsuite–gairai ryōhō no jissai wo chūshin to shite (On Morita therapy–With special reference to outpatient therapy) (in Japanese). *Shinkeishitsu* 2(1) (1961).

[4] Kondō, K.: Tanki seishin ryōhō to Morita ryōhō (Short-term psychotherapy and Morita therapy) (in Japanese). *Shinkeishitsu* 6(2) (1966).

only of absolute, isolated bed rest and work assignments, and there are critics who suggest[6] that it is better also to consider psychological guidance, advice or persuasion from a religious or philosophy-of-life standpoint within the scope of Morita therapy, as a broad therapeutic approach. The author's views on Morita therapy in this instance will be clarified in the paragraphs that follow.

The most basic requirement for carrying out effective Morita therapy for *shinkeishitsu* is having a patient overcome *shisō no mujun* (contradictoriness in thinking), which is the kernel of the symptoms of *shinkeishitsu.* For this purpose, Morita stresses that a patient should leave his or her symptoms alone as they are (to cease all attempts to alleviate the symptoms) and to carry out life in conformity with the condition, obedient to the *sei no yokubō* (desire to live) that the patient possesses.

The basis of Morita's theory and the therapy system on which it rests is contained in the operational procedure of a therapist, and this procedure is given the general name of Morita therapy. However, in general, this procedure consists of inpatient hospital therapy, with absolute, isolated bed rest and work assignments provided. Bed rest is prescribed to elicit spontaneity in a patient by promoting consciousness of the hunger for stimulation; the work assignments develop in the patient persistence and direction for daily life activities. However, it appears that Morita did not strictly adhere to inpatient therapy, often providing psychological guidance. With this approach, even outpatients could accept human nature as it is by means of interviews or diary guidance by written correspondence, on a case-by-case basis, while still adhering to the therapeutic principle.

In accordance with Morita's mode of thinking, we do not provide Morita therapy only to inpatients. For outpatients, however, in line with Morita's therapeutic principle, we apply these alternative forms of therapy. The environment in which outpatient treatment is carried out differs from the environment in which inpatient treatment is carried out, and although there is no stringent rule for the therapeutic procedure, certain points should be borne in mind.

• First of all, outpatient treatment differs from inpatient treatment in that there is no specific environment for therapy for outpatients. There is no surrounding therapeutic environment that incorporates all of a patient's existence, including the neurotic instability that all such patients have. The therapist-patient relationship evolves solely from a one-on-one interview across a table in a medical clinic once or twice a week. (This interview format resembles that of general psychotherapy.) Consequently, a therapist must try, during the interview, to encourage a spontaneous decision by a patient to leap forward out of the framework of neurotic defense that he or she has been clinging to.

• For this purpose, it is necessary for a therapist to understand, as much as is possible, the inner life history of a patient. However, the essential feature of Morita therapy is that, even though the inner problem of each patient is probed in detail, the objective is not to cast dynamic meaning on that problem.[7] Consequently, the therapist must take a stance in which he or she accepts the suffering of the patient as the suffering of a fellow human being with whom he or she coexists, by attaching importance to the rapport with the patient that is developed by the exercise of empathy.

---

[5] Ikeda, K. and Kasamatsu, A.: Morita therapy (in Japanese). *Seishin Igaku* 8 (9) (1966).

[6] A. Kasamatsu considered psychotherapy, in a narrow sense, to include counseling, psychological guidance, advice on the life outlook of the patient and normative discussion of such questions as, "Is life worth living?" Within the scope of Morita therapy.

[7] In Morita therapy, an attempt is made to understand thoroughly a patient on the basis of his or her inner life history, but this understanding does not have a direct bearing on the therapeutic technique, which features *fumon* (refusal to function as a dialogist; see Chapter 17), that is, a form of speech that is sublated and "to be accepted without anticipation" (facing reality). It resembles the "discarding of thoughts and knowledge of the heart, in order to simply sit and wait quietly," as taught in Zen Buddhism.

• Important in an outpatient interview is a therapist's acceptance of a patient. With that acceptance, the patient begins to believe that his or her suffering is understood by the therapist. Eventually, this belief provides an opportunity for the patient to become aware that his or her suffering is produced by and results from his or her direct involvement in living.

• More importance is placed on understanding gained from experience through life activities carried out by a patient than on experience gained from oral communication. Therefore, it is essential that, during an interview, a therapist deal with a patient in such a way that awareness of experience is created. Since absolute bed rest and work assignments cannot be used directly in outpatient therapy, it is necessary to deal with the patient in such a way[8] that he or she does not evade life activities while the therapist relies on the speech procedure. Together with the need for experiential awareness cited in footnote 3, the therapist must bring the patient to an awareness and a decision that only he or she is in a position to accept his or her life situation.

• Consequently, it is necessary for a therapist to grasp accurately the core of a patient's complaints and, at the same time, perceive thoroughly the patient's present condition. The therapist needs to determine what the patient is searching for, what condition he or she wishes to attain and whether that condition can be reached in view of the patient's present condition. The therapist also needs to make the patient understand whether his or her desire will materialize in line with his or her hopes and wishes, and needs to teach the patient that all his or her uneasiness and suffering is not due to an illness. However, the therapist should not force this realization on the patient by using his or her own value judgments or oral persuasion. In this respect, the therapist should have a full understanding of the special character of the therapist-patient relationship in Morita therapy,[9] as Kondō and colleagues[10-12] explain.

• In the process of conducting an interview with an outpatient, a therapist sometimes provides a psychological explanation of *shinkeishitsu* or explains that the patient's symptoms are the result of human nature. The therapist may explain the progression of the symptoms and the treatment policy, but his or her first objective is to establish rapport with the patient. The therapist must attempt to make the patient understand that the success or failure of therapy will depend entirely on cooperation between the patient and the therapist.

• After each session, a patient is obliged to summarize and repeat the insights that he or she has acquired during the interview. At the next session, the therapist asks the patient to explain how he or she applied those insights to his or her daily life activities.

The major points that a therapist should take into consideration when conducting Morita therapy on an outpatient basis are summarized as follows:

1. The therapist must strive to understand a patient's condition as thoroughly as is possible by grasping the patient's inner life history.
2. The therapist must first ask the patient to direct his or her attention to the symptoms by means of his or her life experience.
3. The therapist must then encourage the patient to come to a decision to face life as it is, abandoning the stance of a neurotic defense.
4. At this point, the therapist needs to direct the patient to carry out actual living with a frank acceptance of the facts of his or her life condition as they are (the attitude of *arugamama*).

---

[8] This approach is what Morita often refers to as "plunging into anxiety."

[9] For a discussion of this relationship in Morita therapy, see Chapter 17.

[10] Kondō, A.: Seishin ryōhō ni okeru chiryōsha kanja kankei–Horney ha to Morita ryōhō ni tsuite (Therapist-patient relationship in psychotherapy–On Horney's school and Morita therapy) (in Japanese). *The Japanese Journal of Psycho-analysis* 7 (6) (1961).

[11] Kondō, K.: op. cit.

[12] Ōhara, K., Aizawa, S., et al.: Morita ryōhō ni okeru shomondai–chiryōsha no kihonteki taido wo chūshin to shite (Some problems on Morita Therapy) (in Japanese). *Seishin Igaku* 10 (10) (1968).

5. The therapist then guides the patient to acquire an understanding of his or her condition by use of experiential methods that lead the patient to perceive that his or her neurotic suffering is rooted in his or her life reality (self-acceptance).
6. Last, the therapist encourages the patient to carry out his or her life role (by acquiring sociability).

Therapy does not progress smoothly, without resistance: many patients try to accept treatment by relying on their therapists, but because their desire to obtain a speedy cure is strong, their symptoms may not be alleviated, even if they faithfully follow their therapists' instructions. Such patients may then begin to distrust the therapy or the therapist, wondering whether other methods or other therapists would provide faster results. Morita explains that this attitude signifies that such patients[13] are not placing complete confidence in their therapists. Such patients will not experience uneasiness if there is a guarantee from the beginning that therapy will be effective but, lacking a guarantee, they will begin to feel distrustful.

One reason that many patients do not have complete confidence in their therapists is past experience with various treatments, none of which were effective.

A therapist cannot force a patient to place trust in a treatment. However, a patient does not know what he or she should do if distrust and uneasiness arise, so that gaining the patient's cooperation by engendering confidence in the therapist and the treatment is important. Confidence evolves from an attitude of candor on the part of the therapist. It is basically the same as a scientific experiment: what is important is that the experiment is carried out, regardless of whether it turns out to be successful. What is clearly of concern here is that the treatment procedure is carried out, as such, because there is no way for the patient to progress other than to rely on the therapist and follow his or her instructions for managing *shinkeishitsu*, even if the patient has doubts about the treatment and its effect. An important attitude for a patient in this regard is that of *hakarawanai kokoro* (an open, accepting heart).

However, a change that can be assumed to be a curative mechanism will appear in the consciousness of a patient as treatment progresses.[14] In some cases it occurs slowly, in others rapidly. In both instances however, a patient does not ordinarily have a clear awareness of this change in consciousness at first. In many patients, the will to face life is determined autonomously (by self-determination). As such a patient becomes aware that what he or she anticipated has now materialized to some extent, he or she will become conscious of the inner change.

When that condition arises, resistance to therapy declines and the therapist's explanations are accepted more readily.

Space does not permit an explanation of all the elements of Morita therapy for outpatients, but the author will explain, with a few examples, some approaches that he uses to bring patients to the point of considering the essence of their symptoms. It is most important for outpatients to be made aware of the core of their complaints, to make them understand that their symptoms are fabricated.[15]

Most patients suffering from *shinkeishitsu* have a strong character tendency toward pride,

[13] There seems to be a similar situation in psychoanalysis. A patient tries to cooperate with a therapist as much as he or she can in accordance with the contract, but the patient tends to deny the utility of therapy when he or she finds that his or her efforts do not fulfill expectations. This denial does not mean, however, that the situation is completely negative because communication progresses within a scope of harmony and can be maintained because there is a positive motivation to adapt to therapy. This is quite the same as the situation in Morita therapy.

[14] A therapist must clearly perceive whether a patient's attitude of application is suitable. It is necessary to determine the extent to which a patient can persist and be cooperative with therapy. At the same time, the therapist needs to reduce, as much as is possible, the negative motivation of the patient and must provide suitable emotional participation to some extent, so that a positive motivation is also provided. As a result, the therapeutic negotiation will progress, dissatisfaction and distrust will be reduced in the consciousness of the patient and this result will change the patient's attitude in the direction of self-acceptance.

while being dependent, so that a therapist should not inform a patient that his or her symptoms arise from human nature and are fabricated. Instead, the therapist should have the patient regard himself or herself as having the symptoms in his or her life environment, so that the patient will become aware of the facts. For example, when dealing with a patient who has anthropophobia, a therapist first asks a patient how strongly he or she experiences this fear of people in life situations. The reply will usually be that when the patient faces a company superior, a member of the opposite sex or a large number of people, or when he or she is called on to express his or her opinion in a formal manner, he or she becomes tense, perspires profusely, and cannot look directly at the other person's face or looks away, and if the patient tries to force himself or herself to look directly, he or she becomes flustered and feels that he or she cannot bear to stay there any longer. The patient's face may become distorted, due to excessive tension, so that he or she becomes upset. If the patient gets into such a state, he or she is unable to discern what the other person is saying or conveys very little of what he or she is thinking about. When the patient thinks that someone nearby is looking on while he or she is working, the same reaction will again take place: the patient will be flustered, the hands will shake, the number of mistakes made in the work task will increase and it will become impossible to continue writing.

These reactions are common, everyday experiences in the lives of healthy people in a similar state of mind. However, a therapist should not attempt to explain or persuade a patient that any such state of mind is normal and thus is nothing to be concerned about because it also occurs in healthy people and the therapist, as well, should not tell the patient to be openhearted. Most patients who have such experiences cannot be outgoing anytime they wish to be, and even if they want to feel at ease, they cannot do so. Such patients will adhere to the state of mind and will have a character that has been strengthened because they have forced themselves to seem to be at ease while being deeply worried about their inner condition.

Instead of using persuasive methods of theory or encouragement, a therapist should ask a patient why he or she becomes tense and feels ashamed in front of a company superior or a member of the opposite sex and why he should not feel tense and ashamed and yet tries to relax and be at ease. Such questions are meaningless as such, but they do raise issues that the patient, who has been struggling powerfully to relieve the symptoms, has not considered even once.

When each symptom is considered independently, a patient perceives the symptom as being an obstruction or foreign matter, but when the symptom is viewed within the context of the complete phenomenon of human life, it is no longer a simple obstruction or foreign matter but, rather, something of life meaning entirely different from what the patient had previously supposed. For this reason, the symptoms of *shinkeishitsu* should not be viewed simply as isolated phenomena. There is meaningfulness in having them accepted as phenomena that express a concern for human existence.[16] For example, saliva is neither foreign matter nor a contaminated substance while being carried in the mouth. It is a substance that we require, and we usually swallow it unconsciously. However, once it is outside the mouth, it is foreign matter that has become separated from one's body, and even if it is one's own, taking it once more into the mouth seems unsanitary, and there is a strong resistance to doing so.

A patient frequently admits, with self-scorn, that "it is so meaningless to be captivated by

[15] T. Kōra explains this state as follows: Patients with *shinkeishitsu* find it difficult to look at themselves objectively, as they are, with a cool mental attitude because their judgment is colored and distorted by their hypochondriacal mood. Therefore, the substance of the symptoms of which they complain is often different from what they claim it is. Kōra uses the term "subjectively fabricated nature" to identify that condition of the symptoms of *shinkeishitsu*. (Kōra, T.: Morita therapy. *Nippon Seishin Igaku Zensho* 5 (1965))

[16] T. Masugi explains in his paper "Morita therapy viewed from Gestalt psychology" (*Seishin Igaku* 9, 1963) that the symptoms of *shinkeishitsu* pose a problem in segmenting the background figure of perception from Gestalt theory.

anything so trivial," while still complaining strongly about the suffering caused by the symptoms. The patient needs to discern fully by himself or herself whether the condition is "useless," as he or she claims, or whether, by not taking into account that practical consideration, he or she should decide on the basis of inner feelings that the pain must be relieved and then concentrate only on trying to escape from the discomfort and suffering brought on by the symptoms.

Actually, however, things do not go as a patient might wish, and as suffering increases still further, the patient criticizes the condition with self-contempt, claiming that "it is a useless condition, serving no purpose," as if trying to minimize the importance of his or her uneasiness.

A patient frequently gets lost in pondering the questions posed by a therapist, and will invariably reply, "I feel my ability will be brought into question by another person if I cannot speak as smoothly as I wish," or "I feel I am being slighted by other people" or "I have a feeling that the other person will show an unpleasant facial expression, and that would be painful to me."

The therapist will then sometimes ask the following question: "Is there anyone who does not become tense when facing a company superior or a young, attractive member of the opposite sex?" Or, "If a feeling of tension or shame is not experienced, is the other person, in fact, not a company superior or a young, attractive member of the opposite sex?" Or, "When any such feeling of tension or concern arises, is it not possible to control it or suppress it by exercise of willpower, because even if such feelings do occur naturally, they are not wanted?"

A patient who has ereuthophobia may complain, "Why do I have a stronger sense of shame than other people, and why am I the only one who blushes when other people do not blush and do not act as if they are ashamed? If I were an ordinary person, I could talk as smoothly as I wish in a friendly manner with everybody and could associate with anybody, but I try to avoid people because I cannot do this, and that condition is painful to me."

To reply to such complaints, the therapist might ask, "How do you know the actual degree of the feeling of tension or shame?" The patient is virtually certain to reply that "many people do not blush the way I do, and associate in a pleasant and friendly way with anyone." The therapist may then reply, "Does it really make sense for someone who suffers from such tension and shame to compare only the content of his own consciousness, which can be felt directly, with the condition of a person who seems by outward appearance not to feel ashamed; is it truly possible for you to determine that your feelings of tension and shame are stronger than those of other people only from that viewpoint?"

This question brings the patient to consider the basis of this kind of decision. [Anthropophobia and ereuthophobia (erythrophobia) are characteristic neurotic conditions in Japan but probably are not widely considered neurotic in the Western world; see Chapter 9.]

In another instance, a patient who has a morbid fear of desultory thoughts complains that he or she is having trouble because desultory thoughts do arise. The therapist may reply that such thoughts arise when the patient tries to concentrate on something else, when he or she tries to listen carefully to someone talk or when he or she tries not to think about anything and just rests his or her mind. The patient then complains that desultory thoughts become more troublesome because they occur unconsciously and are unrelated to what he or she wants to do and that when he or she tries to brush them off, they recur even more strongly, the more they are opposed, and he or she becomes captive to these desultory thoughts.

The condition the patient desires (i.e., full concentration on what he or she wants to read, think or listen to, for effort required in study or work) pertains to something he or she views as having great importance, a matter of some consequence. This thing is a matter that needs to be dealt with and that the patient wants to take care of. When the therapist asks the patient to pinpoint the exact nature of the condition in which he or she has trouble with desultory thoughts, for example, while engaged in extremely delightful reading, in which there is no end of interest, a very interesting comic book, a conversation that is so pleasant that one almost leans forward to listen or an activity that comes so easily and effortlessly in a manner similar to thinking about something so fascinating that one feels a natural excitement, the patient responds that the conditions in which desultory thoughts take hold are those that require great effort and hold little enjoyment, or conversations that must be carefully monitored. The patient realizes that it is a matter of something that is not going to turn out as he or she originally wanted it to or that something unrelated to what he or she is hoping for arises in his or her mind, without any relation to his or her desire, and the patient wants to know the reason and also says that he or she has had no such experience in the past. The therapist then pursues the patient's doubts. "Up to now, was there not at least one occasion when you were thinking about something, and you suddenly recalled a task you had to do that was entirely unrelated, and as a result you were able to do something you had forgotten about?" Or, "Even when you were doing something else, did you not think suddenly about something that was not directly related to it?" Or, "Do you always have thoughts directed only by your will?"

The following question may then be posed: "When you strain your ears, you will no doubt hear different noses, though very slightly, but during our conversation have those noises been offensive to your ears?"

The patient replies that he or she had not heard any noise until the therapist directed him or her to listen. "Now that you have been informed about the noise, you will be able to hear the noise without particularly straining your ears. If you try not to listen to the noise because you do not wish to listen to it, will it become silent in line with your wishes?" Likewise, "You believe desultory thoughts have not appeared up to now, but is not that because you had not become aware of them?"

Also, one sometimes comes upon the following example. This is a symptom that can probably be called a morbid fear of not being able to put things in order or the inability to be perfect. A patient tries to dispose of documents that are no longer in use, but a feeling that they may become useful again at some later date may arise suddenly, and as a result the patient cannot dispose of them and suffers from the complication of having the undisposed documents still stacked on the desk in front of him or her.

The suffering comes from worrying about the possibility of disposing of something of value by mistake that may be needed in the future. The papers could be disposed of, and there would be no suffering if that worry did not arise, but the patient interprets this tug of uncertainty as being abnormal. Separating what is needed from what is not needed, without any doubt or hesitation when putting things in order, seems normal to the patient. The patient's notion that there should be no ambivalence becomes the basis for his or her life attitude.

In view of this attitude, the essence of the patient's suffering has already shifted to the uncertainty that arises from his or her attempt to decide one way or the other, with no relation to his or her original intention of putting the documents in order. The patient suffers without becoming aware that his or her intention was impossible. This state of mind is due, in many cases, to the fact that a minor incident, such as having the past experience of an error occasioned by carelessly throwing away something that was needed, or knowing someone who did something similar, comes to the forefront of the patient's awareness, and a neurotic preoccupation is gradually strengthened by his or her attempt to avoid thoughts that arise naturally when someone is putting things in order, with a motive similar to this at the start.

The patient will not become aware that he or she is making an unnatural judgment, from a point of view that is contrary to the human facts of the situation, distracted by a feeling that even slight ambiguity should not be present in one's mind when putting things in order, as a fixed standard.

The therapist may ask a question that will make the patient aware that when some sort of decision must be made by any human being in everyday life, a selection is made in a condition of the mind in which ambiguity exists to some extent, rather than in a clearly decisive state of mind. A similar therapeutic approach is used for patients with mysophobia or acrophobia. Without exception, such patients suffer from an impossible expectation that their sense of uncleanliness will disappear and that they will be able to touch anything they wish, like any other human being. Again their sense of uncleanliness would disappear and there would be no need to wash their hands repeatedly. They will likewise set up impossible expectations that run counter to the facts of the natural human mind if uneasiness is not experienced in high places.

The therapist should have such a patient become aware of how the sense of uncleanliness and the fear of great heights arise from past experiences that formed the seeds of these special sensitivities, all of which are reactions of a natural human mind. The therapist should give the patient examples of various real-life situations, explain to the patient that even if the emotional reaction to such sensitivities is that of a strong, resistant pressure, the original feeling is not something that can simply be discarded. If an attempt is made to discard the feeling, the resistance will increase even further. There is no alternative to conducting life activities in accordance with the facts of a situation, on the basis of self-development, with the resistance left alone to be felt as it is. For that purpose, the therapist should constantly try, during each interview, to make the patient understand how his or her symptoms arise and how they are strengthened.

The question asked by the therapist for that purpose does not have much importance, in itself, but to a patient in a condition in which the issue is serious, it is a question that represents a "dead angle" of thought, something of which the patient had not been aware, revealing a fact of the human mind of which he or she naturally needs to become aware, with a content he or she has not even considered because of his or her lack of awareness.

The patient will start to think about the condition, in which suffering is increased as soon as the meaning of the question posed by the therapist comes to mind, and will try to think again about what he or she is really looking for. The attitude of the patient in trying to look straightforwardly at the problem, by putting a question to himself or herself in that manner, instead of letting loose of the symptoms, puts the patient into direct confrontation with his or her suffering.

When Morita therapy is carried out with hospitalized patients, it begins with a period of absolute, isolated bed rest. Because in this period there is no means for a patient to divert feelings of uneasiness, the patient is placed in a situation of having to experience uneasiness and suffering of mind just as they are. However, the patient is not in a position to decide, with a clear attitude, the exact nature of this uneasiness, nor will self-acceptance appear immediately. When suffering is finally accepted as suffering, with no means to control it, so that it reaches its limit, there will be a complete change in the patient because a strong feeling of boredom will set in.[17]

In the treatment of outpatients, this extreme condition, which necessitates the final acceptance of uneasiness, at least temporarily with absolute, isolated bed rest, does not occur. In the various conditions of the lives of such patients, they must form their own decisions of attitude by their autonomous will, so that the procedure used by a therapist is made more difficult.

A therapist must bring a patient to the point of deciding to let go of his or her old role of

[17] It is believed that this change of mind is due to a deficiency of stimuli that appears in reaction to a kind of sensory deprivation, but this process is not simply physiological because it has, at the same time, meaning from psychological as well as psychosociological standpoints. The self-autonomy (which Morita calls the desire to live) of a patient's healthy character is liberated by producing a condition of a so-called famine of social association by isolating the patient from all human contact. It is interesting to note that this change of mind does not appear easily in hysteric patients whose uneasiness increases when they are placed in a situation of absolute, isolated bed rest. This type of patient is not able to withstand that condition.

avoiding a confrontation with reality because it will make him or her suffer from the symptoms. The patient needs to put into practice a new role of suffering from the symptoms exactly as they are. As long as the patient continues to adhere to the old attitude of neurotic defense, he or she will have to face the fact that nothing his or her "true self" desires can arise from a condition in which no progress is possible.

When Morita says that "there is no way to proceed than to frankly recognize the natural human mind," he is talking about this new kind of awareness. If the desire for self-realization becomes stronger than the neurotic defense, it is natural that mental resistance formed by the facts of reality will also be strengthened. The only path to self-understanding is that of "acceptance of what is, as it is." If a patient with *shinkeishitsu* does not openly accept this fact of reality, his or her neurotic preoccupation is strengthened in the process of trying to avoid uneasiness, as well as the additional uneasiness that arises from doing that. The incomplete feeling that accompanies a sense of self-reproach, owing to discarding the former role of struggling to escape reality, will overlap this uneasiness. Further, the patient's inner feuding over the failure or inability to overcome the uneasiness in facing reality is added to his or her condition, so that he or she must now suffer multiple aspects of uneasiness.

To help a patient who suffers from multiple aspects of uneasiness during each treatment session, a therapist needs to consider and examine how the patient's life activities, which were discussed in a previous session, are developing practically in real life. The therapist also needs to consider repeatedly how the content of instruction for this scheme of activities has been and will be put into practice during the interval until the next session. The therapist does not adopt, as an important topic for each session, the patient's complaints of symptoms.

These few examples have been offered to elucidate somewhat the approach that is used in carrying out Morita therapy on an outpatient basis. The author encounters each of the symptoms that have been discussed in daily clinical work. The author does not make an attempt to discuss the special features of each symptom with a patient but deems it a key point to ask the patient about the symptoms only as a therapeutic means to make the patient aware of what the core of his or her complaints consists of, by calling upon the autonomy of the patient's human nature.

Because of the widespread need for Morita therapy, treatment is not limited to a small number of hospitalized patients, instead being made available to a much larger population on an outpatient basis. Use of the outpatient approach cuts costs, reduces the commitment of time that a patient must make and fosters easier acceptance by family members, enabling more patients who need Morita therapy to receive it and benefit from it.

Group Therapy

It is hardly necessary to mention the effect of group therapy on individual patients. The dynamics of this form of therapy were long ago discussed in a systematic manner in the Western nations. The number of studies on group therapy increased rapidly during the 1940s, and remarkable progress has been made in its application.[18] However, group therapy in Japan is a relatively recent development, being around only 20 years-old. Without immediate concern with its dynamics, Japanese therapists hope to demonstrate the effectiveness of the technique through widespread application.

[18] Dreikurs, R. and Corsini, R.: Twenty years of group psychotherapy–Purposes, methods and mechanisms. *American Journal of Psychiatry* 110:560–575 (1954).

In regard to structure and application, there are different types of group therapy, as well as community care, for example, that allow schizophrenic patients to return to society as healthy, functioning members.[19] Although the benefits of group therapy are universally recognized, this treatment modality[20] did not develop as readily in Japan as did individual therapy. During Morita's lifetime, group therapy was not in general use. Accordingly, Morita therapy was long considered a unique treatment modality,[21] in being a type of individual therapy that provides the basic structure for conducting group therapy. The group structure used in Morita therapy and its inplications will be discussed in this section.

Group Characteristics

Ever since Morita therapy was introduced, it has been conducted in hospitals as a rule. Usually ten to 20 patients undergo treatment as a group.

The patients are, of course, gathered together by chance, and there is no special cohesiveness among group members. Each patient has his or her own relationship with the therapist, and each patient undergoes treatment within a stipulated framework, participating in activities of daily living on that basis.

At first glance, it might appear that going to the same clinic and having the same mode of life while undergoing treatment would tend to make the patients exhibit cohesiveness as members of a group. This is not the case because Morita therapy is a form of individual therapy, and patients thus live their own lives.

Nevertheless, Morita therapy is characterized by a certain grouplike configuration[22] because each patient undergoes the same form of treatment, a feature that tends to draw together members of the group. A therapist has an individual relationship with a number of patients who gradually get acquainted with each other.

Each patient group constitutes a therapeutic community.[23] Further, participating as a group member is equivalent to living as a member of a local community. The purpose of

---

[19] Such therapy consists chiefly of homelife guidance and homelife treatment carried out in mental institutions. A therapist does not delve deeply into the unrealistic world of a patient. Instead, the therapist conducts realistic studies, as representative of the realistic world, to raise the patient's understanding to the psychotherapist's realistic level. The patient then adopts the objective of adaptation to society from a daily life standpoint through a course of practical education. This approach resembles M. Jones's social learning in some respects.

[20] There is no satisfactory definition of group therapy, but from a practical point of view after the definition of R. Corsini (*Method of Group Psychotherapy*, McGraw-Hill, 1957), it is a means of therapy in which the objective is to ameliorate the symptoms of each member of the group to restore his or her social adaptability by a specially controlled process in a protected group that is formally organized. According to this description, however, Morita therapy cannot be considered as being group therapy in the true sense. The reason is that a Morita therapy group is not organized intentionally, and support for the therapeutic process through the group is not much anticipated, although in terms of the results, the group does have an influence.

[21] Morita does not consider the therapy that he developed for *shinkeishitsu* to be a form of group therapy. He opposes group therapy on the grounds that its therapeutic effect cannot be anticipated through cooperative work in a group. He did, however, hold group meetings with patients who had already started to undergo treatment. The meetings were held periodically as social gatherings. However, Morita soon began group counseling for aftercare of patients who had been discharged from hospitals and for homelife guidance for patients who were still hospitalized. He began to use this approach around 1929, but even after his death, many Morita therapists continued to use the same type of group therapy. Morita lectured on topics that involve daily life for about two hours after supper each evening. He also held question and answer sessions and had his patients express their opinions. This was the beginning of the group counseling format called the *keigai-kai.*

[22] The small group that is receiving treatment is in a situation in which the members are gathered together at one location to confront each other, experience individual impressions and perceptions and exert a mutual effect on the group as a whole.

[23] The therapeutic community referred to differs from that of M. Jones. It has no supervisory or any other particular feature and refers only to a small group from a therapeutic standpoint.

Morita therapy is to allow such patients to return to society as healthy, functioning human beings, so it includes social training.

Thus, Morita therapy has a group therapy and social learning structure, with individual therapy as its nucleus. However, even if the therapeutic environment has the feature of a group structure, it cannot truly be called group therapy if that structural characteristic is not intentionally utilized. The problem that arises is how to utilize the dynamics of the group structure in a systematic manner, and this issue is the heart of the matter in extrapolating to group therapy from the principles of Morita therapy, a treatment modality that was developed as a type of individual therapy.

Group Structure

Inpatients have a relationship that can be considered to represent complete life contact with a therapist. However, the relationship is strongly "vertical." Interpersonal sentiment gradually forms among patients who are brought together, and orderly vertical relationships are formed on the basis of character, age, sex, occupation, education, and length of time in treatment. Eventually, a group hierarchy akin to that of society will be formed. The common characteristic of having the same therapeutic purpose is heavily underscored, so it is difficult for patients to form ordinary "horizontal" relationships of near equality.

Nonetheless, a feeling of wanting to have warm relationships with other patients lies dormant in the consciousness of each patient. As a result, the functions of a family-like group begin to appear, owing to the receptive attitude of the therapist[24] and the homelike atmosphere of the clinic.[25] Formation of a family-like group is stressed as a special feature of the environment in which Morita therapy takes place.[26-28] Although a family-like structure has a cushioning effect that relaxes the emotional tensions of a patient, it does not necessarily support the therapeutic process with any consistency. The dual structure of the vertical ranking of patients' relationships with each other and the family-like group relationship must be considered as having therapeutic benefit in helping relieve the symptoms of *shinkeishitsu.*

Symptom Structure of *Shinkeishitsu*

The symptoms of *shinkeishitsu* have a complicated structure akin to the fundamental characteristics of *shinkeishitsu* as such.[29]

The dual structure of relationships can be observed in each patient, who experiences intense uneasiness, tension and fear, but at the same time wishes to participate in a group and

24 Morita and many of his successors personally experienced *shinkeishitsu* to some extent, but they learned to overcome it. This experience increases a therapist's understanding and sympathy toward his or her patients. As was explained in Chapter 6, Morita asserts that patients who suffer from *shinkeishitsu* acquire an understanding that it is not a condition of inferiority vis-a-vis ordinary people, nor is it morbid; it signifies a strong desire to live as a healthy human being. The suffering is caused by ideological and idealistic attitudes. A therapist accepts a patient as a comrade who has come to open the door to the world of healthy human relationships. The patient begins to acquire the awareness of being in a clinic that has a "homelike" atmosphere in which he or she is readily accepted.

25 Morita treated patients with *shinkeishitsu* in his home. He calls this approach "home therapy." This therapy does not have the indifferent atmosphere of a hospital, providing a patient with an environment that is warm and congenial.

26 Fujita, C.: Nihon ni okeru shūdan seishin ryōhō–Morita-ryōhōteki tachiba kara no kentō (Group psychotherapy in Japan–Review from Morita therapy) (in Japanese). *Seishin Igaku* 10 (7) (1968).

27 Aizawa, N.: Morita ryōhō no shomondai-tokuni chiryōteki jōkyō ni tsuite (Some problems of Morita therapy—Especially the therapeutic situation) (in Japanese). *Seishin Igaku* 11 (2) (1969).

28 Uchimura, H.: Morita ryōhō ni okeru "toraware" to chiryō no "ba" ni tsuite (*Toraware* (neurotic captivation) and the therapeutic situation in Morita therapy) (in Japanese). *Seishin Igaku* 12 (9) (1970).

29 In this instance, *shinkeishitsu* is classified as a type of disposition.

acquire adaptability for social living. There is conflict within a patient aroused by the desire to have a social life that is free of uneasiness and tension in opposition to the facts of the situation. In other words, this conflict is one of contradictory suffering brought on by the idealized level of "what it should be" and the realistic level of "what it is, as was explained in Chapters 3 and 8.

The psychological condition that such patients consider as being ideal is one in which tension has been relaxed and there is no need to be concerned. In concrete terms, this condition is the level of consciousness that has developed in a family-like group in which all the members understand one another. As Nakane[30] points out, within the framework of the *uchi* (inner circle) called "the home," there is stable and softening emotionality that tends to seep over into other personal life fields. A strengthening, through group unification, of feelings toward other human beings can be accelerated. However, there is still the possibility of a condition of poor social adaptability due to each patient's thoughts and actions. The symptoms of *shinkeishitsu* develop with that form of emotional dependence, or *amae*,[31] in the background. However, in general, patients afflicted with *shinkeishitsu* hold too much hope and expectation of maintaining a mental condition that will not give rise to uneasiness, tension or disturbance. Such patients desire to have an unstrained state of mind, free of tension in all social activities, similar to that of family life. Moreover, in their belief that a healthy person lives consistently in that tension-free state of mind, they deepen their commitment to achieve that expectation. Nevertheless, because the facts of social life do not conform to their expectations, they worry about this reality and consider themselves subnormal, which is why the structure of their symptoms is so complex.

When this anxiety is observed from the standpoint of belonging to a group, a patient with *shinkeishitsu* reveals an emotional structure of a strong desire to belong to two kinds of group, a primary group and a secondary group, while slways maintaining the same tranquil feeling, and, further, hopes to attain this idealized condition.

When we compare this emotional structure with the dual nature of a Morita therapy group, the environment in which therapy takes place has an important bearing on a patient suffering from *shinkeishitsu*, in that his or her anticipation and desire are accepted, even if only temporarily. There is both passive and active acceptance. The patient's sense of isolation gradually vanishes owing to anticipation that the therapist will understand how much he or she suffers from the symptoms and, at the same time, will become aware of the suffering of his or her fellow patients.

Further, the patient begins to experience mental tranquility as he or she (passively) becomes accustomed to the homelike atmosphere of the clinic. The patient also (actively) discovers in himself or herself the possibility of participating in a cooperative, communal way of life while dealing with inner suffering without evasion. These factors elucidate the group structure in Morita therapy, together with the structure of the symptoms of *shinkeishitsu*, and readily show the effectiveness of forming a group in the therapeutic process. This is the precondition for group therapy, which we will now describe.

Group Method

Morita prescribes absolute, isolated bed rest and daily work assignments as measures that effectively engender creativity and personal autonomy in each patient. These measures mostly

---

30 Nakane, C.: *Nihonteki Shakai Kōzō no Hakken* (Discovery of Japanese Social Structure). Chūō Kōron Sha, Tokyo (1964). (Printed in Japanese)

31 Doi, T.: Shinkeishitsu no seishin byōri—tokuni toraware no seishin rikigaku ni tsuite (Psychopathology of *shinkeishitsu*, especially regarding the psychodynamics of its *toraware*). *Psychiatria et Neurologia Japonica* 60:733 (1958).

relate to the realities of life. However, Morita emphasizes avoiding group activities as much as is possible to prevent the therapeutic process from becoming too formalized. In general, he tries to foster spontaneity and endurance in each patient. Since, however, the final objective is to elicit personal creativity as much as is possible, the author has carried out group therapy for the past decade from the perspective that absolute, isolated bed rest is a situation in which a patient is isolated from group life and in which the personal relationship of "I–we" is emptied of immediate content. It is a period for oneself, for each patient alone.

This period of absolute, isolated bed rest is intended to stimulate a reconsideration of oneself in the relationship of each person called "I" to any group called "we." It may seem that this period is a negative condition, in which human relationships have been cut off, but the importance of this condition is that it offers an opportunity to shift to positive approaches to relationships that oblige a patient of make himself of herself accountable and to foster a genuine sphere of the "I–we" relationship.[32]

Work is a form of participation in group living, in which the self is placed in an "I–we" relationship. It is a period in which the meaningfulness of personal isolation actually becomes apparent. Each patient leaves his or her symptoms as they are for the time being and is relied on by other patients to contribute to group living in his or her assigned role. It is also a period in which a patient is aware of the real fact that something is expected of him or her and that he or she has the experience and the reality of being of service. Varying the quality and quantity of work assignments during this period is a rational approach adopted as a learning process, even in society as a whole.

The objective here is to create a group in which both the form and the content of life among the patients are replete. Group objectives include supervision of dietary concerns,[33] consolidation of the life environment,[34] mutual knowledge and cultural refinement. For leisure, there are sports, games, hiking, various handicrafts, sketching, music appreciation, art appreciation and reading sessions.

Group meetings are held once a week for the purpose of examining these group activities. Therapists and cotherapists participate in the meetings, but the position of chairperson is rotated among all the patients the group.

Participation by Patients

In therapy for hospitalized patients, it is important to consider what responses are shown by patients who begin to participate in a group after they have completed the period of absolute, isolated bed rest.[35] There is no major difference between the therapy group and society, and because the group structure has the dual nature of a family group as well as an ordinary social group, the patients can participate in a more receptive condition than they could if they belonged to a therapy group organized for a specific purpose. Further, the distortion of personal relationships and the evasive way of thinking that are characteristic of each patient are

---

[32] See the discussion on *fumon* (disregard) and "acceptance" in Chapter 17.

[33] As a rule, the weekly menu and the purchase of foodstuffs within the limits of the stipulated budget, with the food prepared under the supervision of a resident nutritionist and cook, are handled by consultation among the patients as a group.

[34] This objective is chiefly a matter of keeping things in order and cleaning indoors and outdoors, as well as devising, improving, inspecting and repairing facilities, utensils, equipment and systems to make life easier for the members of the group. Cleaning the yard and flower garden, looking after birds and weeding and caring for trees and plants are responsibilities assigned by members of the group.

[35] The psychological state of a patient who participates for the first time in a group, after completing the period of absolute, isolated bed rest, is generally complicated. Uneasiness and constraint are experienced in meeting strangers for the first time. There is tension and a feeling of resistance at coming in contact with a new environment. The desire to associate and become friendly with other members of the group, and the anxiety of wondering whether one will be able to get along with the other members, are intermingled.

gradually overcome through participation in work assignments and through a new reality of being able to converse mutually with other patients in the group.

Each patient does not know, at first, what is expected of him or her, how one should behave, and would tend to feel uneasy if a fixed relationship or role were imposed. Therefore, instead of being fixed, work assignments are flexible. (Morita exercised care to encourage spontaneous activity by a patient during the first phase of the work period and provided work that did not require specific guidance.)

A therapist will first have a patient observe the surrounding life environment. As the patient's desire for participation arises, flexible work assignments are given that do not impose a fixed role. As the living condition is gradually understood, the patient becomes conscious of the group objectives, and a new condition that is consensual and suitable will be formed through such group processes as suggestion, approval, correction and negation. Each patient will learn how to harmonize with this new creative process and will become aware of a selfhood process that is not shackled by symptoms.

Until this point, a patient has been enveloped in a condition of receptive, direct reconciliation in a homelike atmosphere, but now a relationship engendered by a role-playing assignment, chosen by his or her will, begins to form. The prior attitude of concentrating only on oneself will be expanded to take in "the whole," with the mind directed toward this wholeness and with actions changed to take into consideration the group.

The patient will desire a role in a social grouping of mutual dependence that confers responsibility and can now state personal views while accepting the opinions of other patients. As a result, a genuine individuality begins to form. A sense of community acceleration by participation in the group will have meaning only when a patient becomes aware of this. The group can become unstable, and the effect of the group on each patient cannot be anticipated, if the experience of each patient is insufficient. This is related to the specific composition of the group's members and will be explained later.

Treatment Conditions and Problems for Therapists and Cotherapists

One factor that has an important role in the treatment process is the presence of the therapist. The scope of activity of the therapist is that of having a role in both group and individual therapy.

The hospital setting in which Morita therapy is carried out is the therapeutic community, and all the patients are the objects of group therapy. It is not a group in which each patient joins together on his or her initiative, as in other forms of group therapy, or a group formed by the patient's will within the framework of a clinic. In other words, it is not a therapy group formed specifically to carry out group therapy but rather, a group in which group therapy is carried out concurrently with individual therapy.[36] In fact, there is no intent to deliver group therapy in the conduct of Morita therapy. Also, as a rule, there is no fixed format for an interview. An interview is conducted on a one-to-one basis or within the group for a fixed period, without taking into consideration this general constraint.

From the standpoint of structuring therapy, the group method that the author uses incorporates activities and discussions. This method consists of individual life therapy[37] in combination with group therapy to which the individual therapy is connected.

A therapist conducts interviews once a week, providing the instructions necessary for moving a patient through the treatment process. The therapist observes the group activities and determines the time at which each patient is ready to perform work assignments after the

[36] Because each patient receives both individual therapy and group therapy, Morita therapy is considered a form of combined therapy (Clifford, J. S.: Combined individual and group therapy. In *Comprehensive Textbook of Psychiatry.* Williams & Wilkins, Baltimore (1967)).

bed rest period, as well as the patient's fitness for receiving visitors or going outside. The cotherapist participates in this procedure and provides guidance for the activities.

The therapy team also includes a pshychiatric social worker, a clinical psychologist, a nurse and other personnel who take charge of the group and assist each patient in life activities, in accordance with the therapist's treatment policy, and who also assist the therapist as necessary. It may be more appropriate to say that the cotherapist lives with a patient and behaves as a coworker who deals with community life much more smoothly than does the patient.

A cotherapist is not a new development in Morita therapy,[38] and this member of the therapy team has been a helpful component of the team. The cotherapist helps stabilize the group and helps the patients handle work assignments, but the need for a cotherapist was not given much attention in the past because Morita therapy was not evaluated from the standpoint of in the past because Morita therapy was not evaluated from the standpoint of being a group treatment modality. In the author's opinion, the role of a cotherapist should be evaluated more carefully, and a cotherapist should be viewed in a more positive light than was customary in the past.

A therapist should continually observe the condition of the group as a whole by maintaining as close contact as is possible with his or her cotherapist. However, the therapist should refrain from giving direct instructions or making comments during activities or discussions, instead conducting individual interviews while remaining in the background.

A within-the-group interview is conducted separately from a regular interview. An important consideration for a therapist who is carrying out group therapy is how he or she handles information obtained from individual interviews and information gathered from group discussions. There are instances in which information obtained from interviews becomes more useful when it is mentioned during group discussions. Conversely, there are instances when a patient's resistance will increase if information gathered from a group discussion is presented to the patient during a regular interview.

Inducing a patient who prefers to talk on a one-to-one basis with the therapist, not in a group, to talk in a group setting is the group method role of the therapist. However, instruction is given in the original mode of Morita therapy to face reality head-on, not to evade it.[39]

This instruction also has validity when given to the group as a whole, for instance, in

---

[37] The term *life therapy* is now commonly used in the field of psychotherapy in Japan. Its definition is not fixed, but from an overall standpoint it is considered to be a daily life training therapy that fosters social adaptability and a return to society. The content of the life therapy that this author includes in the group method is, in summary, a simplification of the complexities of ordinary daily life into simple fundamentals, the aggressive adoption of this approach as a therapy activity within the group and a search for one's controlling function through this type of action. It is similar in some respects to Redl's place of livelihood interview. This is particularly true of the group discussion method.

[38] At the time Morita first carried out his therapy, two or three patients lived in his home and experienced the absolute, isolated bed rest period and performed work assignments there. During that time, Morita's wife cooperated with him to provide the patients with concrete guidance for daily life activities. It is believed that the arrangement of having a cotherapist who has an important live-in role in the special condition of homelike therapy for daily life activities was introduced into Morita therapy in that manner.

At one meeting of a *Keigai-kai* group hosted by Morita, including former patients who had been released from the hospital, one of the patients began to chat with another and said: "When you wish to discuss something, it would be better to talk to the doctor's wife, since the doctor himself is a rather difficult person to talk to." There are records in which Morita's wife had said: "I feel as if the patients are my own children; I shall be very pleased to listen to anything you may want to say." It can be inferred from this comment that the role of Morita's wife as a cotherapist was important. In practice, a Morita therapist, whether male or female, can be said to have a "father-like" or teacher-like role, while the cotherapist has a "mother-like" role. See Records of the 19th *Keigai-kai* meeting. *Shinkeishitsu* 1:238 (1932); Uchimura, H.: *Toraware* (neurotic preoccupation) and the therapeutic situation in Morita therapy (in Japanese). *Seishin Igaku* 12(9) (1970). Aizawa, N.: Morita ryōhō no jissai—chiryōteki kankyō (Practice of Morita therapy—the therapeutic situation). In *Gendai no Morita Ryōhō* (Present-day Morita Therapy, Its Theory and Practice), edited by T. Kōra and K. Ōhara. Hakuyōsha, Tokyo (1977). (Printed in Japanese) talking about the role each patient has in community life. This instruction is meaningful to all the patients in the group, and it has great relevance as a subject for discussion among group members, so that efforts to elicit as much conversation as is possible among the patients, voicing opinions relating to their concerns about daily life, will be welcomed by all the members and serve to promote this kind of discourse. As a result, the anxieties and fears of each patient will tend to abate as they discuss such subjects among themselves.

A therapist tries to guide the conversation away from a patient's symptoms and in the direction of the patient's awareness that matters of concern need to be addressed so that the patient can take responsibility for his or her problems and for his or her participation in group activities and discussions. In this way, the patient learns to understand that there is no difference between his or her value orientation as a person and as a member of the group, and treatment then progresses smoothly.

The chief objectives of a therapist in group therapy are to determine to what extent group life (activities, discussions) affects the stability of a patient and to be watchful continually to determine how the treatment process can be accelerated by means of the group method. In other words, the therapist is obliged to acquire as much information as he or she can in regard to approaches that tend to accelerate group therapy and a patient's cure accordingly.

Group Members

Shinkeishitsu is necessarily the central cohesive factor for a group, especially in that it sets the groundwork for group activities. It is a group method, but it is still based on the principles of Morita therapy, so that its objective is still confined to curing *shinkeishitsu*. However, patients with impure types of *shinkeishitsu*[40] and patients with borderline variants can also participate as members of a group if they do not interfere with stabilization of the group.

Group activity may be hindered by including such other patients, and the group may become unstable. Judicious use of drugs can be effective in stabilizing a group in this situation and in promoting the group treatment process.[41] A group should have fewer than ten members, seven or eight members being the ideal number. In most cases, group life is easier if gender and social class are not taken into consideration, except when all members are of the same sex or, for instance, when all are students.[42] A group functions more effectively if its members are all within a small age range.

Speech and Action in the Procedure for Fundamental Classification of the Group Method

When therapy is considered from the standpoint of the procedure that is employed, speech is generally considered an important aspect of the individual treatment method. However, in group therapy, speech is not as important as a component, particularly in group activities. There is a certain distinction between the role of speech and the role of group life in therapeutic com-

---

[39] Morita frequently uses the term *fuan totsunyū* (anxiety inrush). This expression signifies that the actual life setting should be faced as it is, without evasion, by not opposing such feelings as fear and anxiety. A patient should accept anxiety as such (including its meaning as anxiety) when and as it arises, as it inevitably will, in true life situations. The therapeutic technique places insistence on having the patient face the facts of life as they are, with a spirit of determination to improve oneself, leaving anxiety in a sort of bracketed condition, just as it is.

[40] Takeyama defines a number of impure types of *shinkeishitsu* and classifies them into a schizophrenic type, a cyclothymic type, a psychasthenic type, a hysteric type, a paranoiac type, an exhaustion type, a weak-willed type and an accompanying type. See footnote 1.

[41] Drugs are used infrequenfly in Morita therapy, but there are cases when a minor tranquilizer may be used to relieve various symptoms observed in the impure types of *shinkeishitsu*.

[42] According to the author's experience with therapy for groups of outpatients selected at random, there are many cases in which a patient remarks that it is easier to hold conversations with patients of the same general age or to reach a mutual understanding with patients who have the same kinds of symptoms.

munities in Japan. The relationships between the life viewpoints of the Japanese and their speech patterns have been studied from various perspectives, but the Japanese do not necessarily rely on speech for communication. There are occasions when silence is more important. In addition, the Japanese do not express themselves well with oral communication. This is particularly true of expressing one's inner self.

This observation is related to the poor sense of sociability of the Japanese, but as Nakane[43] points out, the Japanese frequently have little need to converse with one another. There are many situations in which speech is not needed for emotional harmonizing and direct relationship perspectives of a shared awareness. It is difficult to foster sociability under such circumstances. As a result, the Japanese have the peculiar quality of lacking proficiency in oral communication.

Because one objective of group therapy is to foster sociability, the author is keenly aware of the difficulties that lack of effective oral communication can pose. Therefore, oral communication as such must be encouraged as a habit, necessitating that various techniques be used by a therapist.[44]

In general, even patients who speak well in regular interviews tend to remain silent in within-the-group interviews and do not say anything even when called on. This problem makes the group method, which relies on oral communication, difficult.

By contrast, the procedure is made easy if the group method is introduced as a sphere of "action," and this approach accelerates the rate of oral communication among group members. The reason that Morita avoided procedures that required oral communication, preferring word assignments (i.e., action) in a hospital environment instead, is a matter of interest, but he emphasized actions akin to life situations, not actions that are simply mechanical.[45]

This rational approach makes best use of the indigenous character of the Japanese. Activity can be made more meaningful, however, only when it is reinforced by oral communication. What a therapist should strive to derive from the group method is a set of experiences, obtained through group activity, that lead to a recognition of the true meaning of group living through a linguistic procedure of group discussions. This recognition can then be applied to the practice of activity, in reviewing matters of concern.

Speech is an important process for accelerating sociability, but if too much emphasis is placed on oral communication, even if it is increased in a group setting, the sympathy and stability, and the feeling that the perception of isolation has been eliminated, will remain at a shallow level or will not be fully accepted by each patient. Full acceptance will not take place if individual awareness is lacking. It is still most efficacious for a patient to begin with activities to attain the most immediate therapeutic goal.

Comparison of Differences

Comparing any difference in effect between standard Morita therapy and the group method can pose problems.

First of all, the group method has made it easier to accelerate stability and to accept treatment with relatively little resistance, through concrete activities of role playing. Standard Morita therapy was centered chiefly around the therapist. In the group method, the life situation is centered around the patients, which makes it easier for a large number of patients to accept therapy. Even in standard Morita therapy, receiving treatment in a group was a relative shortcut toward acceptance of one's suffering. The group method has intentionally made this effect more certain. The change from the original one-to-one form of therapy to group therapy seems an inevitable step to take in the present era.

---

[43] Nakane, C.: op. cit.

[44] The author has found from the following two experiences that although oral communication is difficult with the group method, the circumstances can become considerably different according to the arrangement of the group. In one experience, one session per week was carried out ten times in 1958, with outpatients suffering from *shinkeishitsu* who also had anthropophobia. Each session was attended by five to 12 group members, with the position of chairperson for each session rotating among the members. At first, the objective was to have the members converse freely among themselves, but because there was almost no spontaneous conversation, the method was changed; each member was asked simply to introduce himself or herself (e.g., by giving name, age and occupation), and thereafter the topics of conversation centered around that patient's past and present condition and wishes for the future. The patient who acted as chairperson for each session did the utmost to talk, but because there was little conversation among the members, the session consisted mostly of questions directed to the therapist and the therapist's replies. As a result, conversation among the members dwindled even further, or even if there was some conversation, it was intermittent, and silences continued so long that sometimes there was even a feeling of awkward tension. Each patient became the chairperson once, and on that occasion, the patient tried to talk as much as he or she could, but the members became completely reserved when they faced each other seated around a table. However, each patient, when face to face with the therapist, tried to give a spontaneous impression of the group meeting. For example, one patient thought that he was the only member who suffered from problems of personal relationships, but his feeling was somewhat relieved when he found that other patients had the same problem. He explained much of his consciousness and feeling, in which he compared the impressions of other patients when viewed from the outside, such as those who suffered in a manner similar to his own. However, the symptoms of those patients seemed to be milder than his symptoms, and when he realized that those patients could talk freely, it did not appear that they were suffering from the same symptoms.

Although some people are fearful of interpersonal relationships, there is no general opposition to make attempts to relate with one another in a group meeting. There were many positive opinions to the effect that the group meetings should be continued. The patients' attitudes as a group and as individuals appeared to be contradictory, but this is actually a manifestation of the dual structure of the symptoms of *shinkeishitsu* and may be ascribed to the fact that, while most patients give an impression of avoiding human relationships, they actually seek out relationships strongly within their minds. In fact, such patients are too timid to face an actual social situation, owing to their idealistic attitudes and their overly keen concern to reconcile themselves to other persons. As a result, the desire for self-realization is suppressed within and the lack of sociability begins to reveal itself even more conspicuously.

In the second experience, a psychodrama session was conducted once a week for about two hours after supper over a six-month period in 1960, with a group of patients suffering from anthropophobia who were receiving Morita therapy as inpatients (see Fujita, C., et al.: An application of psychodrama to the treatment of *shinkeishitsu*, especially anthropophobia (in Japanese). *Seishin Igaku* 3(7) (1961)). The decision to use this method was based on the following considerations. There appears to be a limit, and considerable difficulty, in communication by speech alone in the group method, so that instead of conducting therapy in which only free conversation is carried out around a table, the psychodrama format, even if contrived, brings group therapy closer to life situations. Further, it makes use of speech that has more concrete meaning because of the addition of action. Role action is assigned by participating in the drama, and the so-called crucial regulation of therapy in which spontaneity is aroused by an accompanying sentimental experience is inherent in the process of psychodrama. Regulation of catharsis and reality testing by action gives rise to an emotional catharsis experience by its combination with speech. The dramatic aspect of psychodrama accelerates the spontaneity within a patient and reveals the facts of the patient's condition (see Fujita, C., et al.: The roles of psychodrama in the mental hospital (in Japanese). *Shinkeishitsu* 6(1) (1966)). On the basis of this experience, the author began to use crude psychodrama utilizing a stage setting from whatever was available. Moreno frequently used the monologue and mirror methods, but because the Japanese are essentially poor at lucid self-expression, scenes from daily life that resemble the life situations of the patients were set up as the scenes of the drama to produce scenarios that are relatively easy to express. This approach was tested with the method of changing roles. What emerged clearly from these sessions, as distinct from ordinary group meetings, was that each patient played his or her part with a considerable spirit of self-assertion and delight (although all patients appeared to be shy). Each patient learned that the actions of the other patients, and the acting of the therapists and nurses who participated, in the roles of auxiliary egos did not differ much from their own, and that other patients, too, feel the same tensions and shyness when acting in front of an audience. The patients showed concern and took an interest in receiving direct, candid criticism of their acting from the audience, and they expressed a desire to have the psychodrama format continued in the future.

On the basis of these two experiences, the author has found that there is a great difference in motivation toward oral expression and its effects. Patients are prone to be silent while sitting around a table, and lively conversation among group members in this situation cannot be expected. In the psychodrama format, however, each patient acts aggressively and conversation progresses. In view of this observation, the author has used a therapeutic community that is similar to a life situation to create a living stage. The author has tried to carry out, concretely and assertively, the group therapy explained in this chapter with an interest and anticipation as to how the members will try to fulfill their role assignments, how this format can become an emotional catharsis, what awareness of reality it can bring and how the spontaneity of each patient can be engendered.

What the author has observed through use of the group method is summarized in the paragraphs that follow.

When a person has difficulty maintaining self-identity in modern society, group therapy can have an important role in the eradication of this difficulty. A patient is regulated by the group context to recover his or her true ego identity, and the true ego can be restored chiefly through group therapy. However, only 30 years have elapsed since group therapy was first studied and applied in Japan. This treatment modality still does not have a firm footing in the Japanese social and cultural milieu. The apparent reasons are the difficulty of forming therapy groups and lack of widespread acceptance of such therapy.

The characteristics of human relationships in a group are an important consideration. The objective of group therapy is, from one standpoint, the formation of horizontal human relationships. However, group relationships in Japan are directed toward strengthening the vertical form of social structure and function. It is thus difficult to foster a horizontal format for social relationships. One problem is that many group treatment modalities do not take into consideration this observation, adhering to theory alone.

There is also the problem of procedure in relation to speech and action. In many group treatment modalities, speech becomes the medium because the format of a group discussion is used. However, the Japanese are not skilled in oral communication, particularly in the context of human relationships in which each person has direct contact and an awareness of being a "member of the inner circle," which increases the feeling of being understood without speaking.

Improving the capability for oral communication and sociability through self-expression by means of speech is difficult to achieve as a means of personal growth. A person who has the habit of not placing importance on self-expression via oral communication can, however, with great effort, learn to break that habit. It can readily be seen that such a breakthrough will have a certain effect on that person's thoughts and actions.

The Japanese can be said to have a quasi-neurotic deficiency in oral communication and interpersonal relationships. Group therapy differs from individual therapy in that oral communication among group members is difficult in many cases. This difficulty is particularly conspicuous when a group is composed of clinically neurotic patients. Group therapy can be conducted to fulfill a therapist's expectations only when these facts are taken into consideration.

On the basis of experience with Morita therapy, which was created out of the basic social and cultural milieu of Japan, the group method needs to have a special structure suited to patients who suffer from symptoms of *shinkeishitsu*. Further, even if human relationships in the group are therapeutic, there will be a strengthening of the vertical form of social function. The author does not ignore this fact but, rather, seeks to strengthen independent consciousness by introducing role behavior. To develop this approach, a form of group activity to which it is relatively easy to get accustomed was set up as the main component, and the experience obtained from role behavior through oral communication, called group discussion, was promoted.

[45] Morita avoided the group method and cooperative work assignments when carrying out occupational therapy. The chief reason was that group action tended to become generally formalized and would flow mechanically when work was carried out within a group. No interest in, or attachment to, the work assignment was engendered, and there was no sign of creativity or inventiveness. Morita believes that a patient's spontaneity cannot be cultivated, or his or her persistence in work fostered, when a group approach is used (see Chapter 1).

Experience with and Advisability of Using Drug Therapy as an Adjunctive Measure

There is no doubt that the most basic therapies in modern psychiatry are psychotherapy and drug therapy. In essence, these two treatment modalities can be considered as the two wheels of a bicycle and as being inseparable.

In this respect, there is no drug therapy that does not incorporate psychotherapy. Conversely, a form of psychotherapy that makes use of drugs,[46,47] such as the anaclitic therapy induced by drugs,[48] has been developed. The trend toward an even closer interrelationship between these two basic treatment modalities will undoubtedly continue.

In the past, it was generally thought that these two treatment modalities originated from different conceptions and that they have different focal points of action, mechanisms of action and areas of action. However, on the basis of lengthy experience with drug therapy, the author is not hesitant about using the two treatment modalities in combination, even if the essential theory of psychotherapy is taken into consideration. The two modalities converge with each other, irrespective of differences in concept or in structure, in the sense of therapeutic purpose and effect. They have a complementary relationship that can be anticipated in some cases. However, this observation gives rise to the questions of when and by what method a drug should be administered.

This issue provides unique and worthwhile material for discussion of theory, technique and the effect of psychotherapy. With the present-day situation of psychotherapy and drug therapy taken into consideration, an attempt will be made to discuss the present relationship of drug therapy to Morita therapy, chiefly outpatient therapy, which, for the most part, has been conducted without use of drugs.

Current Status of Drug Therapy in the Management of *Shinkeishitsu*

It is difficult to prevent the use of all drugs in the author's clinic. Ordinarily, the author would not use any drug for the management of neuroses, particularly *shinkeishitsu*. However, the use of drugs has been increasing as is shown in Figure 1. The introduction of numerous tranquilizers for such dysfunctions of the autonomic nervous system as anxiety and its physical manifestations (which represent the fundamental symptoms of *shinkeishitsu*) that are effective and have negligible side effects cannot be overlooked.

Reviewing the use of such drugs for the management of symptoms of *shinkeishitsu* reveals that some drugs have been effective in alleviating symptoms. However, such drugs only relieve the symptoms of *shinkeishitsu*; they do not provide a true cure of the mental disorder. Anxiety can be considered a dysfunction of the autonomic nervous system rather than psychological in origin. The mental conflict observed in many patients with *shinkeishitsu* does not respond positively to drug therapy, which simply makes such patients less sensitive to their intense inner conflict by relieving the nervous tension.

---

46 Nishizono, M.: High dose treatment with psychotherapeutic drugs seen from the psychoanalytic viewpoint (in Japanese). *Psychoanalytics* 5(34) (1964).
47 Nishizono, M.: The anaclitic drug psychotherapy. *Folia Psychiatria et Neurologia Japonica* 19(9) (1965).
48 Azima, H., et al.: Anaclitic therapy induced by drugs (in Japanese). *Comprehensive Psychiatry* 2:281 (1961).

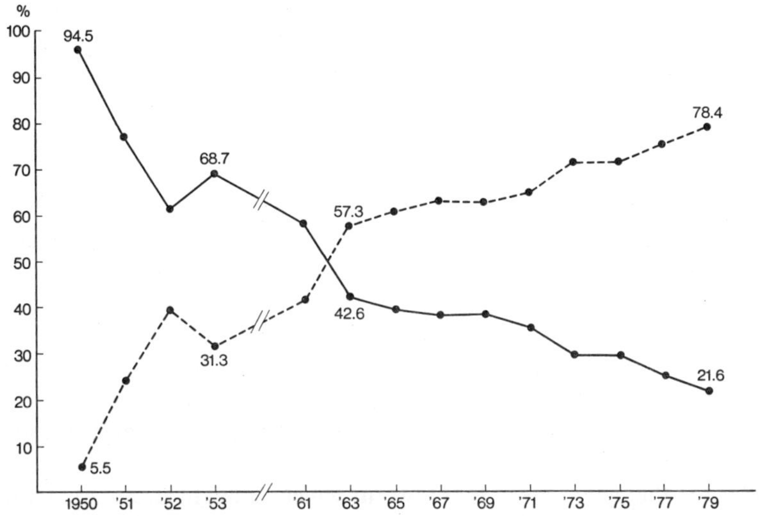

Figure 1. 1950–53: Psychiatric outpatients' department of the Jikei University School of Medicine; 1961–79: Tokiwadai Psychiatric Clinic. ———, Psychotherapy; -------, psychotherapy and drug therapy. All patients were treated on an outpatient basis.

Drugs have no effect on the hypochondriacal attitude that is the basic symptom of *shinkeishitsu.* Drugs only alleviate or shift the relevant somatic symptoms. This is also true of obsessive-compulsive states. Thus, although the scope of application of drugs for the management of neuroses, particularly *shinkeishitsu* as the object of Morita therapy, has been narrow, and although the effectiveness of drug therapy has been mininal, there has been steady growth in the use of such therapy. The reasons for this increasing popularity of drug therapy relate to therapists, on the one hand, and their patients, on the other. Currently, it is almost impossible to conduct psychotherapy carefully, from the standpoint of the time available for the large numbers of neurotic patients who continue to seek treatment, so that therapists, are being compelled more and more to substitute other treatments for psychotherapy, even if only temporarily. What seems most convenient is the large assortment of tranquilizers at hand, and the use of such drugs is perceived as a reasonable option for therapists in the present state of affairs.

The attitude of a therapist who is continually prescribing tranquilizers ultimately becomes a major factor that persuades the therapist to comply with the requests of his or her patients for immediate relief of symptoms. A neurotic patient wants relief from pain and anxiety, and as quickly as it can be obtained, so that his or her livelihood is not impaired by incessant anxiety. To deal with activities of daily living, the patient does not acknowledge the pain and anxiety as being symptoms of a problem in his or her life, and the patient feels no need to deal with the problem head-on. Most patients have great expectations that the causal factors of pain and anxiety will be examined by scientific testing and a cure rapidly obtained. Such patients usually keep their distance from therapists who, they believe, will only conduct interviews and not provide practical medical treatment. If a therapist offers drug therapy in response to their requests, the drugs will seem to be an attractive substitute for such patients.

The use of drugs has been accelerated by therapists in their haste to provide a temporary substitute for psychotherapy and in response to their patients' requests. Thus, psychotherapy alone is being conducted for a dwindling number of patients. Many patients seemingly undergo psychotherapy but actually are being treated almost solely with drugs.

The use of drugs in this instance indicates that such therapists believe that drugs have limited application, but this situation still presents a problem in evaluating more aggressive use of drugs for the management of neuroses. If drugs are useful for managing neuroses only from the standpoint of convenience, such therapists have a responsibility to develop an autonomous therapy plan for the future use of drugs.

The action of drugs and their clinical effects can be anticipated in the instance of tranquilizers, but such factors as the characteristic action of a drug (i.e., drug specific or nonspecific, in which a direct action of a drug is absent) need to be considered Use of drugs that have nonspecific actions involves a number of influential factors: the patient-therapist relationship (i.e., the attitude of a patient toward a therapist), the character of the patient, the psychological condition of the patient (anticipation, suggestion) and the therapeutic environment of living conditions of the patient. Any and all of these factors can complicate the effect of a drug that has a nonspecific action and the evaluation of therapy with such a drug. There is a clear need to develop a system for drug therapy in which the target symptom is amenable to cure by the characteristic action and effect of the drug and in which other influential factors are taken into consideration.

Even anaclitic therapy induced by drugs, in which different drugs are administered in accordance with the various aspects of the symptoms and personality of the patient, is a therapy in which an attempt is made to integrate drug usage aggressively in combination with psychotherapy. It is difficult to expect much from the present array of tranquilizers in terms of permanent effect on a target symptom. Integration of a patient's personality and development of creativity in living through drug therapy alone is not productive.[49] Drug therapy must be combined with psychotherapy, even if this approach is not considered sufficiently positive.

Drug therapy in combination with psychotherapy is characterized by an organic interrelationship, such that combination therapy tends to differ according to how the therapist considers the role of each treatment modality. It thus becomes necessary to discuss this interrelationship by differentiating psychotherapy supported by drug therapy from its counterpart, drug therapy supported by psychotherapy, as Pflanz explains.[50]

In this regard, we probably need to consider how Morita therapy is conducted for outpatients, first by determining whether a therapist is using drugs simultaneously with Morita therapy or whether he or she is supplementing drug therapy with Morita therapy. However, according to the information that the author has gathered, this consideration is an academic one because drugs are customarily administered for immediate relief of target symptoms and because it has become a habit to use drug therapy as a substitute for psychotherapy.

This habit originated in clinical practice as a result of a need to treat increasingly large numbers of neurotic patients under constraints of time and space. Moreover, the development of tranquilizers has made it possible to treat large numbers of patients on an outpatient basis.[51]

Many therapists try to get through their daily practice by using these drugs as a substitute. The use of drugs may seem to be passive, but each therapist, in fact, administers drugs on the basis of his or her experience and his or her appreciation of which drug should be used for which patient and for what purpose.

Therefore, it is important to restudy cases in which drugs have been used. The author has studied experience with drug therapy in combination with psychotherapy. The appearance of a

---

[49] Cole, J. O.: Control of the mind and drugs (in Japanese). In *The Voice of America Forum Lectures*, translated by Y. Sasaki and Y. Ono. Seishin Shobō, Tokyo (1966).

[50] Pflanz, M.V.: Geissen: Organische Verfahren Arzneimittelbehandlung und Psychotherapie; Europädische Gesichte-Punkte, *Handbuch der Neurosenlehre und Psychotherapie*, Band IV; Spezielle Psychotherapie II und Neurosenprophylaxe. Urban & Schwarzenberg, Munich and Berlin (1959).

[51] Kielholz, P.: *Psychische Pharmakotherapie in Klinik und Praxis.* Hans Huber, Bern (1965).

Table 6 a Data from 131 Outpatients at the Jikei University School of Medicine (1953)

	Psychotherapy			Psychotherapy and Drug Therapy		
Number of patients / Number of visits	90 (68.7 %)			41 (31.3 %)		
1	42 (46.7)			10 (24.4)		
2	8 (8.9)			6 (14.6)		
3	7 (7.8)			4 (9.8)		
4	14 (15.6)			8 (19.5)		
5	9 (10.0)			5 (12.2)		
6	5 (5.6)			0		
7	0	2.8	4.5	0	4.2	6.1 (61)
8	2 (2.2)			4 (9.8)		
9	0			0		
10	3 (3.3)			0		
11	0			0		
12	0			0		
13	0			4 (9.8)		

Table 6 b Data from 88 Outpatients at the Tokiwadai Psychiatric Clinic (1979)

	Psychotherapy			Psychotherapy and Drug Therapy		
Number of patients / Number of visits	19 (21.6 %)			69 (78.4 %)		
1	9 (47.3)			11 (15.9)		
2	2 (10.5)			5 (7.2)		
3	2 (10.5)			1 (1.4)		
4	1 (5.3)			2 (2.9)		
5	0			1 (1.4)		
6	1 (5.3)			8 (11.6)		
7	2 (10.5)			2 (2.9)		
8	1 (5.3)	3.3	6.1	5 (7.2)	8.7	11.2 (84)
9	0			0		
10	0			6 (8.7)		
11	1 (5.3)			3 (4.3)		
12	0			5 (7.2)		
13	0			3 (4.3)		
14	0			7 (10.1)		
15	0			4 (5.8)		
16	0			6 (8.7)		

drug use phenomenon, which is contrary to general therapeutic rules, even in Morita therapy, in which drugs are rarely used, is simply due to circumstantial demands.

The intention of the study was to determine whether there is a widespread tendency to use drug therapy as an adjunctive treatment modality in the management of the symptoms of *shinkeishitsu*. With that in mind, the use of drugs could be considered in a more positive light than it has been in the past and can probably provide worthwhile material for evaluating the concepts and techniques of Morita therapy from a new point of view. Before studying representative cases for which drugs have been employed, the author would like to present a comparison of the number of patient visits to hospitals for psychotherapy as opposed to the number of visits for drug therapy. Tables 1a and 1b show differences in the number of visits to hospitals for psychotherapy alone and the number of visits for adjunctive use of drugs in 1953 and 1979.

The number of visits is important to therapists from the standpoint of conducting therapy with both approaches. If visits to hospitals are stopped, therapy is necessarily curtailed, with either method, and information needed to evaluate the therapeutic effect is left incomplete.

It is clear from Tables 6a and 6b that the numbers of visits for psychotherapy alone were 90 (68.7 percent) in 1953 and 19 (21.6 percent) in 1979, but there were 41 cases (31.3 percent) in 1953 and 69 cases (78.4 percent) in 1979 in which treatment was stopped after only one visit, fairly large proportions. In the instance of adjunctive drug therapy, the numbers of cases in which treatment did not extend beyond one visit were 10 (24.4 percent) and 11 (15.9 percent), respectively, so that compared with treatment with psychotherapy alone, the numbers of cases in which treatment was stopped early are considerably smaller.

The average numbers of treatment sessions were 2.8 and 3.3 for psychotherapy alone in 1953 and 1979, respectively, and 4.2 and 8.7 respectivly for psychotherapy and drug therapy in combination, showing that the average numbers of visits for combination therapy were larger in both years. For cases in which more than three visits were made, the average numbers were 4.5 and 6.1 for psychotherapy alone in 1953 and 1979, respectively, but these average numbers of visits increased to 6.1 and 11.2, respectively, in cases in which combination therapy was used. It is not advisable to evaluate the implications of these findings on the basis of these figures alone. However, it is clear that drug therapy has an important role in a patient's desire to continue making visits to a hospital for treatment. The differences in the tranquilizers that were used cannot be overlooked, in view of the increase in the average number of visits to hospitals and the increase in the rate of visits from 61 to 84 percent between 1953 and 1979, in the instance of more than three visits made when drugs were administered.

The appearance of drugs that are considered generally effective for the management of specific neuroses (e.g., meprobamate, chlordiazepoxide, diazepam, medazepam, lorazepam, amitriptyline, imipramine, clomipramine) is one reason for the increase in the rate of three or more visits to hospitals. However, the tendency to prolong the treatment period when such drugs are used is an observation that cannot be ignored. Further, the number of visits to a hospital is larger when the drug is changed from time to time, in line with the symptoms, than when no change is made.

There is also a tendency for treatment to be continued for longer periods when psychotherapy is carried out aggressively while drug therapy is being used. Rickels[52] carried out experimental studies with placebos on two groups; one placebo was used in the first group and three different placebos were used in the second group. Rickels found a difference in the numbers of visits made to the hospital by the two groups. A patient's expectations were bolstered when the therapist stated that at least one of the three placebos was type-specific for his or her symptoms, so that it became a major consideration in the patient's decision to continue treatment.

Apart from the specific action of any drug, the attitude of a therapist and the expectations of a patient can strongly influence the therapeutic relationship.

Clinical Study of Drug Therapy

The author will first explain the specific aspects of the study.

Such drugs as chlordiazepoxide, amitriptyline, parazine, hydroxyziene, opipramol and

[52] Rickels, K.: Drugs in the treatment of neurotic anxiety and tension: Controlled studies. In *Psychiatric Drugs.* Grune & Stratton, New York (1966).

Table 7 a Symptom Structure

Descriptive phenomena of symptoms	Obsessive state Hypochondriacal state Fixed in a specific, limited state (simplified state) Variousness state

Table 7 b

Obsessive state	Sensuous-subjectivity Perceptive-subjectivity Perceptive-objectivity
Hypochondriacal state	Sensuous-subjectivity Perceptive-subjectivity

Table 8 Data from 334 Outpatients at the Jikei University School of Medicine (1963)

Obsessive	138 (41.3 %)
Hypochondriacal	196 (58.7)
Total	334 (100)
Simplified	188 (56.2)
Variousness	146 (43.8)
Total	334 (100)
Sensuous	216 (64.6)
Perceptive	118 (35.4)
Total	334 (100)

Table 9 a Data from 132 Outpatients Undergoing Psychotherapy Alone at the Jikei University School of Medicine (1963)*

Obsessive	71 (53.7 %)	Ratio of all cases of the obsessive state: 71/138 = 51.4 %
Hypochondriacal	61 (46.3)	Ratio of all cases of the hypochondriacal state: 61/196 = 31.1 %
Total	132 (100)	
Simplified	96 (72.7)	Ratio of all cases of the simplified state: 96/188 = 51.1 %
Variousness	36 (27.3)	Ratio of all cases of the variousness state: 36/146 = 24.7 %
Total	132 (100)	
Sensuous	81 (61.3)	Ratio of all cases of the sensuous quality: 81/216 = 37.4 %
Perceptive	51 (38.7)	Ratio of all cases of the perceptive quality: 51/118 = 43.1 %
Total	132 (100)	

*These 132 patients represent 39.5 percent of the 334 treated in 1963 (see Table 3).

Table 9 b

<table>
<tr><td rowspan="3">Obsessive state</td><td>Simplified</td><td>63 (88.7 %)</td><td>Ratio of all cases managed with psychotherapy alone: 63/132 = 47.7 %</td></tr>
<tr><td>Variousness</td><td>8 (11.3)</td><td>Ratio of all cases managed with psychotherapy alone: 8/132 = 6.1 %</td></tr>
<tr><td>Subtotal</td><td>71 (100)</td><td></td></tr>
<tr><td rowspan="3">Hypochondriacal state</td><td>Simplified</td><td>33 (54.1)</td><td>Ratio of all cases managed with psychotherapy alone: 38/132 = 25.0 %</td></tr>
<tr><td>Variousness</td><td>28 (45.9)</td><td>Ratio of all cases managed with psychotherapy alone: 28/132 = 21.2 %</td></tr>
<tr><td>Subtotal</td><td>61 (100)</td><td></td></tr>
<tr><td></td><td>Total</td><td>132 (100)</td><td></td></tr>
</table>

diazepam, which have few side effects and which are convenient for use in the management of neuroses, came into general clinical use beginning around 1963. Patients suffering from *shinkeishitsu* who were treated in 1963 will be the basis for the data that will be discussed.

The symptoms of *shinkeishitsu* are classified from a descriptive point of view, as shown in Tables 7 a and 7 b. When the data are consolidated according to this classification scheme, the results shown in Table 8 are obtained. The experiences of the patients are classified from a descriptive phenomenological standpoint into those that more clearly indicate an obsessive state (138 cases, 41.3 percent) and those that more clearly indicate a hypochondriacal stage (196 cases, 58.7 percent). Further, cases in which the object of the symptom is fixed (in a specific, limited state by fixation, strength, change and shift of symptoms that indicate an obsessive or hypochondriacal state) are differentiated from those in which the object of the symptom is variable, expressing either a simplified state (188 cases, 56.2 percent) or a variousness state (146 cases, 43.8 percent). The cases were also classified as representing a sensuous quality (216 cases, 64.4 percent) or a perceptive quality (118 cases, 35.4 percent), in accordance with whether the objective content indicated a relatively concrete state. Further, cases in which experiences showed an exteroceptive tendency were classified as demonstrating objectivity, and those that showed a proprioceptive tendency as demonstrating subjectivity. Cases in which psychotherapy alone was used and those in which drug therapy was used adjunctively were also compared (Tables 9 a, 9 b and 9 c and Tables 10 a and 10 b).

In Table 9 a, which shows cases in which psychotherapy alone was used, there are 96 cases (72.7 percent) of the simplified state, which account for 51.1 percent of all such cases. This figure is far larger than the 36 cases (27.3 percent) of the variousness state, which accounts for 24.7 percent of all such cases).

In regard to the obsessive state as opposed to the hypochondriacal state, there is an insignificant difference between the numbers of cases, although from the standpoint of percentage of all such cases, the number of cases of an obsessive state is larger. In the classification according to sensuous or perceptive, the number of the cases of the former is larger for treatment with psychotherapy, alone, but from the standpoint of percentage of all such cases, the ratio of cases having the perceptive quality is larger.

There are 63 cases (88.7 percent) in which there was a simplified state as well as an obsessive state (Table 9 b); these 63 cases represent 47.7 percent of all the cases in which psychotherapy alone was used, or nearly half of all the cases being studied. In only eight cases (11.3 percent) was a variousness state encountered in combination with an obsessive state.

By contrast, there are 33 cases (54.1 percent) of a simplified state in combination with a hypochondriacal state and 28 cases (45.9 percent) of a variousness state in combination with a hypochondriacal state; as proportions of all cases in which psychotherapy alone was used, the percentages were small, being 25 and 21.2, respectively.

When symptoms are further classified from a structural standpoint (which will be explained later) as being sensuous·subjectivity or perceptive·subjectivity in cases of the simplified state in combination with the obsessive state there were 25 such cases (39.6 percent) and 26 cases (41.2 percent), respectively (Table 9 c); these cases represent about 80 percent of all the cases. In cases in which psychotherapy alone was used, the structure of simplified·subjectivity in cases of the obsessive state represents more than 50 percent of all the cases.

There are 28 cases (84.8 percent) of the structure of sensuous·subjectivity in cases of the simplified state in combination with the hypochondriacal state, and there are also 28 cases (100 percent) of the structure of sensuous·subjectivity in cases of the variousness state in combination with the hypochondriacal state.

In the structural context in which the obsessive and the hypochondriacal states are respec-

Table 9 c Those Same Patients Classified by Descriptive *Shinkeishitsu* Symptoms.

Obsessive state: 71 (53.8 %)	Simplified: 63 (88.7 %)	Sensuous-subjectivity: 25 (39.6 %) Perceptive-subjectivity: 26 (41.2) Perceptive-objectivity: 12 (19.2) Subtotal 63 (100)	Obsessive-sensuous: 25 (35.2 %)
	Variousness: 8 (11.3 %)	Sensuous-subjectivity: 0 Perceptive-subjectivity: 8 (100) Perceptive-objectivity: 0 Subtotal 8 (100)	Obsessive-perceptive: 46 (64.8 %)
Hypochondriacal state: 61 (46.2 %)	Simplified: 33 (54.1 %)	Sensuous-subjectivity: 28 (84.8) Perceptive-subjectivity: 5 (15.2) Subtotal 33 (100)	Hypochondriacal-sensuous: 56 (91.8 %)
	Variousness: 28 (45.9 %)	Sensuous-subjectivity: 28 (100)	Hypochondriacal-perceptive: 5 (8.2 %)

Table 10 a With Drugs: 202/334 (60.5 %) Cases of Patients Treated by Drug Therapy

Obsessive	67 (33.1 %)	Ratio of all cases of the obsessive state: 67/138 = 48.6 %
Hypochondriacal	135 (66.8)	Ratio of all cases of the hypochondriacal state: 135/196 = 68.9 %
Total	202 (100)	
Simplified	92 (45.5)	Ratio of all cases of the simplified state: 92/188 = 48.9 %
Variousness	110 (54.5)	Ratio of all cases of the variousness state: 110/146 = 75.3 %
Total	202 (100)	
Sensuous	135 (66.8)	Ratio of all cases of the sensuous quality: 135/216 = 62.6 %
Perceptive	67 (33.2)	Ratio of all cases of the perceptive quality: 67/118 = 56.9 %
Total	202 (100)	

Table 10 b With Drugs: 202/334 (60.5 %) Those Same Patients Classified by Descriptive *Shinkeishitsu* Symptoms

Obsessive state: 67 (33.2 %)	Simplified: 52/67 (77.6 %)	Sensuous-subjectivity: 15 (28.8 %) Perceptive-subjectivity: 21 (40.4) Perceptive-objectivity: 16 (30.8) Subtotal 52 (100)	Obsessive-perceptive: 50 (75.0 %)
	Variousness: 15/67 (22.4 %)	Sensuous-subjectivity: 2 (133) Perceptive-subjectivity: 11 (73.4) Perceptive-objectivity: 2 (13.3) Subtotal 15 (100)	Obsessive-sensuous: 17 (25.0 %)
Hypochondriacal state: 135 (66.8 %)	Simplified: 40/135 (29.6 %)	Sensuous-subjectivity: 36 (90.0) Perceptive-subjectivity: 4 (10.0) Subtotal 40 (100)	Hypochondriacal-sensuous: 128 (94.8 %)
	Variousness: 95/135 (70.4 %)	Sensuous-subjectivity: 92 (96.8) Perceptive-subjectivity: 3 (3.2) Subtotal 95 (100)	Hypochondriacal-perceptive: 7 (5.2 %)

tively combined with the sensuous quality and the perceptive quality, there are 46 cases (64.8 percent) of perceptive-obsessives and 56 cases (91.8 percent) of sensuous-hypochondriacs, making it clear that these structures have considerable influence in cases in which psychotherapy alone is used. (Table 9 c)

When cases in which drug therapy was used along with psychotherapy are reviewed, it is found (Table 10 a) that there is a greater number of hypochondriacs (135 cases, 66.8 percent) than of obsessives (67 cases, 33.2 percent) and a greater ratio of all cases of the hypochondriacal state (68.9 percent). From the standpoint of simplified as opposed to variousness, there are 110 cases (54.5 percent) of variousness, which represents 75.3 percent of all cases of variousness. When differentiated on the basis of the sensuous as opposed to the perceptive quality, the proportion of the former is larger. When differentiated on the basis of the obsessive as opposed to the hypochondriacal state (Table 10 b), there are 52 cases (77.6 percent) of simplified·obsessives and 15 cases (22.4 percent) of variousness·obsessives, revealing a large disparity.

From a structural standpoint, there are 21 cases (40.4 percent) of the perceptive·subjectivity combination among simplified·obsessives and 16 cases (30.8 percent) of the perceptive·objectivity combination among simplified·obsessives (Table 10 b). There are 11 cases (73.4 percent) of the perceptive·subjectivity structure among variousness·obsessives. At any rate, there is a large number of cases of the perceptive quality in which psychotherapy was supplemented with drug therapy but no correlation between cases of the simplified state as opposed to the variousness state in the instance of the obsessive state (50 cases, 75 percent). There are 36 cases of sensuous·subjectivity in the instance of the simplified state in combination with the hypochondriacal state, constituting 90 percent of all cases of the simplified state. There is also a large number (92 cases, 96.8 percent) of cases of sensuous·sensitivity among all cases of the variousness state. Thus, the proportion of cases of the hypochondriacal state that show a sensuous quality is large, being 128 cases (94.8 percent), as compared to the proportion of cases of the obsessive state that show this quality (17 cases, 25 percent).

The small number of hypochondriac·perceptive combination cases, irrespective of simplified or variety cases, indicates the partiality of this structure toward hypochondriacal delusion rather than the neurotic state, in comparison with obsessive·perceptive cases. These hypochondriac·perceptive cases were accordingly excluded from this study altogether.

When the above results are summarized, certain characteristic differences in symptom structure can be observed between cases managed with psychotherapy alone and those managed with psychotherapy supplemented with drug therapy. The following structural combinations were more characteristic (although not dramatically so) of cases managed with one treatment modality or the other:

Psychotherapy alone was more often used to manage cases that were

1. obsessive·simplified·perceptive·subjective;
2. hypochondriacal·simplified·sensuous·subjective;
3. obsessive·variousness·perceptive·subjective; or
4. hypochondriacal·variousness·sensuous·subjective.

Adjunctive drug therapy was more often used to manage cases that were

1. hypochondriacal·variousness·sensuous·subjective;
2. obsessive·simplifed·perceptive·subjective;
3. hypochondriacal·simplified·sensuous·subjective; or
4. obsessive·simplified·perceptive·objective.

Relationship between Morita Therapy and Drug Therapy

This study shows that the largest number of cases for which drugs were used in the outpatient management of *shinkeishitsu* were those of the hypochondriacal state in combination with the variousness state that displayed the sensuous quality. The clinical contradiction between this finding and the reason that drugs are rarely used in Morita therapy must now be addressed and explained, perhaps by analysis of the symptoms of *shinkeishitsu.*

Generally speaking, the objective of any therapy is first to eliminate the symptoms. However, in Morita therapy, the symptoms are not supposed to be eliminated because the hypochondriacal judgment of a patient who has the *shinkeishitsu* temperament has certain components, which are acquired by chance. These components are the primary hypochondriacal idea, which is followed by a process of "psychic interaction" (Morita) and "self-suggestive action" that intensifies and fixes the hypochondriacal idea by the "antagonistic actions of the mind," which leads to the development of a secondary hypochondriacal interpretation, "contradictoriness in thinking," and, finally, to the symptoms of *shinkeishitsu.*

The intensifying process of development from the primary idea to the secondary hypochondriacal attitude is not limited to *shinkeishitsu* but can be considered a general psychogenic phenomenon of the same nature as many other secondary developments, which make its form and content understandable. The content of this idea is not essentially of a symptomatic nature, and only the mental attitude of a patient (the structural form in which the primary idea develops into the secondary interpretation) is recognized as a symptom of *shinkeishitsu.*

In Morita theory, the answer to questions of how any such idea occurs, how it develops into its secondary form and how it is fixed as a symptom of *shinkeishitsu* is that all these phenomena result from such mechanisms as the hypochondriacal temperament, psychic interaction and self-suggestive action, and antagonistic actions of the mind.

The appearance of the hypochondriacal humor, which is considered to be the decisive causal presence of the idea, is the condition's characteristic framework; the momentum of its formation comes from the chance factor. Consequently, the content of the idea is not considered to be an illness; it is understood as being a specific manifestation of "general human nature."[53] It is not the direct object of Morita therapy. In fact, the objectives of Morita therapy are to discipline the mental attitude of a patient, which has developed secondarily and become fixed due to the hypochondriacal temperament, and to encourage, maturation of the patient's personality and strengthening of his or her social adaptability.[54]

Drugs are used in the management of many cases, as was indicated previously. Further, specific tendencies can be recognized in the symptom structures, as has been shown. At the risk of seeming repetitive, the author again notes that the hypochondriacal state in combination with the variousness state is the basis of the symptom structure, from a phenomenological standpoint, in cases in which drugs are administered; cases of the obsessive and simplified states are next in order of frequency to be managed with adjunctive drug therapy. In regard to cases of obsession, the symptom structure may be explained by reference to anthropophobia as an example, with such conditions as flushing of the cheeks, blushing, hardening of the expression and palpitation over human relationships considered as being *sensuous.* The symptoms develop from such sensuous conditions as the expression of a crying face, laughter that becomes unnatural and a gaze that becomes scathing. The conscious condition of a patient in trying to accept the symptom and have it clearly explained is considered as being perceptive.

The condition in which these sensuous and perceptive qualities of a patient converge to form subjectivity differs from the condition in which a patient senses that someone else is acting on him or her, such as another person sensing the patient's presence as projectively discomforting or as "being in the way," which is a condition of objectivity.

The phenomenon of the obsessive state, in which drugs are apt to be used for management, indicates the structure of perceptive·subjectivity or perceptive·objectivity. The fixation of a patient's consciousness is, for example, on an expression or gaze that is unpleasant or on the feeling that another person dislikes oneself. This fixation makes the content of the obsessive state more structural and concrete and, moreover, clarifies perceptive·objectivity more structurally than if it is only a condition of sensuous·objectivity. There is also a tendency for the other person's opinion to be absorbed gradually. In the process by which "symptoms of

---

[53] For a discussion of this point, see Chapter 3.

[54] The fact that Morita does not consider *shinkeishitsu* to be an illness does not mean that he considers it to be a healthy condition. The conditions that give rise to *shinkeishitsu* are all facts of human nature, but all the phenomena of *shinkeishitsu* cannot be considered as being natural. It makes more sense to consider Morita's assertion that *shinkeishitsu* is not an illness by placing it within the context of therapeutic technique.

shinkeishitsu" are aggravated secondarily, there are cases in which the process stops with an obsessive structure of *shinkeishitsu* as well as cases in which the process evolves into delusional attitudes and, from the standpoint of the type of symptom, shifts to a condition similar to E. Kretschmer's *sensitiver Beziehungswahn* (sensitive reference paranoid condition).

We need to consider carefully whether all these conditions can be included in the classification of *shinkeishitsu* within the framework of Morita theory. Even if conditions that can be considered as being manifestations of schizophrenia, without doubt, are excluded, the phenomenon common to all the other conditions is an obsessive consciousness of an ego conflict. This internal conflict can be clearly seen in the mode in which the self is involved in objective conception. When these conditions shift to a condition similar to *sensitiver Beziehungswahn*, the obsessive appearance of *shinkeishitsu* can still be observed. The sensitive paranoid condition observed in this form of *shinkeishitsu* is within the scope of conditions to which Morita therapy is applicable, but it is plausible that drugs would currently be used for the management of a large number of such cases, particularly in outpatient therapy, namely, the psychotropic drugs that are available.

The content of the hypochondriacal state, however, differs from the content of the obsessive state because there are many more cases that show the sensuous quality instead of the perceptive quality. Cases that have the hypochondriacal·perceptive structure take on the appearance of hypochondriacal delusions in proportion to the strength invested in supporting the certainty of that consciousness, so that many such cases are excluded from therapy at the very beginning.[55]

In cases that have the hypochondriacal·variousness·sensuous structure, the primary hypochondriacal idea, which has such content as the feeling of a heavy head, occurs and evolves into a hypochondriacal conflict secondarily as a result of hypochondriacal uneasiness. In such cases, however, the process also includes a large number of indefinite, scattered feelings, such as headache, a hazy feeling in the head, flushing of the face, sweating and fatigue, indicating that the process differs markedly from that in which the condition tends to converge on the initial feelings.

In a few such cases, the patient is oriented to focus on a specific part of the body but, instead, indicates unstable and multiple complaints of successive connection to a variety of sensuous somatic phenomena through the hypochondriacal humor. This variousness type of the hypochondriacal·sensuous structure has a process of secondary intensifying and development that is not structurally clear; consequently, the hypochondriacal conflict is not too conspicuous from a phenomenological standpoint, so that the therapist tends to believe that a somatic dysfunction is the underlying cause.

The hypochondriacal humor, which has been directed to a certain sensation, will tend to amplify that sensation, but during this period there are many cases of somatic components of the hypochondriacal uneasiness that a patient has. With that understanding, many therapists tend to make the first objective of therapy the relief of somatic phenomena of which a patient complains, if the symptom structure is of the hypochondriacal·variousness·sensuous combination.

Even in such cases, however, there is no difference in considering the content and form of the idea, which occurs in the psychogenic situation to cause anxiety, such as the "inadaptability anxiety" that Kōra[56] cites, as being fundamentally normal Consequently, the effect of a drug

[55] There are a large number of cases that Morita calls hypochondriasis, or paroxysmal neurosis as one type of *shinkeishitsu*, among the cases that have this structure; a hypochondriacal preoccupation with somatic conditions is conspicuous.

[56] Kōra, T.: Morita ryōhō (Morita therapy) (in Japanese). In *Essays in Commemoration of Takehisa Kōra's Appointment as Professor Emeritus*, 1964.

can be anticipated in connection with the process that develops secondarily, in cases of obsessive as well as hypochondriacal states, which are not inadaptability anxiety but, rather, derive from the adjustment of the somatic or autonomic components that accompany that anxiety.

When considered in that manner, it is believed that drug therapy is best carried out at the initial stage of psychotherapy when anxiety becomes aggravated, sometimes excessively. As a result, the somatic components of the hypochondriacal trait and, in turn, the affective components are adjusted, and together with psychotherapy, drug therapy accelerates the mechanism that moves the patient toward a cure.

It cannot be denied that the action for adjustment (potential strength for effecting a cure) that human beings inherently possess can occur purposively during this process.

In summary, the pure form of *shinkeishitsu* is the one considered by Morita to be "ordinary *shinkeishitsu*" (his so-called chronic pseudo-neurasthenia) from a phenomenological standpoint. Although there is at first no clear, conscious orientation in the developmental process of the symptoms, a shift in several somatic areas occurs sensually by means of the hypochondriacal humor, and the process of gradual concentration of consciousness on a specific area can be observed.

It is believed that drug therapy is used chiefly for managing this undifferentiated process from the standpoint of therapeutic results. However, this undifferentiated process is inferred from the assumption that the phenomena that indicate ordinary *shinkeishitsu* take the basic structure of hypochondriacal·simplified·sensuous.

If an economizing energy consumption, which can be seen in the defensive dimension of anxiety, is a "seeming simplification of the defense mechanism," as Kōra[57] points out, it can be considered that ordinary *shinkeishitsu* is the completed form of expression of any such rationalization. The same can be said for the obsessive state.

Morita says that obsession is a phenomenon that can be explained most easily by his theory owing to the fact that the process of development and of strengthening the orientation of the hypochondriacal humor to concentrate on a specific concept can be easily confirmed as being the development of Morita theory from a phenomenological standpoint. At the same time, it indicates a basic structure of *shinkeishitsu* that is obsessive·simplified. It can therefore be said that cases that display the sensuous quality and those that have the structure of variousness, even when combined with the perceptive quality, are of the shifting type of the process that leads ordinary *shinkeishitsu* or of the variant type that deviates from this pure form of *shinkeishitsu.*

When considered in that light, the questions of which structural form is most often managed with drug therapy and, conversely, which structural form is most often managed with psychotherapy alone can be answered by stating Morita therapy alone is used for the pure form of *shinkeishitsu*, and that drug therapy is used increasingly to the degree that the structural form of the *shinkeishitsu* differs from this form, be it an obsessive or a hypochondriacal state.

A study was carried out on the conditions for which drugs are used by citing, as a reference, 553 patients with *shinkeishitsu* treated by the author and his colleagues at the psychiatric outpatients' department of the Jikei University School of Medicine and at the Tokiwadai Psychiatric Clinic during three periods: 1950–53, 1963 and 1961–79 (see Tables 1a and 4 c.)

The author's major purpose here is to discuss the benefit of drug therapy in the conduct of Morita therapy by examining the kinds of case in which drugs are used most often. In this regard, it is apparent that the structure of *shinkeishitsu* and the nature of Morita therapy should be restudied from the standpoint of adjunctive drug therapy and from the perspective of

---

57 Kōra, T.: Morita therapy. *International Journal of Psychiatry* 1(4) (1965).

whether such therapy may, in fact, be a satisfactory substitute for Morita therapy in the management of *shinkeishitsu.*

It is widely accepted that drugs have a therapeutic effect on mental disorders, and adjustment of problems at the somatic level by use of drugs is one form of therapy. Some researchers hold that combination therapy can simultaneously raise a patient's consciousness to an especially high order of mental integration. The author believes that opinion should be considered carefully, particularly in regard to therapy for neuroses.

Drug therapy is unusually effective in certain instances. There is no doubt that potential drug effectiveness can be tempting to therapists because, from the standpoint of psychotherapy (although such therapy may appear powerless at first impression), the person who becomes most acutely aware of its deficiencies is the therapist. Distrust of drugs is similar to doubts about whether a neurosis can be managed solely with psychotherapy. However, setting aside medical technology, it is true that a patient's personality has a great impact in a purely psychotherapeutic situation. However, this factor has little impact in medical therapy in general.

The limitations of psychotherapy do, however, make the use of drugs attractive for the management of mental disorders, in that drug therapy is considered scientific and quick-acting. In the author's experience, this attraction is limited to the possible promotion of the patient-therapist relationship, and therapists need to keep in mind that the effects of drugs have no direct relation to the objectives of therapy. If therapists act by trial and error in trying to determine whether to use drugs or psychotherapy, the management of neurosis will face grave danger.

Therapists do need to be conscious of exactly what they wish drugs to accomplish. There is no doubt that psychotropic drugs will be further improved and that new, more useful drugs will be developed, to the extent that drug therapy could become indispensable for obtaining cures. However, the issue of whether drug therapy alone can free human beings from mental disorders will remain unresolved, even in the future.

An important reason that this issue cannot be resolved is that drugs suited precisely to each one of us, with our unique individual selves, would seem to be impossible to develop. As Cole[58] explains, the limitations of psychotropic drug therapy are difficult to overcome owing to the difference between the subject and the patient, the difference between the therapist and the brainwasher and the differences between drugs.

The author has found that a symptom has a fixed structural trait by analysis of the situational use of drugs in Morita therapy. However, this finding does not answer the question of whether it is preferable to administer drugs or to use psychotherapy to manage symptoms that indicate any such structure. The management of the distinctively individual forms of suffering that are called mental disorders as a so-called general objective does involve the problem of dealing with the life experience of each human being whose creative thoughts need to be accepted.

Managing a disorder only from the perspective of abstract considerations is a misguided approach. Management of a neurosis progresses only if the therapist comes in direct contact with a patient and places himself or herself in the patient's position. Only in this way is it possible for psychotherapy to provide that heart-to-heart involvement with a human being that a drug cannot provide.

In considering the issue of how psychotherapy for neuroses should be designed, by experience with the treatment of outpatients by use of drugs, and also in considering the role that drugs currently have in Morita therapy, it is clear that drug therapy alone cannot successfully cure the pure form of *shinkeishitsu.*

---

[58] Cole, J. O.: ibid.

Part VI

Concepts of Therapeutic Improvement

20

Definitions of Cure in Morita Therapy

The field of psychotherapy is said to be full of ambiguous terms, expressions and concepts.[1] The word *chiyu* (cure) is one such ambiguous term.

To discuss the "condition of cure," expressions apparently borrowed from somatotherapy are used in psychotherapy, as indicated by the expressions "spontaneous cure" and "symptom relief" (lessening of symptom severity).

In reality, however, the concept of a therapeutic cure in psychiatry is different and by no means so simple. Although a discussion of the definition of a "cure" is important, it is no easy task because there are disparities in therapeutic aims and goals, which are dependent on social and cultural requisites, conceptual views of mental health and illness espoused by therapists and, of course, the general problem of the risks and limitations of psychotherapy.

The conceptual content of what constitutes a cure is exceedingly complicated and diverse. Thus, it is understandable that therapists are profoundly concerned with their goals, with what the public considers a proper goal and with what occurs until the goal is attained. Nonetheless, these issues are beyond the scope of this chapter.

The success or failure of therapy can be assessed only on the basis of the context of its predetermined goal. Success of therapy must be evaluated, in separate terms, in accordance with the content of the therapeutic standard. This content must include, for example, the condition of a patient who is receiving therapy and his or her social and cultural milieu. We need to consider the commonalities and peculiarities of therapeutic goals or conditions, with a basic allowance being made for differences, in principle, that are characteristic of each school of psychotherapy and each therapist.

In the following text, the author will express his views of what constitutes the goal and cure in Morita therapy.

Therapeutic Goal and Cure in Morita Therapy

Morita's Definition of Therapeutic Goal and Cure

The following statements on the subject of therapeutic goal and cure have been extracted from Morita's *Shinkeishitsu no Hontai oyobi Ryōhō* (The Substance of *Shinkeishitsu* and Its Therapy), which is considered the seminal reference work on Morita therapy.

Morita states that ". . . . when considered from the perspective of the substance of *shinkeishitsu* . . . the patient's attempt to cure the disorder by himself has the opposite effect, similar to one's awareness of becoming more mentally tenacious in remembering something the harder

[1] Wolberg, L.R.: *The Technique of Psychotherapy*, Part Two. Grune & Stratton, New York (1967).

one tries to forget it. Although electrotherapeutics and a number of drug injection therapies seem to be effective, all of them are reducible to concealed auto-suggestion and are symptomatic therapies of only temporary effect. This is harmful, because the patient loses confidence in these therapies whenever the disorder recurs. He repeats the former trial and error approach, and this often results in the symptoms becoming deeply fixed."

". . . . This is due to the fact that the patient tries to cure the symptoms by himself. But this effort only serves to strengthen 'the contradictoriness in thinking' which activates the symptoms of *shinkeishitsu* and ends in an outcome entirely different from what the patient expected. . . . In particular, the method of continuing the administration of sedatives, ordering the patient to rest, or having him spend time in self-indulgence during therapy for *shinkeishitsu* is completely contraindicated from the therapeutic standpoint."

Morita stresses that during the therapeutic process, a Morita therapist must not use any measure that affords temporary relief of symptoms, regardless of how strongly a patient pleads for such relief. The factors that constitute obstacles must be eliminated; at the same time, assertive attempts must be made to accelerate the curative process.

Morita explains that ". . . the emphasis of therapy must be placed on removal of the complex psychological conflict, to reduce it to simple pain or fear. The patient is instructed only to 'persevere' and to 'not try to avoid suffering.' Persuasive techniques cited by Dubois and others, such as 'overcome it,' 'stop worrying and forget it' and 'do not entertain any such thoughts' must not be used. . . . It is possible to direct the patient toward a cure, without recurrence of the disorder, only by making the patient attain the mental attitude of plunging into fear, if only just once. The mental state of the patient who is oriented toward a cure by this process is one of 'having been brought to his senses' or that 'dawn has arrived,' as frequently stated by patients. In retrospect, the patient looks back at his abnormal condition of the past and may even feel how strange it was to have been in so agonizing a mental condition. The patient who has been in such a condition will only then understand that the substance of what is existent or non-existent in a dream is non-existent in both existence and non-existence; right or wrong in a state of mental conflict is 'wrong for both right and wrong'."

Morita outlines the major aims of therapeutic action by first noting that ". . . the various symptoms of *shinkeishitsu* (including obsession) were not caused by primary theoretical errors of thought but by the hypochondriacal humor which initiated fear and anxiety, and this induced various errors of thought. Consequently, *feeling* is the basis of *shinkeishitsu* symptoms; thinking is secondary. . . . Therapeutic attention must first be directed to the emotional condition. . . . The method for overcoming the emotional disorder is to live in the state of *arugamama*, based on an understanding that the lives and survival of human beings are not invariable. Human beings need to strive constantly to remind themselves that they can, at any time, succumb to illness. They need to eliminate *shisō no mujun* (contradictoriness in thinking) from their lives, comply with the facts of feelings as they are, endure those feelings, and abandon any attempts to shut out or get rid of their feelings."

In summary, the basic emotional state of a hypochondriac must, first of all, be cultivated and trained; second, contradictoriness in thinking must be eliminated. The final goal of Morita therapy is a condition in which a patient lives in the state of *arugamama* as that of his or her human nature.

Arugamama is an ambiguous term, sometimes being taken to mean the opposite of Morita's therapeutic goal. Its true meaning, as is explained in footnote 3, is formed by Morita's understanding of human nature and his view of *shinkeishitsu*. He says that the onset of *shinkeishitsu* is due primarily to mental conflict caused by the antagonistic inner clash of *sei no yokubō* (the desire to live) with the "hypochondriacal humor," which have an oppositional relationship (in the final analysis, a life and death relationship).

The symptoms of *shinkeishitsu* are discovered in the expression of a person's life. The natural function of the mind has been lost, owing to nonacceptance of the fear and suffering of one's condition and of being in contention with it. Actions are shackled as a result of adherence to this condition; the socializing process is obstructed because the person becomes extremely self-centered.

Morita understood that the *toraware* (mental captivity) of the self is not a deviation from normality. Such a person is not mentally ill, but the potential of reaching a high degree of emotional maturity is clouded. What Morita considers as being *arugamama* is the assertive expression of the self in accordance with living conditions and with "suffering accepted as it is," basing one's actions in *sei no yokubō* and not considering one's suffering as something "abnormal" or "morbid." Morita expresses this condition as one of *arugamama* because "it is a phenomenon which can be observed in the condition that it naturally should be."

This *arugamama* condition was stipulated as one of Morita's therapeutic goals, and its natural manifestation is, indeed, the proof of recovery from the *shinkeishitsu* condition. In Morita's words, "a determined shout, generally speaking, is more essential than words in actual *shinkeishitsu* therapy. And experience is even more important than shouting. Free mental activity in human beings lies in harmonizing the antagonistic actions of the mind. Receptiveness is the mental attitude of withstanding fear and suffering. In conflict with this mental attitude of patient perseverance is the craving for action that arises from the desire to live. Cure of the *shinkeishitsu* condition can be commenced only by harmonizing this desire with endurance[2] to prevent it from recurring."

Morita also says that "a cure indicates a condition in which the disorder has been eliminated. . . . There will be no obsession when the mental conflict disappears. If simply being anxious amounted to obsession, it would be a universal human feeling."

A decrease in conflict appears when the antagonistic actions of the mind are harmonized, and this harmonization can probably be considered the final goal of Morita therapy.

Therapeutic Goals and Definitions of Cure in Post-Morita Literature

Statements have been made by various researchers concerning the definition of a cure in Morita therapy. The author will discuss the most important problems that have been cited. Imura,[3] for example, comments that the goal of Morita therapy is "to carry out a psychological reduction down to a simple attitude of accepting suffering as suffering and desire as desire. When viewed from one perspective, this process of reduction is a liberation of the basic desire for life from an unjustifiably self-protective attitude."

Consequently, he continues, "to endure the training of submitting to the facts of suffering, an attitude of absolute obedience, of entrusting the final outcome to the psychotherapist, must come first. This mental attitude of delegating or entrusting is the major defect, i.e., exactly what is lacking in the *shinkeishitsu* patient, who is much too attached to self. The correct mental attitude is one of placing trust in the therapist and in the therapeutic condition. Guided by the therapist, the patient finally attains a mental attitude of entrusting the facts of his situation and builds up a feeling of trust."

Entrusting one's mind to a therapist by absolute obedience, being both receptive and accepting, is the key to beginning to move forward toward a cure.

Imura's statement is a present-day expression of Morita's therapeutic principle as well as an accurate reexpression. Nevertheless, there is a possibility of misinterpreting these terms—recep-

[2] The harmonizing of these two factors is synonymous with being in the condition of *arugamama*.
[3] Imura, T.: *Shinri Ryōhō* (Psychotherapy). Sekaisha, Tokyo (1952). (Printed in Japanese)

tiveness and entrusting–which calls for further explanation. First of all, it is possible that the condition will recur if it appears to be cured by receptiveness alone.

Morita explains that true recovery cannot take place unless continuous harmonizing of the antagonistic actions of the mind into the natural rhythms of the mind is attained. Likewise, the attitude of entrusting is open to possible misinterpretation.

A patient suffering from *shinkeishitsu* lacks the mental attitude of entrusting because he or she is much too attached to the self. For this reason, absolute obedience to the other person, the therapist, and to the therapeutic situation is essential. This condition of then entrusting everything to one's authentic mind is created in the patient by getting him or her to recognize what entrusting is all about. As Morita says, "the individual human life always passes through difficult mental stages in the process of acquiring this entrusting mental attitude."

What Imura describes as absolute obedience to a therapist, or to the therapeutic situation, is a mental attitude that is almost impossible to acquire as a preliminary condition for therapy, with the exception of special cases, in the relationship between patient and therapist.

The absolute obedience that Imura cites apparently refers to an attitude of assertive receptiveness. If this attitude is interpreted as indicating blind obedience, its meaning is thoroughly different from Morita's intent. Blind obedience to a therapist is a maneuver taken by a patient in a bid to elicit flattery, and such a maneuver is nonreflective.

The therapist's instructions are followed thoroughly, with effort made evident only when harmonizing begins in a patient's mind by means of a complex, painful process to resolve repulsion, resistance, distrust, doubt or perplexity directed toward the person of the therapist and the therapeutic situation.

Receptiveness to the realities of human mentality is created by the patient's awakening to adopt an obedient mental attitude and, further, by daily life activities. In due course, a condition of entrusting everything to one's true human nature will develop. Consequently, there is a basic difference between simple receptiveness or obedience and the special attitude of receptive *arugamama*[4] that Morita defines.

Imura's insistence on absolute obedience and trust, if accepted literally, would mean absolute mental and emotional dependence on a therapist (through submission to the therapist and the therapeutic situation). This dependence is the state of mind of a patient who discards all mental discretion and entrusts the entire situation to a therapist. The shedding of the old self, to become the natural self, has something in common with *jinen hōni*,[5] which means following truth for its own sake (which leads to self-realization) in the words of Shinran,[6] who founded one sect of Japanese Buddhism.

However, if the attainment of this state of *jinen hōni* is a prerequisite for success in therapy, it is obviously too difficult. Moreover, because *jinen hōni* is the supreme state of mind, therapy would, then, be unnecessary. Shinran, it is said, attained this supreme state of mind at the age of 86. Morita therapy is directed toward ordinary human beings.

Ikeda[7] explains that Morita theory does not take into consideration each symptom of a patient; he insists that "renovation of character is not taken into consideration at the beginning of therapy. The aim of the therapist is to remove the vicious circle formed by a certain intellec-

---

[4] What Morita calls the receptiveness of the condition of *arugamama* does not arise from resignation, nor is it a temporary therapeutic expedient. To him, *arugamama* is a phenomenon that is evident in the life activities of a healthy human being.

[5] Shinran (circa 1172–1262); see Chapter 3.

[6] Shinran says that *jinen hōni* is a discarding of discretion by one's own power, to entrust all to the Buddha. However, this self-salvation means to entrust oneself to the Buddha at a point where one has exerted utmost effort, instead of depending completely on other persons.

[7] Ikeda, K.: Morita shinkeishitsu to sono ryōhō (Nervosity (Morita) and Morita therapy) (in Japanese). *Seishin Igaku* 1(7) (1959).

Table 11 Percentage of Complete Cure or Some Improvement

Source	Time Period	Number of Cases	Complete Cure (%)	Some Improvement (%)
Morita[8]	1919–26	124	60.0	33.0
Kōra[9, 10]	1929–37	541	61.0	35.5
Yasuda[11]	1949–52	212	49.1	45.3
Yora[12]	1949–53	406	63.3	16.2
Matsunaga[13]	1955–59	71	40.8	35.2
Suzuki[14]	1951–60	263	71.0	19.8
Iwai & Abe[15]	1972–73	139	50.4	36.7
Suzuki & Suzuki[16]	1963–74	731	61.1	35.4

tual posture and to return the patient to a condition in which his authentic human character, in elementary form, can be exhibited, as it is, in actual living."

Restoration of a patient to this condition leads to his or her recovery. Ikeda goes on to say that "a hypochondriacal personality has the character of being essentially more concerned about detail than the average person. It is a personality that seeks perfection; the individual suffers because of his or her imperfection. The condition which constitutes a *shinkeishitsu* cure is that of the individual's self-image of being someone who lives in the endurance of suffering and anxiety alien to the experience of the average person or, in particular, the optimist."

Ikeda further adds that "the most ordinary cure condition" is one in which there is no *toraware* (mental captivity). Because there is no change in the original character trend of *shinkeishitsu*, the cure can be described as "a self-possessed, quiet mental structure of discovering by oneself that, before one is aware of it, one is free to do what he pleases; one was not able to do this before, even though one has no feeling of fundamental improvement as a direct result of therapy."

What Ikeda means by "the most ordinary cure condition" is one in which, clinically speaking, a patient is not aware of any "fundamental recovery" but has become aware that the shackles on conscious action have decreased, leading to an increase in life activities or of attaining a certain freedom of activity.

The author has observed numerous cases of the "cure-image" as Ikeda describes it. If the term "ordinary," though, is supposed to mean "most numerous or average," the author would not consider it as being the general, most common image of cure in Morita therapy.

According to the published results of several therapists (see Table 11), complete cures are obtained with the highest frequency. However, there are considerable differences in the rate of complete cures, which are reported in about 40 to 71 percent of cases, averaging 56.8 percent. Morita reported a complete cure rate of 60 percent, although there is a subtypical difference. Kōra[9,10] also reported a complete cure rate of about 61 percent.

Each therapist defines a complete in a respective form of expression but there are major

[8] Morita, S.: Yo no shinkeishitsu tokushu ryōhō ni yoru chiryō seiseki (Therapeutic results of Morita therapy for *shinkeishitsu*) (in Japanese). *Psychiatria et Neurologia Japonica* 30(8):526 (1929).

[9] Kōra, T.: Shinkeishitsu no mondai (The problem of so-called neurasthenia) (in Japanese). *Psychiatria et Neurologia Japonica* 42:755 (1938).

[10] Kōra, T.: Morita therapy. *International Journal of Psychiatry* 1(611) : 140 (1965).

[11] Yasuda, M.: Shinkeishitsushō kenkyū hoi (A supplemental study on *shinkeishitsu*) (in Japanese). In *Essays in Celebration of the 15th Anniversary of the Opening Lecture of Professor Kōra* (1955).

[12] Yora, T.: Shinkeishitsushō no yogo ni kansuru rinshōteki kenkyū (A clinical study on prognosis of *shinkeishitsu*) (in Japanese). *Tōkyō Jikeikai Ika Daigaku Zasshi* 75(2) : 306 (1960).

[13] Matsunaga, N.: A psychopathological study on chronic neuroses with the obsessive-compulsive symptoms (in Japanese). *Shinkeishitsu* 1:2 (1960).

[14] Suzuki, T.: Morita therapy of *shinkeishitsu* (in Japanese). *Seishin Igaku* 1(7):497 (1959).

[15] Iwai, H. and Abe, T.: *Theory and Practice in Morita Therapy.* Kongō Shuppan, Tokyo (1975). (Printed in Japanese)

[16] Suzuki, T. and Suzuki, R.: Nyūin Morita ryōhō wo uketa shinkeishō kanja no tsuiseki chōsa (A follow-up of neurotics treated by inpatient Morita therapy) (in Japanese). *Psychiatria et Neurologia Japonica* 81(10):666 (1979).

points common to all definitions, namely, the disappearance of symptoms, restoration of the capability for adapting to daily home and social life, attainment of insight into one's symptoms and continuous mental and physical stability.

The first two of these four standards of recovery pertain to elimination of symptoms and can be expressed quantitatively. For example, although some degree of anxiety remains, the cure condition is one in which a patient with *shinkeishitsu* is no longer shackled by excessive anxiety and can participate in daily home and social life more freely than before. There is a condition of "some improvement" in the category of the next highest degree of cure. The rate of cases in which there is some improvement is lower than that of complete cure, being about 15 to 40 percent according to the figures furnished by these therapists. Owing to differences in the rapidity of the complete cure process, time differences can be applied to ranking the efficacy of the therapeutic result.

The "ordinary cure" condition cited by Ikeda can be considered as being one of some improvement rather than as a complete cure. In this ordinary cure condition, the hypochondriacal tendency continues to be a characteristic of patients, as Ikeda points out. The continuation of this tendency could indicate that there is no complete cure condition in Morita therapy. However, as Morita says, if simple concern were construed to be obsession, obsession would be a universal human attitude.

The complete elimination of conflict could be considered as being indicative of the cure condition. A patient who now has no mental conflict becomes clearly conscious of numerous changes in his or her self-consciousness, due to therapy, from the standpoint of symptoms. Some patients express this new mental state by saying that "it seems as if I've awakened from a dream" or that "dawn has come."

Even in the condition of "not feeling basically cured" that Ikeda mentions, many patients have become conscious of basic differences, compared with their condition before treatment. When their conflicts have disappeared, such patients become aware that their minds are no longer captivated.

There is no real doubt that the cure profile for a patient with *shinkeishitsu* is the profile of "a human being who has to live with a burden of suffering and anxiety not borne by the average person or the optimist." However, the author believes that a patient with *shinkeishitsu* who is in the cure condition can be categorized as being an average, healthy human being. The author does not believe that such patients alone experience suffering and anxiety of a type that does not affect an ordinary person. However, there are differences among such patients in regard to the conditions in which the suffering and anxiety occur.

Whether or not a patient becomes keenly aware of changes in self-consciousness, due to therapy or some other factor, the change in self-consciousness–because of the emotional experience generated by Morita therapy and its momentum–will eventually evolve into a reorganization and reintegration of the personality as a whole. The author believes that this condition can be considered to be the basis of the condition of cure.[17]

Patients' Images of a Cure in Relation to Their Social and Cultural Milieu

The common and primary objectives of all therapies are the elimination, or at least alleviation, of a patient's symptoms and the redirection of the patient toward a better condition of mental health. However, the condition that constitutes mental health is defined by a therapist's principles and view of mental illness as well as by society.

Further, there are differences in the images of a therapeutic result among patients. An image is rooted in the personality or environment of a patient.

A therapist must consider thoroughly the procedure needed to mesh his or her goal with the expectations of a patient. The patient's social and cultural milieu must also be taken into account.

Morita therapy differs from psychoanalysis in that it is not a technique for investigation of the unconscious stratum. Even so, efforts are made to understand the personality of the patient, his or her past life and his or her present living conditions from a therapeutic standpoint.

Many patients display dissatisfaction or repulsion toward their therapists or uncertainty of acceptance. This general resistance of certain patients stems in part from the Morita technique of enforcing absolute, isolated bed rest and physical work assignments. The "captivity" symptom that a patient displays is not understood by him or her as being an expression of personality. Also, the patient does not consider the meaningfulness of his or her symptoms from the standpoint of the symptoms being strictly symptoms, instead considering them as obstructions unsuited to healthy human life.

The goal of Morita therapy is to guide a patient toward a self-assertive acceptance of his or her symptoms. However, attempts to attain this condition generate self-centered, dependent attitudes in patients that lead to a complex inner feeling of repulsion toward therapists and Morita therapy. This feeling of repulsion is also due to the high expectations that patients have of their therapists. This self-contradictory phenomenon tends to reveal patients' images of the anticipated cure.

Some of a patient's major expectations are (1) elimination of sensory suffering, (2) elimination of anxiety and fear, (3) attainment of a healthy mental condition without disquiet, (4) acquisition of the capability for taking self-willed action in all life situations and (5) a shift from introversion to extroversion.

This image of a cure espoused by a patient differs according to the type of *shinkeishitsu* that he or she has. For example, patients with ordinary *shinkeishitsu* or paroxysmal neurosis consider the elimination of sensory suffering to be the foremost criterion of mental health, whereas patients with obsession or phobia consider improvement in character, namely, the third and fifth expectations noted in the preceding paragraph, to be the most important criteria.

A patient always desires to be capable of withstanding all sorts of tension, to overcome discomforting feelings and to have the capability for self-expression without becoming mentally unhealthy in all life situations. The patient, further, looks forward to the realization of those expectations.

---

[17] Nakae says that he did not find any significant difference between a group of patients with *shinkeishitsu* examined at random and a group of healthy subjects, using the Rorschach test as an index, with the exception of BRS, Rej., M. This finding indicates that when BRS is used as an index, its value is increased after recovery (an average of 46 days before and after the test). There was no difference observed between the two groups from the standpoint of an overall image of character integration. Also, W/M shifted toward an adequate condition after recovery, with increases in inner stability, self-approval and responsiveness. F+% and R+% also showed remarkable increases to a level no different from that of the healthy subjects. Redirection of patients toward a realistic, impartial attitude, and away from a self-centered attitude, was observed in testing for perception of reality. FM/M also reached an adequate level, with redirection toward inner stability and internal control by a maturation process. The number of the FC<CF+C type was small among patients with *shinkeishitsu*, with no difference observed in the healthy subjects. These findings differ from those obtained in cases of hysteria. There was no marked problem in self-integration of emotional expression. This finding suggests that the change in self-consciousness is not as superficial as it is generally believed to be. Nakae, S.: Shinkeishitsu shō no Morita ryōhō ni yoru chiryō kōka oyobi sono seishin byōri ni kansuru kenkyū—Rorschach test ni yoru (A study on therapeutic effects reflected upon personality change of "Nervosität" by Morita therapy—by means of the Rorschach test. (in Japanese). *Rorschachiana Japonica* 2:86 (1959).

This is an idealized self-image condition of the first order. However, the patient does not readily become aware that this is only his or her fixed conceptual image of a cure.

The basis of this image of a cure is a comparison of one's past self-image seen from the perspective of suffering in the present, along with a certain view of the other persons who inhabit the patient's world, in terms of a patient's condition. The self of the past actually differs from the self of the present. The patient is also firmly convinced that other persons are different, in not being timid and without indication of mental unease. Other persons seem to remain composed, with no sign of anxiety or fear, under any and all circumstances.

In general, the self-evaluation of a patient with *shinkeishitsu* in regard to his or her character is low, even before the onset of morbidity, and the patient tends to consider *shinkeishitsu* as being a character defect.

However, the expectations of a cure that derive from the desire to become at least a commonplace human being, one who can meet the demands of society without hesitation and with no concern over one's mental and physical condition, being able to do whatever one wishes, saying readily whatever one wants to say and thrusting aside the timid self that also sits and broods, results in an objective state of suffering over the vast disparity between actual self-evaluation and highly idealized self-evaluation.[18]

In many cases, the image of a cure espoused by a patient is prescribed by social prerequisites, particularly from a personality point of view. A patient with *shinkeishitsu* believes that society's standard of mental health and the image of a healthy human being projected by members of the patient's family, place of employment or school environment differ considerably from the personality that is characteristic of *shinkeishitsu.*

The public tends to place high value on such qualities as courage, self-confidence, boldness, aggressiveness, resoluteness and practicality or creativity in facing any and all life situations. The *shinkeishitsu* personality that tries to comply with those expectations becomes ever more passive and timid, always concerned about "things," oversensitive, weak and irresolute. This personality cannot readily open up to other personalities in a candid manner, due to pride, in spite of a strong inner sense of dependence on other persons.

The inadaptability anxiety generated by the inability to express oneself in social situations, because of this character inferiority, leads to the emotional crisis of being ridiculed by people, or of becoming a dropout, and thus of becoming more and more antagonistic toward the present self.[19]

The *shinkeishitsu* personality will try to comply with the expectations of the society to which he or she belongs, but the failure of those efforts will result in a deeper and deeper plunge into inferiority feelings.

This tendency further increases as problems of ability and suitability emerge with ever-deepening involvement with society. Feelings of loneliness and autism are reinforced by each obstruction encountered in the thwarted process of becoming a healthy member of society. The perfectionistic trend increases simultaneously. Acceptance of the inner double-image of the self (actual and idealized) becomes ever more difficult to maintain. Independence in selection is avoided and interpersonal involvements shunned. Consciousness of ego identity[20] in society is weakened the more one tries to assimilate the true self with society.

---

[18] Kōra, T., Fujita, C., et al.: Zen no shinrigakuteki kenkyū (The psychological study of Zen) (in Japanese). In *Essays in Commemoration of Takehisa Kōra's Appointment as Professor Emeritus*, 1964.

[19] The anxiety of the *shinkeishitsu* personality estranged from *seken* (reference group) is essentially due to a disposition that can be generally observed in the Japanese as a whole, although there are notable differences of degree. For example, Yanagida has said that the only natural characteristic of the Japanese is an attitude of toadyism, a human phenomenon comparable, perhaps, to the instinctive behavior of migratory birds, an attitude of tenacious adherence to the cultural and social milieu in which one lives.

[20] Erikson, E.H.: *Identity and the Life Cycle.* International University Press (1959).

The *shinkeishitsu* personality that has progressed to this neurotic condition accepts life's psychological rules and receives advice or encouragement in a negative manner, unlike the mentally healthy personality, which accepts all this positively. As a result, *shisō no mujun* (contradictoriness in thinking) arises, and true human freedom is lost. Thus, the *shinkeishitsu* personality falls into a vicious circle and is strongly shackled by social rules; the *shinkeishitsu* symptom becomes more strongly fixed, and the goal becomes an image of a cure that will enable compliance with social demands. In view of this, what image of a cure does a therapist project to meet a patient's expectations? The patient must embody an image of a cure in the therapeutic process, and the therapist must guide the patient in that direction.

Relationship between the Recovery Process and Patients' Self-centered Attitudes

Doi[21] attempts to interpret the mental attitude imposed by the shackles of hypochondriacy as arising from an attitude toward human relationships that can be considered to be instinctive and basic to human beings. That attitude is called *amae.*[22] Doi also states that the image of the self that is at present isolated from this *amae* attitude, in other words, the consciousness that is called the self, is "perceived in a condition in which there is no self" in the process of therapeutic recovery.[23] The danger of *amae* arising during the therapeutic process comes to the fore, and the consciousness of the self is born with this phenomenon as the turning point.

The author sometimes encounters a patient who has a consciousness that "the present self is not the natural self," but there are only a few patients who complain of a shift in consciousness to a condition "in which there is no self." The condition toward which a patient is directed as the general center of the process in Morita therapy is that of the self-centered attitude.

It cannot be denied, of course, that consciousness of a "self that is not the natural self" is similar to consciousness of "no self," but as we can see in Doi's examples, it is believed that there is a difference from a phenomenological point of view, in that a patient does not become aware of this self during therapy, suffers from the consciousness that this self is not the natural self and considers this conscious feeling to be the main complaint.

At any rate, rather than "the consciousness that there is no self," the thought process of a patient with *shinkeishitsu*, in theory, is that it is difficult to recognize a social mutuality or collectivity that is necessary for human beings to live with one another in social situations. This difficulty arises because a patient becomes egotistical, oversensitive or closed-in due to the fact that the issue of a positive proof of personal safety is strongly concentrated within the self.

We can consider the level of the self observed in the *shinkeishitsu* personality as akin to the immature psychological state that is called the undifferentiation of subject-object when compared, for example, with what Piaget refers to as *egocentrisme.*

Morita theory emphasizes a "discarding of the self" instead of aiming at a "process of strengthening the self," as in psychoanalysis. This emphasis arises from the fact that the approach to the self by a patient, who is overly self-centered, is the actual process of a cure,

---

[21] Doi, T.: Shinkeishitsu no seishin byōri—Tokuni toraware no seishin rikigaku ni tsuite (Psychopathology of *shinkeishitsu*, especially regarding the psychodynamics of its *toraware*) (in Japanese). *Psychiatria et Neurologia Japonica* 60:734–744 (1958).

[22] *Amae* is a psychological trend in which one cultivates continuing contact with another person by continuous kindness or acts willfully with the expectation that the other person will recognize one's good nature or intentions. According to Doi; he defines *amae* as follows: Deny the fact of separation which is inseparable from human existence and aspire to be inclined to sublate hard experience of separation.

[23] Doi, T.: *Jibun* to *amae* no seishin byōri (Psychopathology of self and *amae*) (in Japanese). *Psychiatria et Neurologia Japonica* 62(1):149 (1962).

instead of making a self out of "the consciousness called self that was not present before" as the objective, as Doi points out.

Both of these therapeutic objectives, which appear at first glance to be contradictory, can be said to indicate entirely different phenomena. It is true that the mentality of a patient with *shinkeishitsu* also appears to be immature because it exhibits confusion and vagueness and shows a disposition akin to autistic trends and an insufficient sense of social solidarity between personal actuality and objective reality. However, in Morita theory, this mentality is considered to be a condition of autism of the self that is due to difficulties experienced in manifestation of the overall activities of intellect, emotion and volition, such as creativity and spontaneity. In other words, the mind of the *shinkeishitsu* personality is not easily opened to the outer world owing to the condition of "captivity" caused by contradictoriness in thinking.

This condition differs from the emotionally immature condition in which an emotional disorder that appears to be hysteria, for example, readily arises (see the thesis by Nakae). Further, making oneself captive to the hypochondriacal attitude is understood as being temperamental, rather than as being an inferiority of the self caused by frustration in one's past life.

The conflict and captivity of the *shinkeishitsu* condition are a personality reaction, not a deep-seated biological reaction. This condition is considered to be a mental phenomenon at a high level of personality. A patient has a hypochondriacal tendency (of temperament) that characterizes *shinkeishitsu* as a life reaction exhibited from a personality standpoint due to the uneasiness that arises from a lack of self-realization. The natural human self is motivated by "the desire to live" to exert continual effort for improvement and development of the self. This mental activity naturally flows in the direction of adapting oneself to social conditions.

Personality conflict is caused when it is sensed that this natural progression is obstructed by certain situations, and "the desire for life" gradually shifts to the "hypochondriacal attitude" owing to the relativistic relationships that exist between these two factors within the human consciousness. This is understood in terms of a self-activity that is relativistically involved with the desire for life and the "hypochondriacal humor," which are, in essence, mutually disciplined toward harmonious functioning through continual gradations. In a patient afflicted with *shinkeishitsu*, these gradations have led to a condition in which the hypochondriacal humor has assumed a position of superior influence. This change has taken place because the patient's temperament has become hypochondriacally oriented in response to a chance experiential factor and has thus become a generally disharmonious attitude. This chance experience is an ordinary mental event or everyday occurrence, but its meaning shifts gradually and individually as the *shinkeishitsu* personality comes into closer and closer contact with society.

The *shinkeishitsu* personality then concludes that the actual mental and physical experiences that accompany the self-realization process are morbid and abnormal and not only tries to avoid acceptance of this condition but also tries to oppose it, as an obstacle to adaptation to life. Consequently, consciousness is incessantly preoccupied with this obstruction and, at the same time, is in objective pursuit of a completely idealized self-image.

The self that is captivated by so endless and fruitless an autistic vicious circle strongly seeks social solidarity inwardly but becomes blocked because this solidarity cannot be attained, and the patient begins to assume a self-centered attitude. That is, the *shinkeishitsu* personality has the potential ability to concentrate the activities of the self for expression by means of personality integration, through inward harmonizing, self-approval or sympathy, but because much of this energy is used up, instead, in self-conflict, the process of becoming neurotic is strengthened and the personality becomes overly self-centered.

Let us consider, in this regard, the relationship that exists, from the standpoint of the curative process, between "discarding the self" and "strengthening the self" out of this overly self-centered perspective of a patient during the process of recovery.

When the process of recovery and self-centeredness are dealt with in Morita therapy, it is first necessary to point out that the self is the prime constituent of "all oppositional relationships with society." Such oppositional relationships hold a position of so-called *engi.*[24] This concept is a Buddhist or Oriental view of the self.

The subject of the ego is not addressed directly in Morita theory, but if the concept of the ego is considered from Morita's viewpoint, the self as subject (the phenomenal self) is stipulated as the starting point, on the basis of disposition theory. However, this principle is not self-evident. The ego field is a general psychological condition. At the same time, it is something that is supported by a fluid view of human beings who exist in an expanding space-time continuum that can be said to be limitless.[25]

Consequently, this self has a subjective existence instead of being, for instance, an objectively limited self that is recognized as such. "The original self," or "*arugamama* self," of Morita therapy is not a limited, fixed self, such as an ideal self-image of what one should be (e.g., the image of a cure projected by a patient with *shinkeishitsu*), instead referring to a true self to be developed through experiential practice. The patient will tend to move further and further from reality, chasing the phantom of an idealized self in a thoroughly self-centered way. To contend with this phenomenon, Morita stresses the discarding of all discernment of the self.

This state of mind can be considered as being equivalent to the *mu*[26] (nothingness) of Zen Buddhism, but Morita interprets it in his way by considering *mu* to be something that cannot be cut off. The dignity of the original self is exhibited when all mental discernment is discarded to attain a condition of *arugamama.*

What Morita refers to as *junna kokoro* (authentic or intrinsic mind, pure mind) or *jijitsu yuishin* (only the actual fact is true) is a realization of the self that consists of comprehending that only, and nothing other than, the fact is what is true. In this condition, a patient with *shinkeishitsu* has discarded the discretionary functions of the ego and entrusted the self implicitly to the factual state of his or her mentality. Although this so-called self-negation appears to be nihilistic, it is definitely not so. It signifies a complete severance by the ego of any attachment to the self that is fixed or can be conceived. The transcendence of the ego to a state of the true self from that of self-attachment is concealed.[27]

---

[24] This term is a liberal translation of *pratītyasamutpāda* in Sanskrit, and it means something that occurs by means of its relationship to something else, which is the basis of Buddhist teachings.

[25] Self-awareness of the ego is taught in Oriental ego theory, but the purpose of that self-awareness is approvable only in the sense of a chief role for self-recognition. It should not be summarily concluded that the whole content of the self can be apprehended by self-knowledge of the ego. The self that is apprehended by self-knowledge of the ego is only oneself perceived at a certain moment in the space-time continuum. Momentary recognition of oneself does not solve all the problems of the ego.

The problems of the subject as a personality and the problem of the original self are not solved by any such understanding. The unlimited abyss of the whole self is hidden behind this. If we wish to know the true self, we must confront the hidden self. The self that is objectified is formed if this abyss appears in the sphere of consciousness, but the self that becomes known in any such way is only one portion of the self. The reason is that the whole self may be limitless. The self is difficult to discover. It is not revealed a priori.

[26] It is said that the notion of *mu* was first propounded by Lao-tzu, a Chinese philosopher of the latter half of the fifth century B.C. According to Lao-tzu, a limitless sphere that cannot be apprehended by the limited human being is present deep within all of creation. It is difficult to express this concept in words, so the negative term *mu* is used to express it suggestively and symbolically. *Mu* in this sense is not a relative concept that opposes *yū* (existence) as a negation of *yū*, having, instead, the meaning indicated in the proverb "*yū wa mu yori shōzuru*" ("being is born from nothing"). *Yū* is something that creates *yū*, that is, something absolute and infinite. The *mu* mentioned by Chuang-tzu, a Chinese philosopher of the latter half of the fourth century B.C., is a negation of the knowledge and decisions of human beings, and this term can be considered as representing the ultimate goal of individual ethics rather than as representing a metaphysical point of view.

[27] From the Buddhist viewpoint, the ego is negated while affirmed. The ego is affirmed as a whole, but it cannot be affirmed in our world of practical consciousness. The natural standpoint demands that we negate the ego that is affirmed and move beyond it. The doctrine of *muga* (state of selflessness) teaches self-negation as having that meaning.

The real meaning of this self-negation is none other than a submission of the self to that inner relativistic manner of communication that occurs by its nature, and this indicates the way to have the presence of the self per se come into full concord with *sei no yokubō* (the desire for life).

The transcendent ego throughly negates the wayward self to a degree that one is now conscious of being "in the world of practical consciousness." There can be no actual release from that transcendent condition, even if some artificially subjective affirmation of the self remains. This new condition could be called *muga* (state of selflessness), but in reality the ego has already drawn itself away from any supposedly self-serving theoretical objective and has become thoroughly intuitive in its functioning. This *arugamama* condition of selfhood lies beyond any recognized differentiation of subject-object or self-other, or existence-nonexistence (*yū-mu* or *u-mu*) and can probably be considered akin to a state of so-called suspension of judgment. Consequently, in this instance, the ego has shifted to a completely different mental dimension, by comparison with any functionally oriented "strengthening of the ego" referred to in terms of subjecthood or ego identity, or as ego-consecutive or ego-integrative.

If an attempt is made to explain the relationship between the ego and the process of recovery anticipated by a patient in Morita therapy, the explanation would be that Morita therapy seeks to position the self in a state of mind that lies completely beyond any subjective or objective standpoint, even in pursuit of the subjecthood of the ego as such.

This *muga* self is a thoroughly agnostic self and, at the same time, a self that exists in continuous *engi* (relationship) with society. This relationship goes through mental and physical changes; it grows and develops; it is a form of life in which something that is not the self is continually ingested and transformed into the substance of the self. When this self is accepted as equivalent to *kega* (a form of ego), this *kega* acts in accordance with the facts of the patient's circumstances, and the release of the disordered self from the shackles of the *shinkeishitsu* condition takes place.[28]

---

[28] *Kega* (which may be called the ego) refers to the self as existing in an infinite continuum of interdependent and correspondent relationships. In essence, a human being exists, in both body and substance, by the continuous mutual assistance and complementarity of parts and whole. The self is a part of a larger individuality, while containing within itself a number of individual entities as its parts.

The concept of *engi* (to come into existence by means of mutual relationships as a connective) consists of the two characteristics of each human being, that of "complex" and that of "organic integration" of parts or mutual assistance and complementarity of parts and whole. This concept is applicable to human life. A phenomenon that exceeds the strength of any person or any random number of persons can occur when human beings mutually assist and complement each other.

It can be said that the essence of a person is not changed but that birth and death are both present in the phenomenon of organic integration. Birth is "present now where it was not present before," and death is something later changed to nullity. The person is a phenomenon that was not present before but is present now, that is, born. He or she becomes nil by a dispersion of parts, that is, death. The form in which human beings are present is, for practical purposes, the same. We do not know what precedes birth or what follows death. When we become aware of birth, we have already been born, and no one is born by his or her own effort. Similarly, we are not dead as long as we are alive, and we know nothing of what will occur after death.

At any rate, when we look at our present selves, we see that various parts of the mind and body are integrated and that the parts coexist in complementarity as the personality of the person. An ego that acts self-consciously, isolated from the environment, is present in that particular form of materialization. My sphere, called the "I," is the form of myself that "I" present to you or to anyone else. "I" must be independent from other persons to maintain "I" as myself, but to do so various outside substances must be supplied to me and I must take them in. Continual interaction with my social and cultural environment is the prerequisite for this ingestive process.

A person exists with a position relative to the sociocultural continuum as a personal location. The self that has a natural structure and position is called *kega* in Buddhism. This self goes through constant change, both mentally and physically, and continues to grow and develop. True selfhood is attained because the self is in the *kega* state and can act freely to grow and develop without hindrance or limit. (Hirakawa, A.: Muga to shutai (*Muga* and subjecthood) (in Japanese). In *Jiga to Muga* (Edo and Muga), edited by H. Nakamura. Heirakuji Shoten, Kyōto 1966).

21

The Curative Process in Morita Therapy: Gaining Insight and Attaining the Mental State of *Arugamama*

Almost all psychotherapists have similar opinions concerning standards for a cure. In particular, the elimination, or at least relief, of symptoms is the same as it is in somatic therapy.

In psychotherapy, however, it is still doubtful whether the disappearance of symptoms can be considered to be a condition of cure as such. Inquiry into the personality of a patient is necessary, but differences of opinion may arise among therapists, who make their respective decisions. Further, it is difficult to differentiate a cure from the beliefs, world view or *ethos* that form the standards for a cure in psychotherapy, so that evaluation of what constitutes a condition of cure is actually difficult.

However, the necessary and sufficient condition for a cure is that disappearance or alleviation of symptoms must first be recognized and that a physically and mentally stable condition must then be maintained. Internal stability exemplified by adaptation or cooperation with one's environment must be attained, to make family and social life possible. Subjectivity and creativity needed to facilitate one's life condition voluntarily and assertively are also important and indispensable criteria of a cure.

When considered in this manner, the standard for judging a cure in psychotherapy becomes complex. Not only the elimination of symptoms but also the maturation and development of personality become necessary criteria of a cure.

For this reason, the level of the therapeutic goal is high. However, the condition of cure, in the sense noted previously, is fully acquired, after therapy, in the course of a patient's daily living, so there are many cases in which it is difficult to judge, in a so-called precognitive manner, the true condition of cure in the therapeutic process and to determine whether a cure has accordingly reached completion.

Cases that were managed with Morita therapy are explained with the considerations noted previously kept in mind. In terms of progress, the image of a cure in Morita therapy that therapists usually have in mind will be discussed. The author will also consider issues that have a close relationship with the condition of cure.

The image of a cure, which is the major topic of this chapter, makes more concrete the substance of the comparative human image, based on value orientation, which has been explained in detail in Chapter 6. Although the cases used as references for study may be considered to be impure types[1] of *shinkeishitsu*, the author finds them useful because they have less specificity than does the pure form, from the standpoint of psychotherapy in general.

---

[1] Takeyama, T.: Shinkeishitsu no fujun kei no rinshōteki kenkyū (Clinical study of impure types of *shinkeishitsu*) (in Japanese). In *Collection of Theses in Commemoration of Mourning for Professor Morita* (1938).

The author has previously explained how human beings are perceived by Morita as the basis for conducting psychotherapy.[2] This perception is an important consideration in obtaining a deep understanding of Morita therapy, chiefly Morita's perception of human beings in principle, the value structure of Morita therapy and the human image expected to emerge from Morita therapy, again as has been explained in detail in Chapter 6.

This chapter will include discussion of the goals of Morita therapy, psychological changes observed in patients and, especially, the attainment of self-discernment and the mental state of *arugamama* as an image of a cure, with reference to three representative case histories.

Case 1

This man, 35 years-old at the time of treatment, was a technical official employed by the Ministry of Posts and Telecommunications. Uneasiness and attacks of palpitation began to occur around 12 or 13 years of age due to a weak gastrointestinal condition. For about one month, at that time, he was unable to go to school by himself.

Once, after dinner during the same period, the patient suddenly noticed that the illumination of a certain electric light bulb seemed to feel different from the previous day, and he gradually began to experience physiological changes akin to depersonalization. He then began to have numerous fears, such as fear of catching a cold, fainting, going outdoors and being struck by lightning. This condition continued for four or five years. During all that time, the patient felt that certain changes were taking place in his body. The wish to return to the condition he had been in before he became "ill" more and more occupied the forefront of the patient's consciousness.

The patient received treatment at the neuropathology department of a university hospital, but because no improvement had been observed after two or three months, he discontinued it. He caught a cold about ten days before taking a medical examination, experiencing violent palpitation. These attacks later became so frequent that the patient's fears of catching a cold and of going outdoors intensified, and his anticipation of fear became even more exaggerated.

Life History

This patient was the third child in his family. The father worked for a private business concern, but the family was not financially well-off. His mother was weak-willed, sickly, delicate and nervous, and his father extremely arrogant. The patient had been raised by both parents, but his father had a volatile temperament. (According to statements made by other patients, who had been raised in similar family situations, fear and repulsion were felt in response to scoldings or physical punishments that could not be anticipated in advance.)

Probably as a result of this same sort of response, the patient was shy, as well as intelligent, but he could also be aggressive, could easily be influenced by feelings, indicated strong bias and was autonomic as well as self-reflective.

The patient had contracted pneumonia at the age of two and thereafter was physically weak; his gastrointestinal condition was not good, but there had been no recurrence of symptoms of the illness at that time.

The patient's history indicated middle-school (junior high) graduation, followed by vocational education at a technical communications school. He had a love affair while he was a student and later married the girl at the age of 26. However, because the patient was an extreme stickler for cleanliness and also extremely autonomous, his married life came to an end within

[2] Fujita, C.: Morita ryōhō ni okeru ningen kan (A view of the human being in Morita therapy) (in Japanese). *Shinkeishitsu* 1(2) (1960).

three years, although he and his wife still loved each other. Since then, he had remained single. He loved literature and had been a contributor to a certain literary magazine. The patient had assumed his present employment at the Ministry a few years previously.

Description of Symptoms

The patient's major complaint was that of attacks of palpitation, but catching a cold, which triggered the palpitation, was the direct object of his fear. Going to places where he would experience difficulty if the palpitation occurred, riding in public transport facilities, where it would be difficult to take emergency measures, especially when riding in commuter or express trains, and taking a bath, too, were objects of fear in the same sense as catching a cold. Consequently, riding the train to work was a painful experience. The patient avoided riding express trains as much as was possible because the distance between stops was so long. Returning home in a crowded train did not seem so painful. Going to work on the train was more painful because the patient was moving farther and farther from home.

In the instance of taking a bath, the patient was not disturbed by getting into the bathtub, but his uneasiness increased when he began to soap his body because of the considerable time that would be needed to get ready for emergency treatment, somewhat like his feeling of being trapped on a train between stations. The patient's fear of natural phenomena, such as lightning, was so intense that, at times, his body would be completely immobilized and rigid. In view of that intense reaction, he would experience fear, even at the sight of giant cloud columns similar to thunderheads.

The patient also had a fear of water. This fear pertained not only to swimming but getting into boats as well. The patient's fear of water was so intense that he could not even bear to dip his feet into a stream. However, the latter fears did not occur as often in his life as did those associated with catching a cold, riding trains and taking a bath, and these objects of his fear could be avoided, so they did not have as much of an impact on his adaptation to life.

The patient had also experienced symptoms of depersonalization. This experience can be readily understood by reading the following excerpt from the patient's writings:

"The sky is truly blue and clear. I have not doubted the existence of the sky even once. The colors of flowers are vivid. The leaves of trees are green drops. The morning air is pure. All of these things have actual existence. There is a condition, however, in which these things cannot be apprehended by human senses even though their presence can be acknowledged. They are vivid and pure, but one's own feelings cannot merge with them unconditionally. There is a sense of heavy head, headache, of hazy consciousness, always present like a mist between the subject that sees and the object that is seen. It is felt that these objects do actually exist, but there is nothing I can do about the condition in which I view them. All of these objects are self-acknowledged, as they are, with no doubt within the self of the subject-object relationship.

"A change in my perception of an object might occur when I had a fever, but I acknowledged this shift in perception candidly, as it was. The object usually returned to its original form in my perception as soon as the fever disappeared. However, sometimes it did not return to its original form. I might experience terrible ringing in the ears, and when I sat together with my parents, brothers and sisters around the dinner table while they chatted, my own small self would sink into a world wholly unrelated to all of them, and I would have to continually swing my head sideways in response to changes in the illumination of the electric light bulb. I had to fight against this ringing in my ears every night, when in bed, and examine the condition of numbed sensibility by pinching myself.

"The laughter of human voices did not seem real to me. The voices bounced off me and returned to their source as vain echoes reverberating in a void. A youth like me, 13 years-old, could do nothing but struggle in silence with a cold heart, fearful of sad resignation, lending his ears to the sounds of the lives of those healthy and cheerful people in the world with tears in his eyes."

This patient suddenly became aware of a certain new feeling, never before experienced, obtruding itself between subject and object; emotion had grown cold and did not flow; participation of his human heart in human life was completely shut down. When this condition had continued for six months to a year, he began to feel that some physiological change had taken place in his body. His interpretation was that this physiological change had affected his character and had continued to do so up to the present. It was this conviction that made the patient's uneasiness and fears of catching a cold, going outdoors, riding trains, bathing and natural phenomena become even more firmly fixed.

Progress Through Treatment

Therapy was conducted in such a manner that going outdoors and taking a bath, which had become obstructions in the patient's life, were not avoided. Having the patient engage in these fearful activities was the first objective of therapy. All attempts to alleviate uneasiness and fear were stopped. The patient was guided toward realistic efforts practiced through activities intended to restore his everyday life to its original human form. At the same time, the patient was encouraged to keep a diary and to bring it with him when he visited the therapist. Visits were made once a week, with an interview lasting about 40 to 60 minutes. During each interview, the patient was asked to explain his experiences centered around his life history several times, as in the preliminary interview, as well as to explain in detail the manifestation of his major complaint, how he had been managing to accept the condition and what he wanted most in life.

The first attitude indicated by the patient during therapy was a stuborn one of wanting to have the physiological changes in his body explained to him in medical terms. This attitude was one of strong anticipation that a further physical change in his condition could liberate him from his abnormal sensations and from the uneasiness and fears that had continued to afflict him over the past 20 years.

The patient's notion that proper physical treatment would improve his condition could not be easily modified. Many passages in his diary indicated distrust and uneasiness over modern-day medical science. There were numerous statements that showed grieving over his past life situation and his unfortunate fate.

Treatment lasted ten months. A general outline of the patient's progress follows.

The patient mentioned that the symptoms had become less intense about five weeks after treatment had been started. The lessening of symptom severity was due more to his frame of mind than to any real change in his methods for adaptation to life. There was no change in attitude to indicate whether his symptoms had improved. Much of the diary was devoted to detailed descriptions of each day's symptoms. There were also many statements to the effect that he had been trying to exercise self-control according to his standards.

The patient's use of ideological words and phrases indicating "this and that must be just so" was prominent in his attitude toward his life and his opinion of his symptoms. Complications that could not be resolved were left alone to generate continuing unease and suffering, to effect self-control and to encourage the patient against uneasiness and fear.

After the sixth or seventh week, the symptoms abated, or worsened, depending on one's point of view. The patient exercised ideological self-control but also doubted the efficacy of his attitude and began to think about what he should do to change his attitude, to escape from his chronic frame of mind and his ideological vicious circle. The patient finally indicated some interest in improving his actions in life and suddenly became aware that he could now handle his daily work without feeling uneasy.

The following remarks appear in the patient's diary at about that time:

"I feel fine after I have worked and moved my body. . . . I don't seem to need to have a heavy feeling, in spite of the fact that it is very cloudy today. The view of the trees lining the pond enfolded in mist is beautiful. I suddenly paused when I heard the chirping of birds. Cooking food is also pleasant. At present, I am happier when I am busy than when I take time to complain about fear, uneasiness or tedium."

Subjective relief of the symptoms was clearly evident about seven to eight weeks after treatment had been started. Although due to close self-observation, one change that took place in which the patient had seemingly accepted himself without inner opposition is recorded as follows in his diary:

"When I woke up today and happened to reflect on myself, I became aware of the fact that a very ordinary and natural form of myself was moving in me like a flow of water. it seems unbelievable that I had been scolding myself so earnestly till yesterday with such hard words as 'subject,' 'ideology' and 'realization.' My own self, which I have been trying to apprehend during the past two months while groping in the dark, was an ordinary form and not anything special. The natural way and the ordinary form are the true human life.

"I began to become aware of this. Sometimes I resisted and sometimes I bore a grudge against the sadness I felt that I could not find the real meaning of life by suffering. Going for treatment has been an experience full of ups and downs, but I can now be thankful, with heartfelt honesty, that I have come up to this point without giving up midway. Can there be any more beautiful mingling of human souls than this? I understood the term 'rapid progress' only mentally, but now I am actually able to experience its meaning. I can also appreciate the fact that rapid progress will always occur if one follows the natural way of life. . . .

". . . Even if the feeling of being worried about tomorrow is something deduced from one's past life environment, perhaps naturalness and freedom in the situation of one's present actual life are expanded by changing one's own way of thinking and looking at things. This mental experience can be applied, as it is, to actual life, and when it is made manifest here and now, in reality, it cans be said that one has true human health. There is something very wonderful in a certain kind of human experience. It is not clear to me, at present, what that something is."

The patient reflects that he was able to express his feeling of appreciation so frankly to the therapist for the joy he felt when he discovered what his natural self should be, from his experience of rapid progress. However, he once again portrays himself as someone who has persistent symptoms, after another two or three days.

"I had anticipated last week that the symptoms would show rapid progress and, together with the sort of enlightenment obtained, I would be truly free, but there is still a feeling of pressure in my stomach and palpitations of the heart. When I thought I had conquered one problem, others crop up, one after another, with changed shapes. My present feeling is that I am surrounded by a wall whose nature is unknown to me. The uneasiness I feel over *when* the symptoms will recur has taken hold of me.

". . . Even if my stomach aches, or for other reasons, I must not rely on doctors or medicines . . . I need to prepare myself to face uneasiness straightforwardly. . . . I must trust the power to live which lies dormant within myself and do everything with complete confidence. If the symptoms cause me pain while I am changing in various ways, then let me be content to suffer. No matter what happens, I will not retreat even one step until I am truly healthy. I must bid farewell to that suffering which has been with me for the past 20 years and to that passive, life-negating attitude that has resulted from it.

"I will try not to exert myself to understand it by force of will, since this will cause enervation and failure. . . . I will experience a swiftly consuming greed. But I must look myself square in the face and progress slowly, step by step. Making decisions chiefly due to feelings will increase the burden of life itself."

A conscious attitude of trying to handle a certain instantaneous decision while fighting against pain and uneasiness can be monitored from the patient's inner dialogue, but this attitude is still ideological and idealistic. This condition continued for another three months, but the process, to the patient, could be considered as being a second rapid-progress stage. During this time, the patient returned to his family home, after an absence of five or six years, to attend his younger brother's wedding. He met his father again.

The patient felt antagonistic toward his father because of his own character biases and as a remote cause of his present disorder. It appears that the patient had made a certain decision when meeting his father again. When he returned to Tokyo, he did not say much about the experience, mentioning only that "my father appears to have aged; I felt somewhat tender toward him because he is my parent."

Two days later, the patient caught one of those colds that he dreaded so much and had tonsillitis, putting him in bed for four days with a temperature of 39°C. He received immediate medical treatment, of course. Owing to a rapid lessening of his feeling of uneasiness after being examined, the patient later said that he knew his condition had improved psychologically; after he recovered his physical strength and could go out for a stroll, he suddenly had the same conscious experience as he had when he was a boy, and he wrote about his impression of the incident.

"I went to buy cigarettes within a short distance of some 200 meters away. While I was walking through a patch of woodland, seeing young leaves soaked by the rain while looking inwardly into my uneasy self, wondering whether to go downtown or do something else, I suddenly awoke to myself. I shouted in my heart, 'This is it, this is the color tone!' and I looked around to make certain of it. The atmosphere of that objective world which enfolded myself had not changed one whit. I became aware of the fact that this was entirely the same perception I had experienced during my younger days, when I had changed, and I had grieved that the world had changed; I suffered mental pain and feared unease.

". . . I now have the feeling that I can go straight on to a fresh and wonderful self. I will not doubt that feeling now. Although it may be a trivial matter, this sensation that I am now savoring is invaluable. My heart leaps. The day that I will be released is near at hand. It is wonderful, I can express it only as wonderful. Life is throbbing even in the murmur of the brook. The scenes in the country I used to know during my childhood come back to me very vividly.

". . . The veil which has enfolded me in a melancholic world is being quietly removed. I am not spinning round and round in a world of fabrication. It is not strange that I should have a fever and that I suffer. It is also natural to fear death. Something is opening up within me."

The patient says that this experience was not one of reaching the final exit from a closed-in world, but a feeling that he had reached the first point of egress. He has not escaped from his closed-in world, and is still in the same world, but he feels a sensation of health side by side with a sensation of freshness. There was always the hope within him that he would someday return to his original human condition through some sort of stimulus. The patient said that this original condition was what he now felt. He feels liberated from his symptoms, with his consciousness of a great change within himself as the springboard. He can see and think frankly that "this is it," with no need to reason about it, and this new mental attitude is readily accepted as being natural. Although the patient still experiences suffering and uneasiness, these feelings do not loom as such large obstructions in his life as they were in the past, and a feeling of smooth facility has increased in his activities of daily living.

During subsequent interviews with the patient, the therapist spent more time with him in discussion of his workplace, his home activities and his hobbies, rather than his symptoms.

This frame of mind continued for another three months; the patient was thankful that he had been able to bridge the gap and experience a continuation of that original subjective consciousness he had possessed as a healthy child. However, he has now begun to feel that something important is still lacking in his life. He perceives his work as mere mechanical labor (periodically transmitting observations of weather conditions), and he does not wish to do this kind of work for the rest of his life. He would like to do work of great merit. Something is lacking, he feels, but he cannot explain the "something" concretely. The patient's mental disorder and its psychological complications have been dispelled. However, he now finds himself in a condition that lacks mental satisfaction. His concern over how to live like a human being is still unresolved. He says that "this is my own personal problem, something that no one else can solve," and it will, in fact, be the patient's life problem from now on.

The therapist met the patient, once again, six years after treatment had been completed. The patient explained his perception of the treatment at that time and his subsequent mental condition.

"Since my childhood, an ambivalent feeling toward my father would not leave my mind as a memory of the painful past; it led me unawares to thinking that my body had changed. So I was convinced that my abnormal feelings could be corrected by material means. That intense feeling made me ask the therapist for physiological remedies such as medicines.

"But a large obstacle, which could not be overcome no matter how hard I tried, was always in front of me. I began to experience even an irrational feeling of not being able to do anything about the wall which had always oppressed me. When I tried, several times, to get past the wall, it could not be broken or scaled. When I was finally confronted with that fact, I believed there was no one I could rely on except myself, and became resigned to the fact that I must bear responsibility for myself. But my condition was such that my consciousness had not yet become clear. My wonderful experience in the wet woodland was further transformed into a clear consciousness of myself. It then became a very open feeling of self-acceptance. I had been blocked by feeling that I could do nothing in the past, present of future, but now began to move autonomously and to discover enjoyment. My actions became more positive and I began to consider my environment more realistically. My sense of loneliness as an outsider separated from the world where healthy people live has disappeared. My feeling toward my father now is that I would like to have him live as long as possible. My work is the same, and I do not think even now that it is a mentally challenging occupation. However, I believe there is no other way than to do as much as possible. I do not necessarily think that this is satisfactory, and I will probably suffer about it similarly in the future."

Case 2

Description of Symptoms

This woman, 52 years-old at the time of treatment, was a housewife. Her major complaint was insomnia. She had a tendency toward a neurotic character and easily became concerned about trivialities. In the past, the patient had overcome her condition by taking sleeping pills when she could not fall asleep. She had caught a cold about five months before she came in for examination. At that time, the patient had lost sleep because she was worried about a problem of selling land. She obtained a prescription for a mild tranquilizer from a neighborhood physician, but the medication caused a feeling of heaviness in her head. The patient did not feel well and experienced a constant feeling of not being in good health, which was aggravated by taking sleeping pills. Her condition might, she felt, be harmful.

Life History

This patient came from a wealthy home in the countryside. Her family had been prominent in the area for several generations. The patient was the youngest of five brothers and sisters. Her elder sister had once had an attack of depression, but apart from that there was no hereditary cause that could be specifically considered.

The patient had a sunny disposition and was generous-minded. She was active but also prudent, had mysophobia and was bashful. It appeared that she had a warm, liberal education while living with her parents. It was not a completely noninterferent education because the parents had educated the children by encouraging their preferences, after recognizing the individuality of each child and not forcing anything on them. She graduated from a girls' school with good grades and spent her youth in a carefree manner within a free and genial atmosphere.

Her father's hobby was painting. The patient, too, began to paint when she was still young and continued it after her marriage. The patient married her husband at the age of 20. It appears that the family environment of her husband's home was modest. Her mother-in-law had insisted on maintaining old Japanese customs, with a corresponding home atmosphere, so that the open, sunny disposition of the patient gradually vanished.

However, her husband was a warmhearted person, and because the patient's mother-in-law and other members of the family did not torment her, there was no emotional disagreement or repulsion, although it was a life in which she felt a certain amount of cramped constraint. The patient was somewhat at a loss to carry out wifely customs because she had not had any such household training in her home, having to be taught by her mother-in-law.

The patient became passive in her activities, although she did not lose her cheerful nature. There was no opposition to husband and wife going out together; they were encouraged to go and see stage plays, for example, so that she could feel some degree of freedom within the overall household constraints. The husband said nothing about the home, leaving all such decision-making to the patient and his mother. Even after the patient's mother-in-law died, it appeared that the life attitude of her mother-in-law had become the foundation of the patient's life, through long imposition of custom. She had taken on an externally constrained and reserved character. The patient's active and open nature had vanished, making her more and more aware of her neurotic tendency, although she did not lose her sunny disposition.

The patient had given birth to two boys and two girls. Two of the children had already completed university studies and were living elsewhere; the other two children were still attending universities. Her husband was in good health, and the family was financially well-off because he was a company executive. The husband-wife relationship was excellent. The patient had started to study Japanese painting a few years before, and some of her work had been accepted for exhibition several times, indicating artistic talent beyond the scope of a hobby.

Progress Through Treatment

According to the patient, her gastrointestinal condition had worsened when she started to take sleeping pills, which made her feel mentally and physically fatigued during the daytime. She suffered from distraction, caused particularly by difficulty going to sleep and being easily awakened. She wished fervently to be released from the cares of life, having become disgusted with herself, because she had begun to feel heavily concerned about her mental and physical distress.

When the patient visited the therapist for treatment, a mild tranquilizer was prescribed to calm her nerves and make sleeping easier. This medication released her from struggling to go to sleep by willful intention and permitted her to feel that going to sleep is natural to the entire body; it would be fine if she could go to sleep for a while but natural as well if she could not go to sleep. The patient would go to bed at the usual time, get out of bed at the usual time, regardless of whether she had slept, and start her daily activities as usual.

About two weeks after treatment had been started, it was observed that the patient's attitude was still centered around sleeping, that is, that she felt she must struggle to get sufficient sleep, somehow. Tranquilizers were stopped during the third week, and an attempt was made during interviews to carry on conversation centered around the patient's daily activities. The patient complained that she did not have problems with her daily life, but she continued to be inclined to rely on sleeping pills because sleep was still insufficient. The complaint, however, was not as strong as it had been initially.

After about three months, the patient complained that if she became intensely engrossed in her painting, reverberations of mental strain continued well into the night and she became mentally excited. Also, when the patient suddenly woke up at night and started to think about her painting, she could not go to sleep again. She had thought this problem was simply a sleep disorder, was afraid of it and tried to eliminate it in one way or another. However, the patient had recently begun to consider it a natural phenomenon that occurs in the course of painting; as a result, it was natural that she did not get enough sleep. Even if the patient still had insomnia, it was different because she had changed her attitude to say only that she felt displeased if she could not fall asleep.

The patient was not yet clearly aware of this change in attitude, nor was she aware that the nature of her complaint had changed. She only felt thankful that her daily activities could now be carried out smoothly. The patient did remark on a number of deep feelings.

"I recently began to have doubts about painting. Since I had painted in oils when I was young, I do not hate painting. I paint because I love it, and that in itself should be sufficient. However, after I became a member of various clubs and organizations, I began to have the feeling that there ought to be something more to life than just a love of painting. Difficult human relations should be no different from other social relations. The problem is one of how your mind should be set, or how I should treat myself. Essentially, I need to consider myself apart from my painting, but how to do that is one of my problems."

The patient now complains of uneasiness instead of insomnia. This new complaint was made frequently during subsequent interviews, but it is most likely an uneasiness relating to a basic human need, unlike the problem of insomnia. The attitude of the patient is that "nothing can be done even if I tell this to the therapist, because I myself must solve this problem."

Is this mental attitude the same as that evident in her fear of insomnia? The patient has since lived a normal life as a housewife and as an artist in her own right.

Case 3

This man, 31 years-old at the time of treatment, was a government employee. His major complaint was that his face looked as though he were crying when he faced people or while reading.

When this patient was 20 years-old, he began to live with his aunt and uncle, but his aunt tended to make sarcastic remarks about almost everything. The sarcastic remarks made the patient feel so unpleasant at times that he felt suddenly uneasy when he faced people at his workplace. The patient began to think that people were saying unpleasant things about him when they looked at his face (which, he believed, appeared to be distraught). This feeling had gradually intensified about four or five years earlier, and he began to feel more and more sensitive about it. The patient could not speak freely with people, even his coworkers. The patient's face became sulky, even when he was reading; he had the feeling that his face had become stiff, which made him feel mentally fatigued.

Life History

This patient was the oldest of six children. His father was a retired army officer who was inaccessible because he was extremely stern. His mother was timid and bashful and showed a *shinkeishitsu* tendency.

The patient was mostly brought up by his paternal grandmother through the sixth grade. His grandmother was tolerant. The patient had a bashful, timid character, was insistent on cleanliness and was diligent and intelligent. After majoring in mathematics at a university, he worked at an astronomical observatory for seven years. He had married two years previously and had an infant son. His wife was a school teacher.

About six years earlier, the patient had become aware that he was beginning to experience pessimistic feelings about once a month, continuing for four to five days. He usually experienced exhilarating feelings four to five days before his mood became pessimistic. When gripped by pessimistic feelings, the patient's sense of inferiority was strong, and he sometimes felt laid open to some form of accusation. The patient's major complaint became stronger, but he did not take time off from work because of it.

Progress Through Treatment

These periodic changes in feeling and the patient's major complaint were not considered as having the same pathogenesis. Therapeutic planning took into account the perception that the former change was due to a manic-depressive state and the latter was a symptom of *shinkeishitsu.*

In accordance with this diagnosis, psychotherapy was conducted with simultaneous use of tricyclic antidepressants. It was explained to the patient that his fear of his facial expression could be secondarily aggravated by his feeling of depression. Instruction for dealing with activities of daily living was given once each week, when the patient visited the therapist. He was instructed to monitor his psychological state, exactly as it was, including the symptoms. The patient was instructed not to decide that everything was morbid and abnormal; instead, he was encouraged to attempt to accept these facts, in the exact condition of feeling anxious about them, and at the same time to continue his activities of daily living in a manner consistent with his attainment of his original desires.

From about the third week of therapy, the patient became aware of being able to face people without being self-conscious about his facial expression. The patient sensed his major complaint with special intensity when he was living in a mountainous locale to conduct meteorological observations about once every three months. During that time, he carried out his observations along with continuous human relationships within a confined living area. The patient could not be truly relieved of the suffering caused by his symptoms as long as this daily life in confinement was not dealt with smoothly.

When the patient's self-awareness of his facial expression became less intense, he began to show an attitude of looking forward, to some extent, to his observations of his life, which he had tried to avoid doing until that time. This new attitude was also applied to the fluctuation of his mood, which occurred periodically. However, this condition had been made less severe by the use of stabilizing medication.

About three months after therapy had been started, the patient was no longer particularly conscious of the fluctuation of his mood. This type of symptom, which had exerted so strong an influence on the patients life, gradually became less and less intense. The frequency of his complaints decreased, and this change altered the topics of his conversation during interviews. The patient's complaints now consisted chiefly of contradictions and dissatisfactions stemming from the difference between his specialized university studies and his present occupation.

In spite of having finished a university mathematics course, the patient complained that his present work was concerned only with routine astronomical observations; that is, the work was a fixed, unvarying task. It involved no original research, instead being a daily "grind" that he accepted reluctantly, deriving from it no psychological satisfaction. Although his mental and physical suffering had been alleviated, the patient began to feel that the nature of his work was an important problem in his life. His conversation focused mostly on complaints of that nature for some time, but a short time before he completed his six-month period of therapy, he explained his determination as follows:

". . . I have said a lot of things, but when I think about them carefully, aren't they the same kind of mental suffering that everyone experiences as a human being? I've become aware of the fact that my situation is something that only I myself can resolve. From now on, I will try to find a solution to the problem."

Case Reviews

There are many issues worthy of consideration as problems in all three of these cases, but all of the issues were perceived as manifestations of *shinkeishitsu* from a diagnostic point of view, and therapy was carried out accordingly.

In case 1, the factors of the patient's entire human character formation are contained in the background material, and from the point of view of the patient's life history, we can readily consider these factors as triggering the onset of *shinkeishitsu.*

From a phenomenological point of view, however, the patient's experiences of alienation, such as obstacles to self-feeling, constitute the underlying basis of the disorder. At first glance, the experiences appear to form complex symptoms, but they are actually a secondary posture. The patient's attempts to negate feelings of suffering or instability are the root cause of this secondary condition, and they control the overall content of his consciousness.

It is more appropriate to consider the feeling of alienation, understanding it as a fear of being unable to apperceive rather than as an experience of depersonalization. This feeling is not an effort to see an object as being beautiful but, instead, a conscious process of trying to see the object as something ordinary. That it can be seen as such, and must be seen as such, can be perceived in this case. This was felt more strongly as being an experience of the patient.

When the patient looks at an object, it is clearly perceived, but when he views the object while considering the relationship between his attitude and the condition of the object, his consciousness has already drawn away from the object and is directed toward his self, which is engaged in considering how to look at the object properly, so that the self has not become "one" with the object in a pure sense. In other words, the condition of apperception is lacking.

This attitude of not considering how consciousness, which can be said to be present before perception, should operate, then simply negating the unpleasant feeling caused as a result and wishing it would disappear is the fear of being unable to apperceive. This fear is a symptom of *shinkeishitsu.*

In case 2, the unpleasant feeling that accompanied sleeplessness made the patient become more conscious of her sleeplessness. By struggling to escape the unpleasant feeling, the patient feel into a condition in which she could not let go of the unpleasant feeling. This condition is the mental attitude of *shinkeishitsu.* There is virtually no doubt about this diagnosis.

Case 3 differs considerably from the other two cases and seems difficult to understand from a developmental standpoint in a monistic manner. From a phenomenological point of view, it is not possible to determine at first glance which factor constitutes the "picture" of the symptom, but it seems appropriate to decide the issue on the basis of the patient's subjectivity.

The patient's self-consciousness, so concentrated on his facial expression, and the mental condition of the patient, who suffers from its interpretation, from the natural picture of the symptom when it is examined from the perspective of the patient's subjectivity.

It is probable that lurking in the background is the periodic restless emotion of the manic-depressive psychosis that lies within the "picture frame." The patient's attitude of being concerned about his facial expression, and suffering because of it, can be perceived as being the mental attitude of *shinkeishitsu* as such, not as the pathological basis of a manic-depressive psychosis. The latter condition has relevance only in the sense that it is a pathoplastic factor from the standpoint of whether or not the patient's neurotic consciousness is highlighted more clearly by the rhythms of the emotions that lie in the "picture" background.

Even if there seems to be some difference among these cases from a pehnomenological standpoint, we can understand that the consciousness of each patient, which acts to motivate the symptoms, is absorbed in the attitude of trying to control the self by means of an idealized self-image. This type of consciousness is common to *shinkeishitsu.* From that standpoint, all three cases can be discussed on the same plane.

When the symptoms of these patients are alleviated by Morita therapy, which we will now explain, the suffering over mental inadequacy evidenced by the patients is an interesting phenomenological key to an understanding of the human being. It is also the final objective of Morita therapy.

Conduct of Therapy

In this section, the author will discuss the role of Morita therapy in the process of recovery from *shinkeishitsu.* Detailed descriptions of clinical situations from a therapeutic point of view, or the manner in which the therapist issues instructions to the patient, will not be included. The overriding concern, as this point, is to make it clear that Morita therapy is the basis for the procedure used in all three cases that have been described.

Morita therapy usually refers to a method of absolute, isolated bed rest. However, therapy can be conducted satisfactorily even if this method is not used (see Chapter 19, section titled "Outpatient Therapy").

Morita therapy is a unique experiential method, but when it is classified according to its ordinary method, it can be said to belong to a direct, instructive school of therapy. It is, therefore, readily understandable that instead of being a standard, fixed technique, the therapeutic situation differs from patient to patient; in other words, the therapeutic situation is modified in accordance with the inner life history of a patient, the patient's life environment or the various factors that control the patient as a unique human being.

A therapist must clearly perceive what his or her patient really wants. To conduct therapy in response to the request of a patient, as much as is possible, and to elicit with precision the true abilities of the patient, the therapist must have the zeal and devotion to participate, along with the patient, in the process of treatment.

This attitude on the part of the therapist is of utmost importance in conducting psychotherapy in general, but it is seen to be particularly important in Morita therapy. The reason is that the principles of Morita therapy are such that a patient is instructed by a therapist to observe his or her life situation *as it is* and to accept it *as it is.* This instruction is a form of behavior training in which the purpose is to have the patient accept, as it is, any fact that is experienced as a fact, and not to consider the phenomena that take place in his or her mind and body as being in any way abnormal. To make the patient attain this attitude of acceptance, the therapist must have the stringent attitude of agreeing to conduct treatment in full participation with the patient.

The procedure, conducted in this way, with the full cooperation of both parties, is a salient feature of Morita therapy. The method by which this principle is put into practice, even though it may not include absolute, isolated bed rest, is definitive to Morita therapy. In the therapeutic process, the therapist considers each of a patient's symptoms but leads the patient toward a reconstruction of his or her life so that the patient recognizes authentic human nature while still suffering from the symptoms.

It is a therapy in which a patient exerts effort to build a self that is not confined in a framework, by sublating (*Aufhebung*) the symptoms while still being restricted within the bounds imposed by the symptoms. A therapist's request that a patient take an attitude of accepting, as it is, whatever suffering of mind and body is present in the process of attaining this new selfhood cannot be realized if the therapist does not have a proper understanding of the patient or a precise comprehension of the therapeutic situation.

If those factors are not present, the therapist's view of life and normative values will be instilled in the patient; the therapy will suffer setbacks and end in failure. In that event, Morita therapy will be erroneously evaluated; it will be criticized as being authoritarian and as imposing a futile state of resignation on the patient.

Morita therapy was conducted in the three cases that have been described, with the results being as stated. The method of selecting topics for conversation and the method of giving instructions to the patient differed in each instance, but all three patients continued with activities of daily living while in confrontation with mental and physical suffering and discovered the capability for accepting pain as pain and, at the same time, the capability for transcending the suffering in the conduct of their later lives.

Process of Cure in Morita Therapy

When a patient's symptoms of *shinkeishitsu* are viewed from the perspective of the patient's subjectivity, the first consideration is that the symptoms constitute massive obstacles to the conduct of life as the patient wishes it to be. Consequently, the patient's awareness that something must be done to remove these obstacles is strengthened. For this reason, the activity of concentrating attention on the therapeutic procedure will occupy the larger share of the patient's time; roles and activities in daily living, and the conduct of living, will become secondary concerns.

The condition of a patient's life in which an element that should be subordinate replaces an element that should be superior is probably due to the patient's attitude toward life. The greater part of energy for living is consumed by activities intended to eliminate symptoms, so that a patient's life is reluctantly placed outside his or her central interest. As a result, unsatisfied desires become prominent. This phenomenon, together with the uncomfortable emotion that arises from it, and the use of neurotic defense mechanisms that end in failure each time, cause the patient to use of neurotic defense mechanisms that end in failure each time, cause the patient to suffer.

Nevertheless, these neurotic defense efforts that do not succeed are repeated even more intensely. Although the symptoms of *shinkeishitsu* function in the outside world out of a strong original desire for self-improvement and development, the various difficulties and resistances of mind and body that pursuit of those desires engenders cannot be accepted by a patient as phenomena that are normal. The patient isolates himself or herself from the outside world, against his or her will, to aim at some ideal level of human life. The patient struggles against existing resistances and continues his or her complicated life-style in confinement within his or her self.

Patients who continue this contradictory, feigned, autistic mode of life do not know how they can return to an original human life-style, and they are completely unaware of the meanings of their actual roles and activities. When the process of curing such a condition as *shinkeishitsu* by use of Morita therapy is observed macroscopically, it can be roughly divided into the following elements:

- A patient will become aware of his or her behavioral role and actions even with no change in subjective attitude. The patient will become aware that activities that lie outside the framework of his or her interest up to the present are now commonplace to him or her in dealing with the outside world. Although the patient knew of the existence of his or her role, which he or she had not been able to fulfill ideologically, the patient reluctantly remained in his or her shut-in world, with the road to the outside world closed because he or she had concentrated attention on trying to defend himself or herself against feelings of uneasiness. The patient's actions have ended as shriveled sprouts within himself or herself. The patient then becomes aware that his or her actions can assume a common place in the outside world only by his or her decision. It is possible for the patient to correctly evaluate himself or herself objectively because no change has taken place in the subjective, idealistic attitude to which he or she adheres.
- In the next stage, the patient will begin to show an attitude of evaluating his or her actions as having a common place along with the actions of people in the outside world. This attitude is one of subjective self-evaluation conducted simultaneously with objective self-evaluation, and it is a transitional attitude in which self-examination is possible at a certain mental distance. It is also an attitude in which the patient doubts the self that he or she has been observing subjectively.
- In the final stage, the patient's mind has already been opened to the outside world. The inclination to resort to the use of neurotic defenses has diminished, and realistic, spontaneous actions have become more prominent. This attitude is not one of fixed subjectivity. Rather, it is one in which the patient has changed back to his or her original objective before becoming aware of this change. The patient has changed from someone who is shut in to someone who is in a common situation with people. This change in attitude can be observed from the perspective of ordinary subjectivity as well as from the perspective of objectivity during the process of Morita therapy for *shinkeishitsu.* Although the patient continues to experience suffering as a result of the symptoms, he or she can work assertively and can recognize the capability of participating in his or her everyday life. At this stage, the patient can exert an effort to develop a realistic life-style, in conformity with his or her life situation, and can thus recognize that his or her attitude toward his or her life, until the present, has been a trial and error effort to attain a goal that cannot be realized. Even if this change of mind is observed, the symptoms in which the patient has been enmeshed will continue but will be milder. The patient will sometimes still experience attacks of uneasiness, however, that he or she might slip back into the condition of the past painful life.

When a therapist sees these changes in a patient, can he or she positively say that the goal of Morita therapy has been achieved? What degree of cure can be attained with the therapeutic mode of action considered to be effective for managing *shinkeishitsu*?

A general description of the goal of Morita therapy and its value orientation has been given in Chapter 3 and in this chapter. The various curative changes that take place through the system of procedures called Morita therapy have been discussed in the instances of three cases. The changed attitude indicated by the patients, up to the final stage, is one of unavoidable self-confrontation. This new attitude will be discussed as the key to achieving self-transcendence. The attitude of looking directly at the self is the key that permits a patient to grasp his or her essential character.

Interpretation of Mental Health

Understanding the uneasiness indicated by a person who has the *shinkeishitsu* characteristic is one means for understanding the curative process in Morita therapy for *shinkeishitsu*, so it is pertinent to clarify the author's point of view in regard to mental health.

It is often said that human exisence is composed of a biological existence and a psychological (or mental) existence. One can also refer to an individual existence, a social existence or a historical existence. However, these expressions do not signify that a human being consists of these individualized phenomena. Rather, these expressions are stipulations for conveniently defining various aspects and phases of human life, and they only serve to indicate phenomena relating to the fact that a human being is alive.

It is not proper to suppose that human beings afflicted with pain or uneasiness in direct connection with their lives are uneasy about their biological existence per se; similarly, it is not reasonable to suppose that human beings who suffer from psychological conflict are uneasy about their psychological existence per se. Both the biological standpoint and the psychological standpoint must be placed within the entire range of phenomena and situations in which human life is lived, and these standpoints should be considered as being more than direct reflections of body or mind.

Uneasiness in human life differs in accordance with the self-consciousness of the person who becomes aware of it. However, self-consciousness in this instance is an awareness of value orientation. Objectively, it is understood as the attitude toward life that has been adopted by that person. At the same time, it is an existential consciousness of one's attitude as indicated by oneself in correlation with other human beings.

From that standpoint, when one apprehends oneself in some from of correlation with other human beings, a significance factor will be born in terms of human life set into a fixed order, that is, a psychological climate that derives its meaning from one's space-time perspective. If all expressions of attitude are expressions of one's inner self, systematized by one's inner life history, each human being will have a fixed mode of existence. The condition in which a patient with *shinkeishitsu* is seized by uneasiness can, then, be considered as being one of these fixed forms of human existence.

Arugamama Mode of Living

If a realization of the value of association between oneself and any other person means making the most of oneself in a fixed mode of existence, the *arugamama* mode of living is none other than free expression of oneself. It is a means of carrying out one's role of association with another person on one's responsibility, with a free and natural self-expression that is more expansive than intentional control. Life ordering is a matter of a certain system of inner logic and discipline in which one functions for living. However, each human being confronts, as a person, all the varied phenomena that occur within that life-ordering framework. Let us examine this issue by citing commonplace examples.

Let us assume, for instance, that you are going to meet someone. A feeling of tension may arise naturally, to some degree, but its intensity will differ in accordance with the sort of person you are meeting. If that person is a close friend, the degree of tension may be slight, but it could be stronger if the person is in a superior position. There may also be certain differences in the degree of tension according to the conditions of the meeting or the subject to be discussed, the atmosphere at the time and the objective. Any human being will, thus, experience self-acceptance and self-understanding in line with his or her emotional "motions" within that life-ordering framework whether or not he or she likes it.

A person in the mental state of *arugamama* will act on his or her responsibility in a personally natural manner. Morita says that authentic human nature consists of the desire to improve and develop oneself (*sei no yokubō*). It is human nature to obey that desire. However, the expression *sei no yokubō* can be easily misunderstood. If accepted at face value, it may give the impression that authentic human nature consists of some type of instinct. Such an instinct is not Morita's intent. Rather, Morita is saying that living in obedience to our authentic human nature, as it is, also includes our relational role to the life ordering system in which we live, which is also natural.

His remark "*shizen ni fukujū shi, kyōgū ni jūjun nare*" (obey nature and submit to circumstance) refers to this condition. Self-understanding of the conditions in which one lives is *arugamama.* It includes the meaning of taking into consideration ethical conduct on a broad scale. It must be emphasized that life ordering does not consist of only a rational discipline. Life ordering is based on the psychological "climate" of any human being, and it has content that is meaningful to all human beings and meaningful to a greater extent than mere rationality or irrationality.

The "nature" to which Rousseau refers in his famous call to "return to nature" because "only nature is good," in defiance of a decadent modern culture, was not simply the nature of an idle pleasure opposed to rationality, nor was it the Nature of the natural world. An affirmation of intuitive life, which includes irrational and nonhistorical factors, can be apprehended in this sense of "nature."

Is not the developmental realization of oneself within a broad life-ordering framework set up to protect, support and enhance human existence the most meaningful concept of authentic human nature? Morita's expression "*sono mono ni narikiru*" (to be true to oneself) is both a realization of human nature and a self-realization of *arugamama.*

This also pertains to discovering oneself in and through interaction with other human beings within a life-ordering discipline. The self, which is separate and disparate, is also placed within the context of a large number of other selves. The meaning of human existence consists of the two faces of consciousness: of not losing one's authentic self and of having the responsibility to correlate oneself constantly with other selves. This is not the fatalistic view of the human being propounded by the one-time psychologisms.

The process of awareness, exemplified by the three cases that have been, described, continued after the completion of Morita therapy to change the self that was uneasy and obsessed with itself to a self that coexists with that disorder and, in turn, to a self in which the elements of disorder no longer exist. The three patients were, at first, engaged in a feud between an autistic self-consciousness that had lost its connection with the outer world and the authentic self. The self was not fully functional by involvement with other selves. It was in a sort of isolation booth and had lost sight of its authentic nature.

This phase was followed by one in which true self-discovery began to take place through involvement with other persons. This phase is a period of conscious control, that is, a period in which an attempt is made to convince oneself that life must be this or that while self-control is being exercised. The third phase is one in which the authentic self is discovered for the first time. This phase is a period of acquiring true self-autonomy and responsibility.

This process of change can be described as a form of transcendence from an existence in which one tries to seek pleasure and avoid displeasure as the controlling principle of one's entire life, that is, an existence that has lost all correlation with past and future from a temporal standpoint, clinging to an awareness only of the immediate present, and with no awareness of the importance of relationships with other persons from a life-space standpoint.

The therapeutic process in all three cases, in particular the patients' experiences, is one in which the patients became aware that something that can satisfy their authentic human selves underlies the performance of their roles in their involvement with other persons beyond the experiential mode of their present point of view.

Their therapeutic experience is also a new understanding that mere acquisition of pleasure or the elimination of uneasiness is not their true human objective. They go on to discover an authentic selfhood that acquires its value orientation from a dimension that is appreciably different from the one that they have experienced in the past. The suffering about their mental lives that is indicated in the process of recovery from symptoms in all three patients while they became truly adapted to daily life was, for each patient, an earnest problem of life. Even if their expression of it is artless, in comparison with their prior neurotic suffering, their suffering can now be considered as existing in some other dimension.

It is the same human being who suffers, but new effort to solve freely the problems of living with a consciousness of the responsibility of one's self being present in active participation with another person, that is, with one's subjecthood fully involved, must be considered to indicate, in reality, the way that human beings need to live. Their new determination to solve their problems by themselves is entirely different from their prior mode of consciousness, in which a dependent attitude was constantly present due to an autistic existence, behaving as though attempts to secure pleasure and eliminate uneasiness were their only real problems.

Their new attitude is related to an inherent ethic of acting out of one's responsibility. The mental condition that Morita signifies by the term *satori* (discernment or insight) is not derived from a logically thought-out conclusion, referring, instead, to a human condition created constructively through a process of practical experience.

What Morita Therapy Denotes

The disorder by which the authentic self-realization of the *arugamama* state of mind is not possible because a patient's self has been isolated and taken into captivity is the central problem. Releasing the patient from that condition is the most immediate objective of Morita therapy.

Morita stresses the importance of actual living, that is, practice in living. He considers the symptoms of *shinkeishitsu* as being a quantitative enlargement of a basically normal condition, not a mental illness in qualitative terms. He initially considered the primary underlying cause of *shinkeishitsu* to be the hypochondriacal basic tone, as was described in detail in Part III.

With that factor as his keynote, he developed his theory of the hypochondriacal basic tone. This concept was the principal support for Morita's theory from the beginning, but he later began to reconsider the matter from the standpoint of the mental attitude of self-improvement and development and then came to consider *sei no yokubō* as the other face of the hypochondriacal basic tone and the true underlying factor that triggers the onset of *shinkeishitsu* (see Part III).

These two factors do no differ in substance, instead coexisting in a dual relationship. What Morita defines from a phenomenological standpoint as being the hypochondriacal humor exhibited by a patient with *shinkeishitsu* is a matter or hypochondriacal behavior. The factor that supports the phenomenon is *sei no yokubō*.

Morita's initial objective was to understand and consolidate the constellation of symptoms of *shinkeishitsu* until the principles of *shinkeishitsu* could be established. His recognition that hypochondriacal behavior is common to all types of *shinkeishitsu* was farsighted. However, an intuitive insight into the hypochondriacal basic tone as being the manifestation of the basic life force that human beings possess cannot occur easily on the level at which the disorder is examined clinically.

What Morita understood from this insight was that *shinkeishitsu* is in keeping with a normal human condition rather than an illness. The reasons for this consideration, and of why the expression *sei no yokubō* was introduced in explaining the principles of Morita theory and therapy, cannot be readily understood except in the course of clinical practice. Consequently, the change made by Morita in shifting emphasis from the hypochondriacal basic tone to *sei no yokubō* can be considered as being far more meaningful than a simple change in nomenclature.

When that relationship of the two factors is taken into account, we must start with *sei no yokubō* to discuss the curative mechanism of Morita therapy. This subject is the same as the issue of why *shinkeishitsu* is caused by *sei no yokubō.*

In the onset of *shinkeishitsu*, a certain accidental (chance) factor exerts power and direction on the consciousness of a person, triggering an inevitable momentum. However, the onset is not an inevitable result that is self-intended.

By contrast, in the curative process, the chance factor is transformed into a requisite and accelerative curative opportunity within the context in which it is therapeutically schematized. This opportunity penetrates the self in the same way as the original chance factor, but its inevitable role as an opportune factor is determined, on one hand, by the process of the therapist-patient relationship and, on the other, by the interaction between a patient and the environment in which the patient has lived. Even when these situational relationships take on momentum as an inevitable curative process, the strength that the patient invests in the curative process will have great bearing on the outcome.

Morita places emphasis on *sei no yokubō* for no reason other than this strength that a patient with *shinkeishitsu* manifests. How is this *sei no yokubō* manifested in a patient's consciousness?

Morita's reasons for considering *sei no yokubō* as being a mental attitude of a high level called the desire for self-realization, development and improvement, apart from biological desire, have been explained in detail in Part III. This desire is manifested in the phenomenon of human life. A human being becomes conscious of the self whenever this *sei no yokubō* is manifested. The ego acts to satisfy desires, and the phenomenal substance formed as a result of this ego process is called the self, from the standpoint of the phenomenological school of thought.

Concept of Spontaneous Remission and Self-transcendence

Considered in this manner, the curative process in psychotherapy is a phenomenological process of actions taken by the ego as the motive factor of *sei no yokubō.* The changing process of this ego consciousness is first spurred on by the therapist-patient relationship (including its structure and its therapeutic mechanism) and, second, by means of a spontaneous remission that cannot be isolated from that process.

Spontaneous remission consists of various curative processes that occur within a patient, but such processes are often overlooked when therapy is carried out aggressively. The notion that a therapist's mission is to determine how to provide assistance to a patient's inherent curative capability dates back to the time of Hippocrates ("what cures illness is nature") and has continued to the present with the supports of increased theoretical input.

The natural homeostatic mechanism that Meares[3] discusses is also considered to be a manifestation of this idea. Morita's reason for considering *shinkeishitsu* to be a type of neurosis was that, although it is a disorder, he tried to cure it by thinking of it as a condition in which continuity with a formerly normal condition has been cut off. He recognized that the most important curative factor is *sei no yokubō* (which has the great power to stimulate a spontaneous remission).

For this reason, Morita often used the expressions "*sei no yokubō* per se" or "to become wholly *sei no yokubō*" in his therapeutic approach. The structural features of the technique used in Morita therapy include the mechanism called the therapist-patient relationship and the patient's life experience, acquired in living: both features have important clinical implications.

At the same time, various factors believed to have roles in the relief of symptoms of neurosis, such as spontaneous remission, are also closely related to the life experience or the life environment of a patient. Although it is possible, theoretically, to distinguish the processes that are intrinsic to the therapeutic mechanism from the process of spontaneous remission, it is not possible to differentiate them precisely in clinical practice. It cannot be denied that the former process has an important role in the latter process.

In 1960, Yora[4] discussed Morita therapy in his study on the prognosis of *shinkeishitsu*. A total of 406 patients treated on an outpatient basis are described in his paper; the average number of visits for Morita therapy was 1.9. When the patient's conditions were examined five to nine years later, it was found that improvement (including changes relating to behavior and reconstruction of personality) in capability for social adaptation and the elimination of symptoms had occurred in 257 (63.3 percent) of them. When patients who had shown "some improvement" are included, the success rate rose to 79.5 percent.

A change in attitude that frees a patient to participate assertively in social life has taken place. Yora says that, although insufficient by itself, Morita therapy is an approach that is useful in effecting a cure. Yora's study is one evaluation of Morita therapy for outpatients, and although there is no doubt that it has relevance for investigations of the prospects of this form of therapy, it also points out factors of great importance for spontaneous improvement.

Wolberg[5] describes in detail how a spontaneous cure functions as an extratherapeutic (nonspecific) healing aid; he also provides a chart for evaluating therapeutic results (using various approaches). In his rating of areas of change for various types of spontaneous improvement, he assigns values of 60 percent for relief or elimination of symptoms, 40 percent for behavioral change and 10 percent for reconstructive personality change.

Although there is a difference in the extent of the effect of symptomatic and behavioral improvements when the results ascribed to therapeutic situations are compared in this chart, it can be said that the effect ascribed to spontaneous improvement is high. The studies of Yora and Wolberg cannot be compared from the same standpoint, but they both show that it is necessary to take into consideration the phenomenon called spontaneous cure when discussing the curative mechanism. An analogous situation is the fruitless attempt to separate the medicinal effect of psychotropic drugs from the clinical effect of such drugs. Extraneous effects that intervene in these processes need to be taken into account in psychotherapy as well.

However, the situation in psychotherapy is more complicated, so it is difficult to distinguish clearly the characteristic effects of a technique from noncharacteristic effects that are not related to the technique.

For example, if a therapist has full confidence in his approach, accepts the suffering of a

---

[3] Meares, A.: *The Management of the Anxious Patient.* W. B. Saunders, Philadelphia and London (1963).

[4] Yora, T.: Shinkeishitsushō no yogo ni kansuru rinshōteki kenkyū (A clinical study of prognosis in *shinkeishitsu*) (in Japanese). *Tōkyō Jikeikai Ika Daigaku Zasshi* 75(2) (1960).

[5] Wolberg, L. R.: *The Technique of Psychotherapy*, 2nd edition. Grune & Stratton, New York (1967).

patient sympathetically and participates with sincerity, the patient will begin to be infused with hope and confidence in response to the therapist's attitude, and the therapist-patient relationship can thus promote to the cure process to some extent. A therapist's attitude may not be a scientific technique, but it is one facet of his or her professional activity and thus can be said to be inseparable from technique.

Even if we suppose that effective conditions are generally involved in the process that promotes a spontaneous cure, it is natural that this phenomenon alone cannot be considered to be a therapeutic process. Similarly, the decreased incidence of neurosis observed during the war in Japan, and the disappearance of symptoms of neurosis during military service, probably stemmed from factors that prevented emotional disorders or that functioned as mechanisms for relief of symptoms under special wartime conditions, but few investigators would conclude that such factors and mechanisms are akin to the processes of psychotherapy. In the daily life conditions that generally surround neurotics, it is not rare for conditions that promote cures and opportunities that accelerate cures to appear as outer world phenomena within the context of various kinds of human relationship. However, even if such chance factors crop up, they are lost, in spite of the fact that a patient may have a strong desire for a cure, exerting full effort constantly in a fight against symptoms. Psychotherapy is a means to change the attitude of a patient so that the opportunity for a cure can be utilized to the fullest extent possible.

As a rule, the phenomenon called spontaneous improvement is not limited to mental disorders. Almost all common physical illnesses can be eliminated through this process of spontaneous remission. In most cases, a physical mechanism originally present in a living body, such as homeostasis, is utilized in the process of recovery.

This is a performance of the living body that can be called an unconscious property of matching the objective. By contrast, the spontaneous cure that takes place in the instance of mental disorders, such as neuroses, not only is a physical mechanism but also makes it possible to anticipate a more conscious and human character effect.

Needless to say, this unconscious mechanism is not only a biological and bodily defense but also a defense that acts advantageously in regard to human life or adaptation to life at the point of contact with psychological concerns. However, we are less interested in the cause and effect properties of unconscious bodily regulation than in the process of spontaneous remission, which should occur in a more apperceptive context.

Guidance is carried out in Morita therapy so that "chance" experiences relating to the life of a patient can become the momentum that moves the patient toward a cure. This is the most effective force that a patient possesses for obtaining a spontaneous cure.

In the therapeutic process, psychoanalytic therapy, which stresses correlations between technique and changes in symptoms, takes into consideration only the therapist-patient relationship. The process, that is a part of Morita therapy is excluded from psychoanalysis because it is considered to be an accidental phenomenon that has no relevance for achieving a cure. The curative process engendered by the therapeutic mechanism will probably be considered as a separate spontaneous cure or as an effective phenomenon in the nontherapeutic situation. Consequently, it is natural that an attempt is made to introduce a spontaneous cure into this mechanism so that it has a therapeutic effect.

It is true that from the standpoint of analytical therapy, the effect of the technique and the effects of factors that have no direct bearing on the therapeutic mechanism should be differentiated, as a rule, but in the flow of continuous consciousness called the daily life experience of a patient, numerous difficulties are encountered in differentiating these factors from each other in any meaningful way. It is far more difficult to do so in a therapeutic modality, such as Morita therapy.

In viewing the entire character of a patient, it is more accurate to say that the therapeutic processes are started in the patient's life processes. The life of a patient is selectively involved in the curative process through various experiences that the patient has, and these experiences function to create a momentum in the direction of a cure.

These two factors overlap. If an attempt to trace the precise relationship between the therapeutic mechanism and the cure is based solely on general principles, and with the framework of the scientific nature of psychotherapy and its development, before we are aware of it we have fallen into a mistaken supposition that we can manipulate and cure human disorders by a pure exercise of technique. As a result, the contradiction inherent in postulating the true goal of psychotherapy to be that of fostering an independent way of life (human existence) for patients, while actually attempting to manipulate them in a manner similar to handling the controls of a machine, has cropped up.

Actually, however, a patient makes his or her selections, or decisions, and moves on to become involved with other persons and to have an independent way of life by overcoming his or her symptoms. The therapist must never forget this basic fact of human nature.

The author has discussed the spontaneous remission process, which can take place without any direct connection to the therapeutic mechanism, as a rule, and the importance of this remission process in the curative mechanism.

In therapeutic structures or techniques, such as those of Morita therapy, the processing is not limited to therapy alone, that is, the therapist-patient relationship. The mechanism of spontaneous remission becomes an important factor in our introduction of a therapeutic approach that discerns material correlated with the curative mechanism present in the various daily life experiences of a patient.

In particular, *sei no yokubō*, on which Morita therapy places so much emphasis, does express the mental desire of a patient to maintain his or her health and to improve and develop himself or herself. The therapist tries to foster, as much as is possible, this *chiyu e no chikara* (force for cure) to have it comply efficiently with the objective(s) of the therapeutic system. Consequently, the goal of Morita therpy is to have a patient restore himself or herself to the original selfhood. Only in that way can the patient achieve self-realization freely by his or her responsibility.

In all three cases that have been described in this chapter, the patients were enlightened by the therapeutic system to strive constantly for consistency, stability and self-improvement while still in a condition of being threatened by self-doubt, distrust, uneasiness and suffering due to an idealistic mental attitude. The patients displayed phenomena of self-perception, self-strengthening and self-transcendence by means of an internally constant negotiative process of self-questioning.

The case that best exemplifies this process is case 1. The author believes that it is possible to understand from this patient's life history how he created the problematical concept and evaluation of himself, but his most characteristic difficulty was that of having any consistency or stability of the ego constantly menaced, with any improvement of his ego condition always suppressed. The patient's ambivalent attitude toward his father had considerable relevance to his distorted evaluation of himself. Good ego functioning cannot be expected when we take into consideration the developmental condition of such an ego as this patient had. Free self-realization cannot be anticipated in a situation of a negotiative process that has the patient's *sei no yokubō* manifested so powerfully. The patient's consciousness, during the early stage of therapy, was overwhelmed by a self-consciousness that had dramatically changed in quality; his desire to escape such intense ego pressure was also powerful. He craved release from that intense pressure by somatotherapeutic measures, but this craving was merely a heteronomous attitude of attempting to change and transcend himself by depending on a disparate medium (medicine) that lies thoroughly outside the scope of change attainable by force of ego pressure.

Searching for a means to strengthen the ego by use of somatotherapy alone would leave the ego unchanged; the turning point toward a true cure for this patient would not be reached.

If, however, this patient is placed in a situation of being cut off from his strong dependence on chemical substances and is allowed only to carry out activities of daily living within a therapeutic framework, such as that provided by Morita therapy, it is inevitable that the concerns and interests of the ego will be gradually reoriented in that direction. This interest, at first, is only that of an ideological trial of *kaku araneba naranu* (this and that must be just so) and stems from an anticipation of being released from ego pressure. During the process, however, the patient feels the strength to live and, further, becomes aware that although the reason is not clear, the only one he can truly depend on is himself. This awareness does not signify that there is no other way to have the ego seek to accomplish this objective ideologically. It is, rather, a self-recognition acquired by internal necessity, a requisite attitude created by internal dialogue, repeated over and over. However, this self-recognition arises only when the patient has been placed in the critical position of not being able to rely on somatotherapy any longer, so that the only road left open is that of having to face reality on his own, even if his mental condition remains unstable. Only at that time will *sei no yokubō* act to motivate the patient's original human strength and value orientation. *Sei no yokubō*, that is, will serve to revert the patient's self to his original human selfhood, precisely at that critical juncture in which it most palpably poses a threat to the patient. From that critical turning point, *sei no yokubō* motivates the process of action for which the original self truly strives and develops further into a self-recognition of being in the *arugamama* state of mind.

This *arugamama* state of mind is one that must be readied by internal necessity. There are instances in which patients have clear awareness of that state of mind as well as instances in which patients have little awareness of it. The patient in case 1 had a relevant emotional experience, which he described. This experience does not signify that normal feeling had been restored; rather, it was a feeling of fresh recollection juxtaposed with a feeling of having been normal at some time in the past, seemingly as recently as the previous day.

This patient acquired a clear-cut trust in himself, with this so-called physical and psychological experience acting as the springboard for the curative momentum. When this experience took place, the patient began to create an autonomous life structure out of this ongoing process of self-negotiation. This process spread out, later, to widening areas of negotiation with other persons. The patient's attitude of facing up to his problems to seek an authentic ego formation became more prominent accordingly. Any intention of trying to alter his ego heteronomously no longer existed.

What can be observed in this case is a process of autonomous self-transcendence and a self-realization of *arugamama*, which is the objective of Morita therapy, a condition in which the mind, no longer threatened by the self or by the subjectively threatening presence of other persons, has reached the precondition needed to open outward to the world and to become freely adaptable to the facts of life.

Part VII

Position of Morita Therapy in the Genealogy of Psychotherapy

22

Morita Therapy and Logotherapy

Positioning the theory and technique of Morita therapy in relation to other psychotherapies is useful for gaining an understanding of Morita therapy. The background of Morita therapy was explained in detail in Part I, but it is probable that Morita made use of the theories and techniques of other investigators in developing the therapy that bears his name.

Dubois's persuasion therapy and Binswanger's life regulation method had a certain relevance to Morita. Hypnosis was also incorporated in his studies of suggestibility. Comparisons with psychoanalysis from a theoretical standpoint were frequently made during the early period of Morita therapy.

Morita was probably interested in Freud's early work. What he found worthy of consideration from the perspective of critical and comparative homologous studies was that enhancement of the *toraware* (mental captivity) of patients with *shinkeishitsu* was the result of a vigorous regimen of conscious self-persuasion (to build, for example, confidence in oneself or to have courage or not to be overly concerned).

Enhancement of *toraware* can also result from a mistaken sense of discretion (intended to alleviate or eliminate symptoms). Overcoming that discretion was Morita's goal for dissolving the *toraware* condition. He decided that suggestion, theoretical persuasion and a workload regulated only by a fixed schedule have no therapeutic effect and tend to aggravate a patient's problem. He concluded that Weir Mitchell's treatment regimen (enforced bed rest and a high-calorie diet), Dejerinne's or Neisser's isolation or bed rest method, Kant's diversion method and Ziehen and colleagues' tandem regimen of mental work alternated with exercise only confer mental tranquility or distract attention.

Morita did obtain useful insights from these forms of psychotherapy, but the originality of his conception surpassed all of them. Isolated bed rest and work therapy as applied by Morita led patients with *shinkeishitsu* to discover "self-authentication" by reversing a negative trend (symptoms of *shinkeishitsu*) to a positive trend that directs patients toward self-improvement and self-development by eliciting the *sei no yokubō* (desire to live), which is concealed from their awareness in the *shinkeishitsu* condition.

Morita's technique of absolute, isolated bed rest and work therapy is a means for a patient to discover the true self by cultivating the basic creativeness, endurance and spirit of service required to reveal oneself in human life, rather than by eliminating the various symptoms one at a time. The goal of Morita's method was not included in psychoanalysis or other paychotherapies of that time.

The goal of many modern schools of psychotherapy is not solely the alleviation or elimination of the symptoms of a neurosis, including as well the strengthening of a patient's ego, reintegration of his or her personality or mental arousal. From the standpoint of measures that are used to treat a "human being rather than a symptom," it can be said that Morita therapy is a pioneer form of contemporary psychotherapy. However, the major differences between Morita therapy and Occidental psychotherapy are that unconscious psychodynamics are not analyzed, the content of a symptom is not interpreted but accepted as it is and emphasis is placed on action rather than on speech.

In this chapter, Morita therapy will be compared with logotherapy to bring the characteristics of Morita therapy into bold relief.

Victor Frankl first used the expression "existential analysis" as a concept of logotherapy around 1939. This form of psychotherapy became widely used in Japan during the 1950s, after Morita therapy had become better known throughout Japan and Western Europe.

Existential analysis, or logotherapy, gained a firm clinical foothold in Japan, particularly after the publication of *Aerztliche Seelsorge* and *Theorie und Therapie der Neurosen* in their Japanese translations.

Frankl's concept of treating patients by leading them to recognize their suffering as being their responsibility and to accept it in their lives without evasion or without shifting responsibility to other persons became the opportunity for reperceiving that this concept closely resembles Morita therapy in this regard. Considerable interest was shown in the similarity between logotherapy and Morita therapy. Responsible for that trend were the American styles of psychiatry that flowed into the Japanese field of psychiatry rapidly after World War II. Of particular interest was the fact that persons regain tranquility after any excitement as a result of psychoanalysis. And the time was right to discuss that issue.

Interest in Morita therapy also increased, for the first time since its introduction in Japan. The complex, mentally traumatic experiences that psychoanalysis holds are the causes of neuroses seem to be universal. If that is true, however, a convincing explanation of why some people become neurotic while others do not, under much the same conditions, has yet to be advanced. Explanations of all human actions by means of a biology-based causality theory, coupled with the assertion that only a biological manipulation can be efficacious as a special therapy for curing neuroses, formed the opportunity for reexamination and reassessment of Morita therapy as a form of therapy for neuroses, with respect to anxiety and the "desire to live."

What made that opportunity possible is that logotherapy went beyond any previous psychology-based theory of treatment in considering human life as having a unified, totalistic structure. Neurotic suffering was deemed an expression of the struggle human beings go through to infuse meaning into the substance of human life. This was an attempt to cure neuroses through psychotherapy from a noological standpoint, and it made logotherapy a worthwhile subject for comparison with Morita therapy.

There have been several reports on the strong similarities between Morita's and Frankl's theories and therapies for neurosis. The author not only will examine the similarities but also will highlight the special features of Morita therapy, while noting the dissimilarities between the two types of therapy.

First of all, how do the two theories compare in explaining the root causes of neuroses? Both theories assert that a neurotic person's attention is first directed toward a transient psychosomatic phenomenon that is objectively harmless. However, the symptom thus engendered is gradually aggravated, culminating in a neurosis developed by a fixed process. Morita does not interpret the suffering of a neurotic person as constituting evidence of abnormality or heterogeneity because he does not view a symptom as being permanently fixed but, rather, as being a temperamental tendency that can lead to the development of the *shinkeishitsu* condition. A neurotic person forms an introspective conclusion about his or her mental and physical reactions (which are subjective realities in the manifestation of his or her human nature). These reactions pertain to various mental states that are part of human life, which are natural phenomena and harmless. The neurotic response is to interpret such mental states as being abnormal and as representing obstacles to adequate living. A neurotic person will try to break down the obstacles as much as he or she can but is finally enmeshed in the anxiety and mental conflict that arise because it is not possible to eliminate the obstacles.

The symptoms of a neurosis do not arise from a condition that is abnormal. The basic concepts and feelings are normal at the beginning, in most cases, but become intensified by overly anxious reactions that finally tip a neurotic person over into a condition of "captivation." By observing that process, Morita considers not only the symptoms but also a patient's attitude toward his or her condition as being most important. Basically, Morita does not believe that there is a factor that is heterogeneous to the character of a degenerate person or a factor that is fatalistic or fixed. The factor is thoroughly human and, as such, both homogeneous and fluid.

Frankl, however, insists that human action is not impelled only by the libido or by willpower, as psychoanalysis and individual psychology assert. He recognizes suffering in the noological dimension that underlies a patient's symptoms by viewing human life from a standpoint of dimensional ontology as a consistent, unified and totalistic field of existence.

Questions of the meaning of life are one of the most fundamental components of Frankl's theory as motivational factors. These factors are not only the question-motivators that unfold typically in adolescence but also may be formed by a certain experience that radically shakes a human mind. None of the psychological suffering or the mental struggles of human beings who strive to infuse meaning into their lives is pathological in nature, just as questions that arise in adolescence about the meaning of life are not signs of mental illness. This perception of neuroses is embedded in the therapeutic process and is consistently evident in Frankl's interpretation of how neuroses originate.

Frankl's observation that "on all occasions, the psychological problems of any individual human being cannot be dismissed simply as symptoms" is of great interest in comparison with Morita's conception of neurosis, in which the suffering is not considered as representing an illness but simply as constituting suffering as such, with acceptance of *arugamama* (leaving the symptoms alone as they are and leading life exactly as it is) as the proper procedure to achieve a true cure. This similar conception of neurosis that both Frankl and Morita have gives rise to further similarities in their concepts of the development of symptoms of neuroses and in their concepts of therapy as well.

Morita[1] describes the process by which symptoms develop by referring to the "desire to live," the hypochondriacal temperament, antagonistic actions of the mind, psychic interaction, autosuggestive activity and anticipatory anxiety. Frankl's mode of thought is similar, although his terms and expressions are different. According to Frankl, a person's attempts to escape from anxiety and to struggle with obsession confine the person within a ring of neurosis that is hardened by self-observation and anticipatory anxiety. A desire that is too strong will make what the person desires impossible to attain, and an attempt to escape will bring about the realization of something that is an object of fear. Frankl[2] explains this phenomenon by saying that "any clinician who does not have a preconception knows that it is not rare to have anticipatory anxiety as the essential etiological cause within the overall etiology of neurosis. Anticipatory anxiety concentrates the patient's attention on the symptom and thus fixes the symptom, whcih would otherwise remain floating and harmless. The fixing of the symptom gives rise to a corresponding phobia, which then aggravates the symptom. The aggravated symptom further increases the patient's mental trend toward incessant repetition of the symptom. The patient is

---

[1] Morita, S.: *Shinkeishitsu no hontai oyobi ryōhō* (The substance of *shinkeishitsu* and its therapy), 1928. In *Morita Shōma Zenshū*, Vol. II. Hakuyōsha, Tokyo (1974). (Printed in Japanese)

[2] Frankl, V. E.: *Theorie und Therapie der Neurosen.* Urban & Schwarzenberg, Wien (1956). (*Shinkeishō* I, translated by T. Miyamoto and M. Oda), Hakuyōsha, Tokyo (1960); (*Shinkeishō* II, translated by T. Shimoyama), *Frankl Chosakushū* 4, 5, Misuzu Shobō, Tokyo (1961).

finally confined in this fully completed vicious circle, sealed into it in a manner similar to that of a silkworm sealing itself in a cocoon."

Frankl cites the following case as a concrete example: "There was a certain young physician who came to our clinic suffering from a severe sweating phobia. His vegetative nervous condition had been unstable since birth. He one day shook hands with a superior and observed that he was sweating profusely. At their next meeting, he experienced anticipatory sweating. Anticipatory anxiety had roused a cold sweat in the pores of his skin to complete the vicious circle. Hyperhidrosis had caused a sweating phobia, and the phobia then fixed the hyperhidrosis into a fixed condition."

Frankl's approach[3] was to have a patient abandon the desire to be normal or to escape a condition that is abnormal so that the patient could move away from that paradoxical process of psychological entrapment. Morita, too, noted the phenomenon that arises from any such paradoxical psychological process (which he calls contradictoriness in thinking), and it is this process that motivates the vicious circle that produces and aggravates the symptoms of *shinkeishitsu.* Morita's method of treatment was to lead a patient away from contradictoriness in thinking by placing emphasis on dissolving the grip of the vicious circle. The phrase that Morita often used is, "Saying it should be 'thus and so' is still falsehood and is not *arugamama* (living with the symptoms or facing the pain and accepting it as it is)."

This is the "truth" that explains the process used in Morita therapy. What Morita considers as being most important is not the intellectual understanding of a patient but, rather, the emotional experience acquired through his or her behavior. He expresses this concept by using the term *taitoku* (realization from experience) in plain language. This term denotes the awareness that is attained by performing actions by oneself and through the experience of doing so. By contrast, intellectual understanding is an abstract knowledge that deduces by reasoning whatever "should be" or "should not be." According to Morita, this concept is the same as the theoretical persuasion method employed by Dubois, in which natural feelings and facts are often ignored and the patient sinks deeper and deeper into perplexity and error.

Morita opposes the use of any persuasive approach that tries to appeal to intellectual understanding, from a therapeutic standpoint, because the frequent disparities between thought and reality (contradictoriness in thinking) increase a patient's suffering and have harmful results. Correct understanding and realization of facts finally come into agreement, but during the therapeutic process up to that point, especially in the activity of severing the vicious circle, that agreement is not possible. Morita insists that a patient undergoing therapy should pursue a livelihood that is based on the natural factor of the "desire to live" or the "facts of feeling" and should leave the symptoms alone as they are.

Frankl[4] places similar emphasis on emotionality and tried to guide patients to learn how to pull themselves free from their symptoms by relying on their sense of humor. He advised patients to satirize their symptoms, explaining that "the patient must learn to face anxiety, nay, to ridicule it in its face." He adds that "there is no making a distance between oneself and some situation like humor, so one learns to satirize, at last to overcome the symptom of neurosis." Actually, humor is the lively feeling that indicates a basic opposition toward tragic feelings or toward the life anxiety of a neurotic patient.

The emphasis on emotional experience stressed by both investigators is intended to make a patient learn how to look at his or her neurotic condition objectively by facing the symptom, not turning away from it, or by ridiculing the symptom. Frankl and Morita agree that a

[3] vid. do., paradoxe Intention, pp. 47, 132, 151.
[4] vid. do., Humor, pp. 161, 162.

patient's symptom is not the true object of therapy; the objective is to change the patient's attitude toward the symptom.

Frankl places emphasis on liberating a patient from self-observation, excessive self-examination or tenacious attention. He explains dereflection, one of his logotherapeutic techniques, by citing an example of sexual neurosis to stress its necessity. Excessive observation or self-reflection can frequently obstruct the process of normalizing life functions. For example, self-reflection on the sexual act is compounded with a forced intensity of sexual desire, and both conditions are etiological, characterized by excessive intention and attention. For example, when the sexual act is carried out in a manner similar to sleeping, excessive intention will have a detrimental effect completely similar to excessive attention. However, the basis of both conditions is an anxious anticipation of obstacles to fulfillment. This anticipation gives rise to an unnatural desire for a functional process that is not obstructed and also brings about a similar compulsive self-observation focused on the obstacle that is the object of fear. This self-reflection usually becomes the obstacle that thwarts normal functions unconsciously and automatically.

Frankl points out, for this reason, that it is more important for psychotherapy to put an unconscious stop to a certain problem to return a patient to normality unconsciously or to free the patient's attention from the symptoms in which excessive attention is concentrated as a focal point. Paradoxical intention, he says, gives a patient the strength to make satirical remarks about his or her neurosis, so that the patient will be able to disregard the symptoms by a process of dereflection; in other words, what makes for authenticity in a human being is not to be rationalistic but to be emotive, which is unconscious or nonreflexive.

It is clear from Frankl's remarks "to be rationalistic is not to be too rational" and "unconsciousness and non-reflection make a wise man" that he ultimately stresses "trust in the unconscious mind" and "trust in the wisdom of the mind." His logotherapy would be called existential analysis from that standpoint, but let us return to Morita before going any further.

Morita strongly emphasizes absolute, isolated bed rest as his most characteristic method of therapy, to bring a patient to an objective observation of anxiety, but because this method is based on Morita's anthropological concepts, the author will delve into that topic later. Morita also used a method that resembles Frankl's paradoxical intention, but Morita's method is more objective and more concrete. For example,[5] a middle-aged woman with paroxysmal neurosis (which is much the same as anxiety neurosis) had suffered from attacks of palpitation for about four to five years. The seizures usually occurred at night, and when they did occur, the woman could not lie down due to anxiety. She would sit up and lean back against the bedding, to wait until the pain disappeared. If a seizure occurred, a similar seizure would occur within three to five days.

At the time Morita examined this patient, she had experienced a seizure during the previous night and was in a state of strong anticipatory anxiety concerning the probability of a seizure the following night. Morita said: "When you go to bed tonight, lie down in the exact position in which a seizure occurs most frequently, and try to will the seizure to occur, endure the suffering of being in that position and cooperate with it, by observing earnestly and in detail the entire process from the time the seizure takes place. This will give you a clear awareness of the nature of the seizure by your experience and will also become the basis for your future therapy. Even if violent pain occurs tonight, and makes you stay awake all night, the pain will be worthwhile if the anxiety and suffering you have been afflicted with for so long are thus relieved."

The patient promised that she would do as Morita had instructed. When Morita examined her the next time, she said: "I did what you told me to do that night, but I could not

---

[5] Morita, S.: vid. do.

will the seizure to occur; I began to fall asleep within five minutes and slept soundly till morning with no awareness of anything."

After that, the patient did not experience any seizures. What made this happen was the patient's change in attitude of resolving to observe the symptoms objectively, resigning herself to suffer the pain of a seizure, and when this change took place, the anticipatory anxiety experienced until that point faded from the foreground of her awareness.

Morita expresses the attitude of this patient as "plunging into fear itself." His explanation is that the suffering of the patient was increased because of a mistake made at the beginning on where to focus attention. The seizures were anticipated, and an attempt was made to bear them without becoming aware of doing so. Mental confusion arose in trying to escape the condition, but this approach served only to exacerbate the anxiety and the pain. That is why Morita stressed the importance of changing the patient's attitude. He also cited the expression *junna kokoro* (authentic or intrinsic mind, or that one accepts the fact of feeling as it arises in nature, entrusting to it without avoidance or diversion)[6] and adopted this approach as his chief tool for liberating the patient from *hakarai* (devising all sorts of strategems), to oppose suffering or to free herself from captivation by sublating self-observation and reflection. Morita took the position that the patient is not supposed to oppose the symptom while being aware of it and should let it be just as it is.

In Frankl's existential analysis, a human being has an existence that is directed toward a focal point. Consequently, a neurotic person needs not only to divert attention from the symptoms but also to learn to shift direction. Life continues and problems retreat into the background of experience if one entrusts oneself to a single focus from a standpoint of recapturing a new objectivity that can provide meaning and value in one's life.

Morita similarly stresses *ishiki no tai-mokutekisei* (immediate object orientation of human consciousness)[7] and disregard of "the fact of feeling" (see Chapter 5) as being in error, a form of "false wisdom" that obstructs the natural flow of the mind (see Chapter 5). A patient should, instead, have a *junna kokoro* (authentic or intrinsic mind) rather than false wisdom and should strive to attain a condition of "will-less attention" (see Chapter 14), characterized by *kokoro no mama ni ikiru* (to live as the intrinsic mind directs). He explains this concept as follows: "I try to guide the patient during therapy in such a way that he will become aware of *junna kokoro*, as well as *jiko honrai no seijō* (one's original human nature), and shift into a state of mind which is not self-deceptive. *Junna kokoro* signifies our innate nature, and the strict reality of that nature should not be negated or deceived. We begin with this fact as the basis; it is not an idealistic principle of determining standards of morality and propriety, and then acting accordingly, nor is it *kibun hon'i* (feeling-centered) [see Chapter 6]. When we get to work, we will naturally devise ways to simplify, accelerate and validate whatever task we undertake, if we begin with the mind

6 It indicates the case, for example, in which a patient with a noise phobia tries to shut out a certain sound because it is irritating and becomes captivated by the sound the harder he or she tries to shut it out. However, if the patient accepts the noise as it is, without opposing it as an irritant, and continues to do whatever he or she is doing, he or she will become engrossed in that activity and the noise will fade away into the background of awareness, creating a situation of not being attentive to it, even though it is still within the range of hearing. Kōra describes the Zen Buddhist expression *seiju fuju* (accepting something as it is exists in nature is the same as not feeling anything at all about it).

7 Morita explains this point: One's attention or consciousness acts centrifugally toward the objective only. On that occasion, one is generally not aware of anything else. For example, when one throws or catches a ball, one merely directs attention to the ball. One is not aware of how the hand moves. Morita calls this nature of attention or consciousness *ishiki no tai-mokutekisei* or *ishiki no masshōsei* (peripheral nature of consciousness.). As a result of *ishiki no tai-mokutekisei*, one is prone to perceive inversely the process of cause and effect. For example, one is apt to think that brachial biceps muscles swell as a result of bending an arm. In reality, contracting the muscles bends the arm. People frequently become aware of such a routine mental fact. Morita attaches much importance to such facts in connection with *shisō no mujun* (contradictoriness in thinking).

as it is, even if the work is troublesome. . . . . An idealistic person thinks he must make an effort to work or endure it, and thinks he should not consider the work as abhorrent or troublesome, even if it is, and his mind is consequently preoccupied with an impossible attempt to negate his genuine feeling, leaving no opportunity to progress in the direction of unfolding his authentic self. . . . Such being the case, the consciousness of the difference between *junna kokoro* (pure mind) and *akuchi* (false wisdom) cannot be acquired by verbal explanation alone but must be truly experienced."

It is clear from this explanation that human life is a natural phenomenon. Basically, a person can actuate spontaneous action of the mind and body if he or she does quickly what he or she can do, in accordance with the proddings of the mind, which occur naturally if one acts "as a natural human being." This spontaneous action is characterized chiefly by acting for improvement and development of oneself and not for any self-destructive purpose.

The similarities between Morita and Frankl include their theories of the origins of neuroses and their therapeutic principles. The difference between these investigators lies in their application of technique. Both investigators often use characteristic nonmedical terms when explaining their theories. Morita uses Buddhist, particularly Zen Buddhist, terms or terms that have been in widespread use in Japan since ancient times. Frankl makes skillful use of Christian and existential philosophical terms to communicate his message. However, such terms are nothing more than formal similarities. There are considerable differences in cultural content.

Both investigators agree that a human being should be considered as being a monistic entity, not a composite of a disparate mind and body. However, Frankl views a human being from the standpoint of dimensional ontology as consisting of a noological-personal dimension and a psychosomatic dimension.[8] Human spirit, he believes, has the power to resist both mind and body; a human being can always break away from the present self, can transcend that self. Accordingly, a human being can always progress and develop infinitely. A human being is involved in constant change and will not remain unchanged in the future. A person will not always be as he or she is in the present moment, as neurotic persons believe. The intention of existential analysis is to make a patient "become conscious of the unconscious, intrinsic human hunger to express and develop the self."[9] Frankl says that a therapist must bring into conscious action a patients's unconscious potential. The purpose of this action is to reestablish unconscious habit. The therapist needs to reestablish the patient's reliance on the self-evident fact of unconscious, purposeful activity.

Morita's concept is that a human being is a natural phenomenon manifested by the actions of the mind and body. A person cannot change his or her nature artificially. All the person can do, even in spiritual action, is "to compile ideas by grasping a fixed concept" from the "association of ideas which occurs naturally." Life as being natural is composed of ordinary activity, but the mind "always flows and changes correlatively between the inner world and the outer world." Mind is not fixed. Further, a human being naturally has a "desire to live," which includes a desire for self-development and advancement, together with concern for self-preservation. A person progresses and improves infinitely by moving along with the "flow of life" when he or she "obeys nature absolutely." Morita therapy could be called a "natural therapy in which a spirit of submission to the dictates of human nature is acquired."

Both theories posit that human existence is engaged in constant progress, in a never-ending growth process, but there are still considerable differences between the two theories. Yamamoto definitively points out the differences as follows[10]: "The first difference lies in how

---

[8] Frankl, V. E.: vid. do. (*Shinkeishō* I).
[9] Frankl, V. E.: vid. do. (*Shinkeishō* I).

the subject is perceived as being involved with the world. When Frankl says that human existence is 'something which always produces,' he is thinking about the 'defiant power of man's spirit.' According to existential analysis, human existence contains the three basic phenomena of spirituality, freedom and responsibility."

Freedom is the substance of what is opposed to impetus, heredity and environment. A human being can place emphasis on his or her subjectiveness and naturalness while defying those three factors. Therefore, even though Frankl views a human being as a being-in-the-world, he stresses that the problem lies in how one should establish one's naturalness while defying those three factors to overcome them. A human being is never a mere product of heredity and the environment. In that fact lies decision-making power, which allows one to decide for oneself.[11]

Morita, by contrast, always stresses *nature* in connection with the fact that life "is evolving and eternally advancing." According to Morita, human beings become inconvenienced because they always view the world and nature as self-adherent. Because human beings belong to nature, any attempt to arrange oneself as one wishes because the natural "fact of mind" is seen to be inconvenient is already functioning under illusion. If a human being entrusts the self to reality, by accepting one's natural desire, temperament and the facts of one's human nature as it is, and thereby conquers one's environment, "a free and unrestricted mind" will flow out in response to stimuli received from the outer world, so that one's natural "desire for improvement and progress" will be motivated and one's natural human nature manifested. For Morita, the problem is one of how a human being can discard artifice, return to reality and manifest natural human character.

Another difference between Frankl and Morita is that of how a human being perceives the method of involvement with the world. Frankl relies on paradoxical intention, whereas Morita relies on the therapeutic technique called *kyōfu totsunyū* (plunge into fear). Frankl taught patients to experience the irrationality of their symptoms, and, in turn, the fact of their minds and bodies, by the opposite course of accepting their symptoms, by looking at their irrationality objectively with humor and a spirit of satire. A patient will thus learn to let go of the symptoms, will gradually discern his or her irrational mental interaction and, finally, will be freed from the symptom.

Morita instructed patients to "confront the symptoms and fears," "willingly accept the condition of one's mind and body and live in conformity with the facts" with a "frame of mind of self-abandonment." A patient is led to discern that these facts of life apply to himself or herself, then to affirm the factual nature of his or her self and, finally, to learn to accept it. In that process, the patient will learn to obey "the truth of nature" and, as a result, will attain "the state of perfect freedom."

Still another difference is that of the orientation of a human being. Frankl frequently uses the expression "will to meaning"[12] in his numerous theses on logotherapy. He explains that the "meaning orientation of the human being is misinterpreted by psychoanalysis, and the characteristic of human effort to acquire values is simply deformed into effort to win physical satisfaction. Individual psychology perceives a person who suffers from a so-called inferiority complex as a neurotic, and has overlooked the fact that the person is suffering from the meaninglessness of existence. Individual psychology fails to notice that the patient is not a person who suffers

---

[10] Yamamoto, I.: *Die Japanische Morita-Therapie im Vergleich zu der Existenzanalyse und Logotherapie Frankls.* Sonderdruck aus "Abendländische Therapie und Ostliche Weisheit." Ein Tagungsbericht; Herausgegeben von Professor Dr. med., Dr. phil. Wilhelm Bitter. Ernst Klett Verlag, Stuttgart.

[11] Frankl, V.E.: vid. do. (*Shinkeishō* II), Entscheidung, 67.

[12] Frankl, V.E.: vid. do. (*Shinkeishō* II), Wille zum Sinn, 116.

only because he feels inferior in value; he also suffers from the fact that his existence does not have 'any meaning'." Frankl[13] criticized the misunderstanding of extremist depth-psychologists by stating that "in the framework of the human image–actually a human being is not 'formed' by a concatenation of impulses, as it may seem if we look only at the impulsive aspect of the human being," because spirituality is not engendered only by impulse. He insists that a human being is not "shoved around" only by impulses but, rather, has an existence that is "guided" by "meaning." A human being must not always be freed "from" something, also having the freedom to "face" something. Further, a human being has responsibility not only "with regard to" something but also "toward" something. Each human being must discover the "meaning" of self in its "freedom," and that is possible only as a "responsible existence" facing "toward" God. He further explains that the interlocutor of the soul, called "thou–God," is always present beyond the human superego.[14]

Morita advocates "nature." What he means by "nature" are the facts of human life, and nature thus consists in seeing life only "as it is." He says that "one should realize that life can be painful for other people as well as for oneself, and should suffer 'suffering,' fear 'fear,' and rejoice in 'joy.'" Further, Morita stresses that life consists in action. He states[15] that "life is creation" with the meaning that "the livelihood of all human beings is action" and that in this action there is "always progress and advance." The acceptance of the fact of life "as it is" is natural, including the phenomenon of the human mind and body. "Even moral sensibility is something which appears naturally as innate to human nature." Negating this "fact" by intellectualizing is inherently impossible. Morita insists that "if we do not artificially value our feelings, learn to ignore idealistic propositions of right and wrong, good or bad" (discard false wisdom) and live only by conforming to "immediate day-to-day realization," we will naturally accept and acquire "truth." He emphasizes the idea that "a man welcomes with delight something which preserves him but avoids with fear something which threatens him. This is the innate feeling of a man who strives to maintain and advance his life. These joys and fears are the basis for the formation of mental obedience. Because a man seeks to maintain and advance his life, he obeys God, he obeys nature, he obeys humankind, and he obeys himself. Because he obeys himself, he discerns his true nature and does not try to exceed it. He takes care of himself with conviction, he practices constant self-examination and is too prudent to be entrapped by egotism. He fears the damage he can inflict on himself and others by giving vent to his desires and thus exercises self-control. Because he submits himself to others, he can accept the strong points of others to supplement his own shortcomings, and he can study the good points of others to cover his own weak points. Because he obeys nature, he steeps himself in the realization of the vast universe, yearns for the perfecting and completion of all that is in the universe and in the spirit, and is not shackled by the bias of ego. Furthermore, because he reveres God, he is led to supreme heights, is enfolded in the riches of human charity, and is saved from taking the wrong path by his recognition of strict authority."

Even from a therapeutic point of view, Frankl advocates the discarding of meaningless "self-observation" and self-sacrifice to devote oneself to "something which is truly worthy of self-sacrifice," while Morita emphasizes only to "obey nature and be submissive to circumstances as *arugamama*, and become self-absorbed in immediate day-to-day activities."

By comparison, one of these two investigators develops theory from phenomenological and theoretical points of view, while the other investigator develops it from descriptive and intuitive points of view. Both investigators penetrate the dimension of mind to discern

[13] vid. do., Triebe, 60.
[14] vid. do., Freiheit, 70.
[15] Morita, S.: vid. do.

neurotic vicious circles and "captivation" in the psychosomatic dimension. The differences between the two investigators appear in how they view the dimension of attitude.

Yamamoto[16] remarks that "the postulate that lies behind Frankl's existential analysis and logotherapy is that the condition of the world depends solely on the existential philosophy based in the Western European tradition, which relies on self-planning by the individual subject, with that subjecthood defined by the Christian concept that the intrinsic self will be developed only by the guidance of God. What lies behind Morita therapy is the postulate that the condition of the world inheres in obedience to the 'truth of the universe and nature,' including human nature, and further insists that this truth is the awareness of *mu* (nothingness). (See Chapter 20.) Human subjecthood is engendered by discerning this truth and bringing oneself into unity with it. This is Oriental philosophy: only if one empties oneself and casts the self into the *mu* of nature can the authentic subjecthood of self be realized and the state of freedom attained, as advocated by Buddhism, particularly Zen Buddhism."

The preceding text provides a general explanation of the differences between the theories and therapeutic methods of Frankl and Morita. There are important dissimilarities between their techniques and the anticipated human image to be the result, notwithstanding the many similarities in their views of a human being, taking into consideration the differences of thought that their respective backgrounds created.

---

[16] Yamamoto, I.: vid. do.

23

Morita Therapy and Behavior Therapy

It is a well-known fact that the term "behavior therapy" came into use as a general description for a clinical approach that is based on the point of view first espoused by H. J. Eysenck in his landmark study *Behavior Therapy and Neurosis* in 1960.

Morita therapy was developed 50 years before the term behavior therapy had been proposed and, for this reason, the terms "learning therapy" and behavior therapy are not used in the explanation of its principles. Nonetheless, the author will discuss behavior therapy in this chapter because even though there is a general difference between Morita therapy and behavior therapy from a conceptual standpoint, there are numerous similarities in the techniques of these two forms of psychotherapy. Again, the characteristics of Morita therapy can be brought into bold relief by comparing them with the characteristics of behavior therapy.

There are differences relating to theoretical composition and cultural background. A simple comparison could detract from a correct understanding of Morita therapy, but the two schools of thought share the feature of not deeply pursuing the cause of the symptoms beneath the conscious level. Eysenck clarifies the position of behavior therapy by comparing it with mainstream psychotherapy, which is based primarily on psychoanalysis. He stresses that behavior therapy is both rational and efficacious.[1]

The author adopts a similar approach for comparing the principles, objectives, goals and techniques of Morita therapy with those of behavior therapy.

Therapeutic Principles

Behavior therapy is a general term used to describe a clinical approach to neurosis taken from a behaviorist standpoint. It is a method of inducing and strengthening adaptation behavior and, at the same time, of weakening and eliminating inadaptation behavior by applying various principles of learning that have been established experimentally.[2] The activities of a patient are regulated and oriented toward the direction that a therapist wishes to pursue by manipulating various conditions for the transformation of inadaptation behavior. One technique is to induce a response that a patient did not have in the past by placing the patient in a new situation; another technique is to prevent a response that is likely to take place in a certain situation.

The first technique concerns conditioning, or the learning process, whereas the second technique concerns the effect of extinction of the response.

In Morita therapy, behavior is controlled for orientation toward a natural direction consistent with authentic human nature by manipulation of various conditions that support the inadaptation behavior of a patient suffering from *shinkeishitsu*. In abstract terms, there is no

---

[1] Eysenck, H.J.: *Behavior Therapy and the Neuroses.* Pergamon Press, New York (1960).
[2] Wolpe, J.: *The Practice of Behavior Therapy.* Pergamon Press, New York (1969).

difference, in principle, between the two therapies. However, the transformation process in Morita therapy affects reasoning by means of emotional experience and has a close correlation with life-style. It provides a philosophy of life and of nature and a world view.

By contrast, behavior therapy has a mechanical simplicity common to animal training.

Therapeutic Objectives

The objective, in the earliest period of behavior therapy, was solely the management of simple phobias, tics, stammering and, in childhood, enuresis, and management of these conditions with behavior therapy then was only in a trial stage. Recently, however, the conditions for which this therapy has been used have been expanded rapidly to include alcoholism and other addictions, sexual perversion, autism, behavioral disorders, compulsion, schizophrenia and mental retardation.

This wider variety of conditions for which behavior therapy is now considered effective is the result of clarification of the pathological basis of problem behavior as an abjective state, with the connections formed that directly link learning theory, therapeutic technique and therapeutic goals, resulting in the formulation of a more integrated model of behavior therapy. Many symptoms regularly encountered in clinical practice have complex structures. When such symptoms are roughly classified, theoretically, into those that indicate that inadaptation behavior has been learned as opposed to those that indicate that learning of adaptation behavior has been insufficient or is lacking, it is evident that most of the reinforcing factors of the symptoms are sociocultural in origin.

From a patient's standpoint, there are many factors, such as constitution, temperament and character trend, that are not clear. These numerous concealed factors, which are difficult to clarify, become complementary, reinforcing factors that motivate the formation of complicated symptoms, whose management may be relatively simple in terms of the goal of an effective therapeutic approach.

Morita therapy is clearly effective only for the management of certain neuroses, particularly Morita *shinkeishitsu.* The phenomenon of *shinkeishitsu* has a pathological basis that is elucidated in Morita theory and that is amenable to successful management with the techniques used in Morita therapy. Patients who receive this therapy are mostly young people who have not formed intellectual obstructions, who genuinely want to respond to therapy and who manifest the "desire to live."

Therapeutic Goals

With the pathological basis of the conditions for which behavior therapy is effective clarified on the basis of behavior theory and learning theory, therapeutic manipulation is always closely focused on a patient's symptoms. Behavior is manipulated in the direction selected by the therapist by controlling the inadaptation behavior of the patient, in line with the goal of treatment, to promote adaptation behavior.

The initial therapeutic goal is to remove the obstructions that hinder adaptability. As a result, a patient's internal confusion is dissolved and he or she has become ready for orientation toward adaptation. By contrast, the most salient feature of Morita therapy is that manipulation is not applied directly to a patient's symptoms. For this reason, Morita therapy is said to be a *fumon* approach.[3] A therapist does not consider symptoms to be the objects of Morita therapy, instead carrying out manipulations to encourage a patient's behavior to move in the direction in which the patient wishes to move and not evading symptoms but simply accepting them as they are.

The compliance of a patient in accepting the symptoms as facts lies in the anticipation of going through a process of autonomous strengthening. However, a therapist's understanding of a patient with *shinkeishitsu* (based on Morita theory) has an important bearing in this regard. A symptom that stands as an obstacle to a patient's adaptability is the hypochondriacal phenomenon that originates from the "desire to live," which is common to all healthy human beings as well as persons with *shinkeishitsu.* (From the standpoint of structural analysis, the symptoms have both physical and personality aspects.) Even if the symptoms are painful to a patient as fixed phenomena of *shinkeishitsu*, they are not pathological or abnormal, being an exaggeration of a state that is normal.

In other words, the symptoms of inadaptability that are characteristic of *shinkeishitsu* are the personality responses of persons who have the temperamental tendency called *shinkeishitsu.* With this understanding, a therapist directs manipulation toward the natural formation of an awareness that a symptom of *shinkeishitsu* is not a heterogeneous "growth" that needs to be removed but, rather, a normal, homogeneous "growth" that needs to be accepted self-assertively.

The problem is the part played by the personality of a patient with *shinkeishitsu* in developing and fixing, as a symptom, something that is homogeneous. Morita therapy is not aimed directly at a patient's symptoms, being directed, instead, toward a cure through training the patient's personality to eliminate the factor that provokes the development of the symptons.

Therapeutic Techniques

Many techniques in Morita therapy are similar, in principle, to those of behavior therapy. A few such techniques will be discussed at this time for the sake of comparison.

In most cases, relaxation reduces and eases fear and anxiety. In behavior therapy, this phenomenon is called reciprocal inhibition. Wolpe[4, 5] points out that relaxation is an effective therapy for neuroses in the sense of being a therapeutic principle. Systematic desensitization and self-assertion training are included in this approach as representative treatment modalities. With the first method, fear and anxiety are overcome by repetitive submission of a patient to conditions ranging, in graduated stages, from weak stimulation by the factor that arouses anxiety to increasingly stronger stages until the patient suppresses the anxiety psychologically.

---

[3] *Fumon* in this instance refers to a therapist's stance of not responding specifically to a patient's complaints about a symptom and of not asking anything about it. The therapist's attitude or response is, rather, that of *fumon* (disregard). The therapist's objective is to have the patient open up *ma* (space) between himself or herself and the symptom to interpose an attitude in which the symptom is examined objectively and to restore a natural emotional rhythm in the patient's mind, which is gripped in artificial tension and anxiety. This approach imposes a characteristic psychological distance between the therapist and the patient. The therapist's human relationship with the patient is one of unity in the attitude of *fumon* created by the therapeutic process. In the diagnostic stage, before therapy is started, the therapist will, of course, listen to all of a patient's complaints to comprehend the structure, content, motivation, progression and mode of involvement between the patient and his or her symptoms (see Chapter 17).

[4] Wolpe, J.: *Psychotherapy by Reciprocal Inhibition.* Stanford University Press, Palo Alto, Calif. (1963).

[5] Wolpe, J.: Basic principles and practices of behavior therapy of neuroses. *American Journal of Psychiatry* 125:1242 (1969).

The second method is one in which a patient is directed toward adaptation by resolving internal confusion and eliminating symptoms in a process of shaping the confronting responses of a group of patients, who sulk, evade and act out physical and mental symptoms, because the attitude of warding off opposing pressure from their surroundings does not develop.

Wolpe decided which symptoms are amenable to management with self-assertion training by using a patient's life history and personality rating scale. Tendencies to be upset easily, to be bashful, to show constraint toward superiors and to be overly self-conscious are tested. Persons who have these tendencies are afraid that they may hurt the feelings of other persons and thus pay too much attention to people around them, restraining themselves from self-expression even when people do something to them that they do not like.

Wolpe applied the muscle relaxation method in such instances as a reaction that opposes anxiety, the underlying principle of the method being that a stimulus that causes anxiety can be suppressed completely, or at least partially, by having it coexist with a reaction that opposes the development of anxiety, so that the connection between the stimulus and anxiety is weakened. The muscle relaxation response is learned, and the systematic desensitization process that is induced by the technique is based on that principle.

Flooding is the complete opposite of the method that begins with the weakest degree of a stimulus that causes anxiety. In flooding, the strongest degree of a stimulus that causes anxiety is introduced at the beginning of therapy. This situation will bring a neurotic patient to experience intense anxiety, but the patient becomes composed and anxiety is not aroused once he or she recognizes that the stimulus will not create a condition of danger. With this method of manipulation, the symptom is eliminated by repeated presentation of the stimulus or by convincing the patient to acknowledge that the anticipated danger will not arise even if the stimulus is presented and not evaded. Mental relaxation follows and accelerates discontinuation of evasion as a direct reward.

Operant conditioning is another method that is worthy of comparison. Skinner[6] states that the crux of this method is the principle of strengthening, meaning that what has been learned is what has been strengthened, in other words, a response that is basically controlled by a stimulus that occurs in accordance with the response. There are both positive and negative factors in any such stimulus, for example, rewards and penalties, and the response is controlled by manipulation of this combination.

In the conditioning method, a movement that is inclined in a certain direction is weakened by addition of a negative strengthening action, with a positive strengthening factor also applied to a desirable action to strengthen it.

Negative practice is also a beneficial technique. With this method, an involuntary neurotic activity, such as a tic, is transformed into a conscious, voluntary activity and, as a result, the involuntary factor is eliminated. The underlying principle of this method is the creation of reactive inhibition by reciprocation, without strengthening any conditioned response, in other words, the induction of a condition similar to a sense of fatigue. Another method is conditioned inhibition by a new conditioning of not responding when the response is brought to an end as a result of this reactive inhibition.

The author has selected and briefly explained the forms of behavior therapy that merit comparison with Morita therapy. The author will now examine the techniques of Morita therapy from a behavior therapy viewpoint in relation to the techniques of other behavior therapies.

It is true that a patient is controlled heterogeneously, but he or she is also controlled auto-

[6] Skinner, B.F.: *Science and Human Behavior.* Macmillan, New York (1953).

nomously, in a certain sense, in regard to conditions of anxiety, tension and fear, which cannot be eliminated or evaded during absolute, isolated bed rest in Morita therapy. However, the patient acquires the experience to withstand his or her condition and accepts it, with the guidance of the therapist, letting it become a kind of operant response (a method of weakening and eliminating the behavior by continuing to ignore it, without applying positive or negative measures to strengthen the behavior, coupled with a positive reward: acceptance by the therapist).

The bed rest condition also induces a relaxation response and, as a result, acts as a competitive factor that alleviates fear and anxiety. In the ensuing work therapy period, a patient is confronted by work assignments in a life environment that has both qualitative and quantitative stages. (This method resembles *in vivo* desensitization, or flooding.) Anticipated dangers do not occur, even when work situations are not evaded. Moreover, comments made by the therapist at opportune times and appropriate evaluations of practical behavior gradually strengthen the orientation of the patient toward elimination of the habit of evasion.

This process also promotes deep, materialistic concern and a genuine interest in living. In Morita therapy, the principle is that a therapist takes the attitude of *fumon* (disregarding a patient's symptoms during the bed rest and work periods as well as during interviews).

This attitude functions as a kind of extinction technique that has the effect of weakening a patient's complaints. Further, the patient is prohibited from taking measures to reduce or evade fear and anxiety throughout Morita therapy. Techniques for confrontation (plunging into fear) are the rule. However, a therapist sometimes includes training to have a patient objectively observe the inner self, which is so gripped by fear and anxiety, by creating situations that provoke fear and anxiety by use of methods similar to the paradoxical intention technique of logotherapy.

For example, the blushing or palpitation that arises from tension when meeting people is so natural that a patient blushes self-assertively or suffers palpitation with the use of a method similar to that of so-called negative practice. Directing a patient with *shinkeishitsu*–who tends to consider his or her suffering as something that is not experienced by other persons and who also has the prejudgment that it is abnormal to accept his or her condition–to overcome those stumbling blocks by observing and listening to people in the community is a technique of social learning.

The behavioral transformation of a patient that is accomplished with the techniques of Morita therapy may be summarized by use of the terms and expressions of behavior therapy. In Morita therapy, a therapist can manipulate heterogeneous behavior by inhibiting existing responses through regulation of positive and negative strengthening factors during the initial period of therapy (absolute, isolated bed rest and work therapy), by disregarding undesirable responses that are recognized as existing and, at the same time, by providing strengthening factors to create new responses that constitute the goal of therapy, or by reinforcing new forms of behavior that compete with prior responses (bed rest or work) to inhibit old responses.

Elimination of symptoms is not the direct therapeutic goal; the procedure accelerates the manifestation of a patient's desire to live. Work assignments are altered qualitatively as well as quantitatively until the stage is reached that conforms best to a patient's real-life situation. A new response of manipulating one's responses is formed voluntarily and independently. A process of self-reinforcement takes place to sustain the new response that has been created.

A number of differences between the principles, objectives, goals and techniques of Morita therapy and those of behavior therapy have been discussed briefly. The major differences can be summarized as follows:

	Morita Therapy	*Behavior Therapy*
1.	The essence of a human being is the natural and coordinated harmony created by *sei no yokubō* (the desire to live, for life improvement and progress) and the hypochondriacal trait (self-preservation), based on descriptive phenomenological and intuitive perspectives.	A human being is viewed in terms of behavior theory and mechanical theory.
2.	The natural exercise of that human essence induces harmony.	Numerous, secondary inducements become the motivators for causing tension-reducing behavior (Barret-Lennard, 1965).
3.	Systemization based on clinical observations.	Systemization based on experimental studies.
4.	Symptoms are considered to be proofs of contradictions and conflicts motivated by the "desire to live" and the hypochondriacal trait, which have an inverse relationship.	Symptoms are considered to be proofs of mistaken learning (Eysenck and Rachman, 1965).
5.	Symptoms are due to "contradictoriness in thinking," the obstacle of an artificial intellectual posture.	Symptoms are considered to be inadaptable conditioned responses (ibid.).
6.	Discard mental discretion, and place emphasis on authentic selfhood.	The concept of selfhood or ego is not used (Barret-Lennard, 1965).
7.	Management of *shinkeishitsu* disorders can be correlated with the *shinkeishitsu* temperament, which readily shows a hypochondriacal trait; present intellectual posture and past life history are not irrelevant.	Management of neurotic disorders is correlated with contemporary sociocultural customs; historical development is largely irrelevant (Eysenck and Rachman, 1965).
8.	Therapy is carried out by training the hypochondriacal temperament and by overcoming contradictoriness in thinking; individual symptoms are not directly treated.	Therapy is carried out by managing the symptoms.
9.	Management of symptoms will not lead to genuine recovery; mere alleviation of symptoms will recur frequently.	Management of symptoms leads to permanent recovery, provided that automatic as well as skeletal conditioned responses are extinguished (Eysenck and Rachman, 1965).
10.	The value of personality maturation, or improvement and development as a human being, is a point of concern.	No concern for normative issues.
11.	Close correlation with self-discernment.	No correlation with self-discernment.

A methodological comparison of Morita therapy with behavior therapy shows that manipulation techniques that have been formulated theoretically are used freely. However, only the behavior manifested by a patient is approached in behavior therapy. (It might be said that the mind is neglected.) In Morita therapy, however, a patient is guided to attain the experience of "things as they are" by means of therapeutic manipulations, such as bed rest and work assignments.

Both bed rest and work assignments serve to establish heteronomous situations created by a therapist for a patient, but because these measures are manipulations carried out under experimental conditions correlated with living conditions, and in direct connection with the life of the patient, it is the patient who ultimately decides to adopt the independent attitude of perceiving a symptom as being a problem characteristic of the world of mind, and it is the patient as well who is called on to propose how he or she should live.

It can thus be said that, methodologically, Morita therapy is a form of existential or humanistic therapy in which a human being is guided to work out the meaning of life independently. In that aspect, Morita therapy can be considered as being a treatment modality that has certain similarities with behavior therapy, with the principle of therapeutic manipulation as the support, as well as a treatment modality that guides the mind of a patient to approach the world through the existential communication that exists between the patient and the therapist.

Part VIII

The Future of Morita Therapy

24

Past Criticisms of Morita Therapy

Morita had made an attempt to introduce his theory to the German Psychiatrics Society but was unable to do so during his lifetime because it was too difficult to understand. However, later investigators in Europe, the United States and other countries began to indicate deep interest in Morita therapy after World War II; with this expanding interest, Morita therapy began to attract greater attention in Japan than had ever been paid to it since its inception, and although the author believes that true anticipation and criticism of Morita therapy must be present in any such situation, he is bewildered to see that after more than 50 years, the same theory and therapy are now considered in a much different light.

Investigators in various countries showed a sudden interest in Morita therapy in the early 1950s, but with few exceptions there was almost no difference from Morita's lifetime in regard to the depth of understanding of foreign investigators. In Japan, the renewed interest in Morita therapy was much greater than that seen during Morita's lifetime,[1] but its popularization and application were not as extensive as its prominence as a topic of discussion. Morita therapy is still carried out only by a small number of investigators and therapists. To develop Morita therapy for universal application, there is a need to depart from simplistic educational explanation and exposition and carry out aggressively original studies of Morita theory and therapy. Some studies have already been carried out, of course, and they include several excellent ones, but it is regrettable that few studies have been performed to date. Representative studies, in chronological order, are discussed in this chapter.

Shinfuku[2] stresses that the "force causing *toraware* (mental captivity)" is a conflict between instinctive human fear and intellectual activity, and he explains this observation in psychoanalytical terms (1954). Kawai[3] says that the symptoms of *shinkeishitsu* form a constant defense for attaining stability (provisional stability) against anxiety, but it is a nonproductive stability with excessive consumption of psychological energy. Experiencing liberation and exercising intrinsic human consciousness, which is obstructed and clouded by the excessive protective action of superficial consciousness, are activities that take place during Morita therapy.

Kondō[4] tries to bring into bold relief the characteristics of Morita theory that relate to *shinkeishitsu* and psychoanalysis, particularly the neurosis theories of Freud and Horney, by

---

1 To know such situation, refer to the following article, for example, which reviews the literature on Morita therapy published after 1945 in Japan: Miura, M. and Usa, S.: A psychotherapy of neurosis, Morita therapy. *Yonago Acta Medica* 14(1):1–14 (1970).

2 Shinfuku, N.: Toraware no seishin byōri to Morita setsu no tachiba (Psychopathology of *Toraware* and position of Morita theory) (in Japanese). *Psychiatria et Neurologia Japonica* 55:737 (1954).

3 Kawai, H.: Shinkeishitsu shō ni taisuru Morita ryōhō no seishin-byōrigakuteki kenkyū hoi (Psychopathologic supplement of Morita therapy concerning *shinkeishitsu*) (in Japanese). *Tōkyō Jikeikai Ika Daigaku Zasshi* 74 (1958).

4 Kondō, A.: Shinkeishō ni kansuru seishinbunseki gakuha (Freud oyobi Horney) no riron to kore ni taihi shite mitaru Morita no shinkeishitsushō ron (Morita's theory of *shinkeishsitsu* compared with the psychoanalytic theories of Freud and Horney on neurosis) (in Japanese). *Tōkyō Jikeikai Ika Daigaku Zasshi* 73:2077–2133 (1958).

comparing them from a comparative mental-medical point of view. Doi[5] tries to grasp the meaning of the *toraware* characteristic of *shinkeishitsu* by associating it with the human emotion called *amae*, which is, in a sense, both basic and instinctive. He discusses *shinkeishitsu* anxiety as being formed for repression of the desire for *amae* (instinctive desire for dependence) from a psychoanalytical viewpoint. Kondō[6] attempts to discuss the characteristics of *shinkeishitsu* and Morita theory from a transcultural standpoint in relation to the essence of the phenomenon common to both, even if there is a cultural difference.

Although not in chronological order, there is another thesis that should be mentioned at this point, that on the *shinkeishitsu* personality written by Shimoda,[7] who opposes the concept that the *shinkeishitsu* trait is inclined excessively toward predisposition theory and proposes instead, an environmental theory of placing importance on education because the condition is formed a posteriori by the type of parent-child relationship that exists during infancy. Shimoda's thesis is full of suggestions for the development of Morita theory.

Each study that has been cited is an important one, but what is most important for providing a path for the future development of Morita therapy is the popularization of Morita therapy in foreign countries; in other words, the need for investigators not only in Japan but also in countries having different cultural conditions to take a fresh look at it. For this purpose, it is meaningful to reexamine the extent of interest that investigators in Europe, the United States and other countries have shown in Morita therapy, especially their criticisms and expectations of Morita therapy, dating from the peak period of interest in the 1960s.

The academic perspectives of foreign investigators have been diverse, and there has been a broad range of opinion in their understanding of Morita therapy. Some investigators immediately indicated strong interest in Morita therapy during discussions with Japanese therapists, and they commented on this therapy from their own different points of view. Other investigators read only one or another thesis on Morita therapy and criticized it deductively on the basis of their own methodology. Accordingly, it is not possible to note all the comments of those investigators in one breath, but a general explanation will be given in chronological order on the basis of information currently available. First of all, the period of Morita's lifetime until several years after his death (until about 1945) will be considered. This period can be called the "barren age" of Morita therapy. Next is the period that started about 15 years after World War II (to about 1960); this period can be called the "cradle age" of Morita therapy. This period is the time when Morita therapy began to attract great attention from foreign investigators. The third period began about 1960 and can be called the "developmental age."

During the initial period, it was not unexpected that investigators in foreign countries would know nothing about Morita theory or therapy; even during this period, however, the basic characteristics of this new methodology were communicated to German mental hygiene circles through the efforts of Morita. However, as has been mentioned, introduction of the theory in its complete form was not possible at this time because it was too difficult to understand. Nonetheless, in 1938, the year Morita died, a request was received from Professor Göring, then director of the German Psychoneurology Society, for an article on Morita therapy to be published in *Zentralblatt für Psychotherapie und Ihre Grenzgebiete.* The article was, in fact, published in this journal in 1940[8] through the efforts of Professor Naka of the psychiatric

[5] Doi, T.: Shinkeishitsu no seishinbyōri–tokuni toraware no seishinrikigaku ni tsuite (Psychopathology of *shinkeishitsu*, especially regarding the psychodynamics of its *toraware*) (in Japanese). *Psychiatria et Neurologia Japonica* 60:734–744 (1958).

[6] Kondō, K.: Morita ryōhō no bunkateki sokumen (Cultural aspects of Morita therapy) (in Japanese). *Seishin Igaku* 17:1348–1354 (1975).

[7] Shimoda, M.: *Seishin Eisei Kōwa* (Lectures on Mental Hygiene). Iwanami Shoten, Tokyo (1942). (Printed in Japanese)

[8] Morita, S.: Der Begriff der Nervosität. *Zentralblatt für Psychotherapie und Ihre Grenzgebiete* 12(1):1 (1940).

department of Kyūshū University. The article did not attract much attention in Germany, supposedly because Japanese neurosis theory and psychotherapy had no special interest for investigators in other countries at the time.

In the next period, after World War II, mutual cultural exchanges gradually increased, following the restoration of diplomatic relations with Europe, the United States and other countries, and interest in Morita therapy came to the fore as a result. This interest was initiated by the late Karen Horney's visit to Japan in August 1952.[9] After stating that a comparison between Morita therapy and psychoanalysis was much too premature because of insufficient knowledge of Japanese culture, she explained, with utmost care, her views on some features of Morita therapy.

Because of the social and cultural differences that exist between Japan and the United States, she mentioned that the trust that a patient invests in a physician is much higher in Japan. The difference of opinion between the two countries concerning the ego is pronounced. However, she indicated strong interest in the approach of placing weight on emotional experience, rather than on intellectual understanding, to overcome the self-centered personality of neurosis in Morita therapy. She further stressed the acute need for mutual exchange of opinions between Japan and the Western countries in the future on therapy for neurosis and said that exchanges need to be based on a thorough understanding of the differences in cultural characteristics, philosophy and religion.

In the same year, Jacobson[10] and Berenberg[11] published theses on Morita therapy from a psychoanalytical point of view. According to these investigators, internal discernment of a patient by means of changing his or her attitudes, without considering the dynamism of conflict, is anticipated in Morita therapy. Because the method of Morita therapy is one of conscious operation, the impression that this therapy is authoritarian and nondemocratic is strong.

Morita therapy is also perceived as being a religious therapy, in reference to its subject matter that is associated with Zen Buddhist experience, and its psychological motivation does not satisfy the various standards for proper psychological treatment conditions. The perspectives of the latter critics differ from Horney's critique and conclude with simplistic comparative theory. For example, concerning the discernment of a patient in Morita therapy, it is claimed that true discernment is not attained because the dynamism of his or her conflicts is not clarified, and only a change in the patient's life attitude is desired. The conclusion is that the instructive activity of the therapist is authoritarian and nondemocratic.

These critics have apparently overlooked the process by which the discernment of a patient is formed gradually by overcoming the patient's self-centered defense mechanisms because the instructions on actual or relevant actions provided to the patient in Morita therapy place emphasis on the emotional experience brought about by those actions. Further, the instruction that is intended to induce change in the life of a patient is not directed to constrain the patient's subjectivity; the therapist wants the patient to live well in society and urges the patient to discover his or her authentic human nature by discarding his or her role imposed by the inferiority complex that shuts himself or herself off from people in a hypochondriacal manner and, at the same time, to act forcefully for self-realization.

The opinion that Morita therapy is authoritarian and nondemocratic is superficial and not in the least correct. Again, Morita therapy is not a religious therapy and does not motivate a patient toward Zen Buddhist thought. Wendt points out that Morita therapy operates in

---

[9] Kōra, T.: Kōra's Introduction to Horney's "A lecture on developments of new psychoanalysis" (in Japanese). *Nihon Iji Shimpō* 1491 (1952).

[10] Jacobson, A.: Japanese psychiatry and psychotherapy. *American Journal of Psychiatry* 109:321 (1952).

[11] Berenberg, A. W.: Japanese psychiatry and psychotherapy. *American Journal of Psychiatry* 109:321 (1952).

a dimension entirely different from that of Zen Buddhism. The only feature that Morita therapy and Zen Buddhism share is that, during the therapeutic process, the therapist places emphasis on a patient's experience as a result of his or her actions; however, the patient is not placed in a position of direct, intellectual, heavily influenced dependence by means of instruction or persuasion. Several years later, Kelman,[12, 13] an associate of Horney, also visited Japan. At that time, he concluded that Morita therapy is not applicable for use in the United States and that its influence is bound to decrease in the future, even in Japan, with Japanese young people becoming more Westernized and thus less responsive to authoritarian appeals. He also noted that if a fruitful dialogue between psychoanalytical thinking and Oriental perspectives can be achieved, the development of thought at the intersection of these two systems would be important to psychotherapy in the future. It is believed that this opinion was the consensus of investigators specializing in mental science around 1960.

The Western trend of interest in Oriental philosophy had risen rapidly at the time as one conceivable means for overcoming the stalemate of rationalistic thinking. This interest took in the realm of Oriental psychiatry as well, with interest in Morita therapy engendered by that general trend. The initial thrust was in the direction of obtaining a deep understanding and discernment of Oriental thought, by means of comparative cultural and transcultural studies incorporating philosophy, religion, social psychology and cultural anthropology. Representative studies specifically concerned with Morita therapy include those of I. Y. Wendt and W. Caudill.

The activities of these foreign investigators extended over the period from the 1960s to the present. It appears that both Wendt and Caudill had a considerable interchange of opinions with their Japanese counterparts. Wendt[14] approached Morita therapy by comparing it with Zen Buddhism, concluding that Morita therapy is conceptually based on the ascetic practices of Buddhism, particularly Zen, as its concrete model. However, the Zen exercises originate from a desire to materialize certain spiritual potentials that lie deep inside the human mind, whereas Morita therapy for *shinkeishitsu* has as its objective the treatment of patients who are alienated from ordinary, healthy human life, apart from any deep mental considerations. People who aspire to the Zen experience are in the same state of mind as the Buddha himself,[15] who decided to "forsake his father's home" when confronted with the sufferings of this world.[16]

By comparison, a patient suffering from *shinkeishitsu* is confined in his or her self-centered shell and must be brought back once again to "his or her father's home." A patient who has acquired a vital creative power after a long period of suffering probably has more awareness than a person who has lived without an experience of neurotic anxiety. However, this neurotic experience is merely comparable to the *satori* (discernment or insight) of a Zen Buddhist priest. A Zen priest starts his ascetic exercises in a mentally healthy condition. However, for a patient afflicted with *shinkeishitsu*, this healthy condition is the final goal of therapy.

It should be noted that many Western therapists who show an interest in Zen cannot differentiate between these two states of mind. Wendt clearly states that someone who tries to compare the principle of Zen Buddhism directly with the principle of psychotherapy is thereby

[12] Kelman, H.: Eastern influences on psychoanalytic thinking. *Psychologia* 2(2) (1959).

[13] Kelman, H.: Psychotherapy in the Far East. *Progress in Psychotherapy* 4 (1959).

[14] Wendt, I. Y.: *Zen, Japan und der Western.* Paul List Verlag, München (1961). Translated by S. Nakamura. Misuzu Books, Misuzu Shobō, Tokyo (1963).

[15] Morita formerly interpreted the suffering of Buddha as being due to obsession from a psychiatric standpoint. That is, Gautama Buddha was captivated by the sufferings of this world, entered the priesthood and spent six years practicing an ascetic life-style. After experiencing the most extreme degree of mental and physical emaciation, he became disconnected from suffering and attained the states of *satori* (insight) and *jōbutsu* (self-realization). In this experience, Morita sees a form of thought that is common to contemporary youth in seeking liberation from the captivation of obsession, rediscovering oneself and returning to society in the serial type of life process.

[16] In Buddhism, the basic causes of suffering in this world are the four factors of life, old age, sickness and death.

considering psychotherapy to be a substitute for religion. Wendt also states that it is not possible to compare Japanese methodological psychotherapy with Western psychotherapy, and even the possibility of its application to Western peoples cannot be studied concretely because Westerners have neuroses for which psychoanalysis is the only effective treatment modality.

Wendt further states, however, that there are other types of patients in the Western world for whom the principle and method of Morita theory and therapy would be more effective, if applied after obtaining a patient's consent. For example, certain people cannot carry out their chosen roles in their professional lives, and if no other means of help is available, they may as well become stupefied (*Betäubung*) and forget the problem, or if they begin to realize that the only way left open to them is to ingest the vital force provided by a physician or therapist, a new sphere of living will open up to them, once they realize that happiness cannot be achieved without effort, without the willingness to bear suffering by themselves and without recovering the vital creative force within themselves, which is the objective of Morita therapy. The discovery of the authentic self by means of Morita therapy brings about the vital creative power cited by Wendt, and this power is an important matter that will be discussed again later.

• The patterns of Japanese culture and national character from an anthropological standpoint have been discussed by R. Benedict in her book *The Chrysanthemum and the Sword.* Caudill[17, 18] also conducted a comparative practical study of model personality that examined differences in conversational relationships between mother and child in the United States and Japan. He further investigated the correlations between Japanese culture and symptoms of neuroses in patients with Morita *shinkeishitsu.* However, he does not discuss Morita therapy in much depth.

At the beginning of the 1960s, Hoskovec[19] referred to Morita therapy as a Zen Buddhist system. Discussions of Morita theory in the context of Zen Buddhism have frequently appeared in the past; examples are those of A. Jacobson and A.W. Berenberg. However, such studies differ in viewpoint from those of Wendt because Jacobson and Berenberg, among others, apparently were impressed by the surface similarity of the various phenomena that appear in Zen and in the process of Morita therapy, generalized from this similarity to incorporate even the principle of therapy and discussed Morita theory and Zen Buddhism as having the same root. Czerny[20] also discusses Morita therapy in relation to Zen. He attempts a comparative discussion of the *arugamama* state of mind in Morita therapy with that of *satori* or *gedatsu* and proceeds to investigate the possibility of incorporating absolute, isolated bed rest and work therapy into Eastern European psychotherapy, as equivalents of *zazen* and *samu* (miscellaneous activities in daily life).

• Another prominent development in the 1960s was the interest redirected toward Morita therapy from the standpoint of behavior therapy. Leonhard,[21] in particular, discusses in detail the similarities between Morita therapy and behavior therapy in relation to his own therapeutic experience. For example, he tried to desensitize an object of fear by making a patient confront the fear, and he used the method of relearning how to live while in a state of painful endurance. This approach is equivalent to the experience called *kyōfu totsunyū* (the plunge into fear) in Morita therapy. Leonhard comments on *arugamama* by noting that a simple explanation,

---

17 Caudill, W. and DeVos, G.: *Achievement, Culture and Personality: The Case of the Japanese-American.* Holt, Rinehart, New York (1961).

18 Caudill, W. and Schooler, C.: *Symptom Patterns and Background Characteristics of Japanese Psychiatric Patients.* East-West Center Press, Honolulu (1969).

19 Hoskovec, J.: Psychotherapeuticke aspekcy systemu Zen. *Psychiatry* 69:406 (1963).

20 Czerny, Y.: Zu den psychotherapeutischen und philosophischen Fragen der japanischen Neurosen; Psychotherapie nach der Morita Konzeption. *Akt. Fragen Psychiat. Neurol.* 6:66 (1967).

21 Leonhard, K.: Die japanische Morita Therapie aus der Sicht eigener psychotherapeutischer Verfahren. *Archiv für Psychiatrie und Nervenkrankheiten* 209:185 (1965).

given to a patient by a therapist who conducts Morita therapy, that anxiety will disappear as a result of taking action is mistaken. What is important is not to make a patient feel at ease but to make the patient endure unpleasant feelings for a certain period to lead the patient into a condition of submitting to fate. Whether or not anxiety will eventually disappear is disregarded.

Anything that human life confers on oneself is accepted as *arugamama* by Leonhard. This view differs considerably from the previous and prevalent mode of thought that *arugamama* signifies compliance with moods or that it represents resignation. Leonhard's concept is a step in the direction toward correct interpretation.

We can see from this discussion that Morita therapy not only has characteristics confined to the Japanese sociocultural milieu but also has a universal character that can be understood by people of different cultural roots, which the author believes is the result of basic acceptance of the facts of human nature, as is inherent in Morita therapy.

Morita, for instance, says that snakes and caterpillars are unpleasant creatures to healthy-minded people, but this feeling is an expression of the human mind that is similar to feeling fear when standing at a great height. It is a natural human expression, much the same as feeling cold in winter and hot in summer. Not expressing a feeling of fear when something is feared or expressing an unpleasant feeling when something is felt to be unpleasant is a factor of the natural fluidity of the mind, and spontaneity and creativity are exhibited only when the mind is in this condition.

From that understanding of human nature, *arugamama* signifies an aggressive attitude of frank acceptance of facts as they are, as opposed to the passive life attitude of submissive resignation toward whatever happens, without acting when appropriate to oppose it. Leonhard mentions that "it is probably difficult for the German people to take on such a mental attitude. A German patient wishes to have his illness cured, but dislikes being directed toward acceptance of a given condition as something which cannot be changed." This comment can be construed as failing to grasp thoroughly the attitude of *arugamama*. In other words, *arugamama* is recognition of a fact as it is, without subjective selection by likes or dislikes or by wishes to accept or reject. This attitude is different from submission and is clearly not resignation. It is an absolute acceptance or "this is, indeed, what it is."

The difference is not based on any difference in mode of thought between East and West. The difference between the mental attitude of *shizen ni fukujū* (obey nature), with the integration of subject and object characteristic of the Oriental perspective, and the conquest of Nature, with the opposition of subject and object characteristic of Western peoples, is only a problem of the extent to which the facts of human nature have been observed, at least for a correct understanding of *arugamama* (see Chapter 22).

Leonhard says that the rationalist attitude, for example, may be that "life is always exposed to danger at all times. Therefore, if one thinks that he must resist all unpleasantness, suffering will only be increased." However, this notion is a departure from a correct understanding of *arugamama.*

In rationalistic thinking, the correct understanding is that of the dual relationship of the pleasant excitement of a ride in an airplane accompanied by feelings of danger or of the heroic feeling of exploration into ultimate conditions or unknown substances accompanied by actual danger. The relationship here is one of contradictory concerns that apply equally to the dualistic mentality (ambiguity) cited by Frenkel-Brunswik.[22]

Direct confrontation of this contradictory condition of the mind is a characteristic of a mature human being and is, indeed, the character of *arugamama.*

[22] Frenkel-Brunswik, E.: *Intolerance of Ambiguity as an Emotional and Perceptual Personality Variable.* Eloge de la Philosophie L'oeil et L'esprit par M. Merleau-Ponty (translated into Japanese by S. Urashima and G. Kida. Misuzu Shobō, Tokyo (1966)).

After this dissertation by Leonhard, approaches to Morita therapy were made by Reynolds[23] and Elzinger[24] from their respective points of view. The latter investigator discusses the subject by making analogies with behavior therapy. Reynolds directs his attention to Morita therapy from the standpoints of comparative anthropology and behavior therapy, noting that there are many forms of Morita therapy that resemble behavior therapy but that Morita therapy does not simply eliminate symptoms. He considers the intrapsychic shift that occurs in a patient through acceptance of the facts of human nature and tries to pinpoint the essence of the human aspects of Morita therapy and the therapist in relation to Morita theory, with its deep roots in Oriental philosophy or Zen Buddhist thought.

In outline, Reynolds points out that in spite of contrary assertions by behavioral therapists, it is apparent that psychotherapy not only eliminates symptoms but has a broader influencing power. Psychotherapy reaches the deep truths of the human being, and therapists as such understand how people should live, whether or not they are aware of it.

Reynolds has apparently treated patients in the United States by incorporating the Morita approach in his practice. He remarks that Morita therapy has provided physicians in Europe and the United States with a ready means for distinguishing healthy persons from persons afflicted with *shinkeishitsu* and that this therapy also indicates how to deal with a patient's suffering, or what kind of therapeutic procedure to apply. Further, through the application of Morita theory, suggestions can probably be developed for new theories and therapies in the field of mental hygiene supervision.

Morita therapy, he goes on to say, provides a truly humanistic viewpoint or mode of thought concerning the suffering occasioned by the extreme difficulty a patient has in differentiating the boundaries of health and illness, normal or abnormal. He also remarks that Morita therapy is universal in teaching human beings how to live from day to day productively and substantially.

Kim,[25] of South Korea, stresses the implications of Morita therapy for synthetic psychotherapy. He praises the encounter between a Morita therapist and a patient from a psychodynamic standpoint. Concerning the specific problems of the adolescent period of self-discovery and the development of a mature self-temperament, he stresses the real, immovable relationship of "thou and me," in which a therapist does not permit a patient to become dependent or pugnacious and, at the same time, encourages to patient to comprehend the reality of "here and now," rather than regressing to the past.

Kim considers this therapeutic encounter as constituting one goal along the road to naturation of personality. He concludes that Morita therapy is an aggressive method for reintegrating elements of a mental disorder that, when brought into correlation, point a patient toward the true therapeutic goal of manifesting and developing the temperament of the natural self. This is, indeed, what psychotherapy in general aims for, and in that respect, Morita therapy has made a substantial contribution as a pioneering therapy.

When we look back again at the latter half of the 1960s to take note of still other studies of Morita therapy, we find theses published in 1965 by Kumasaka,[26] Levy[27] and DeVos.[28] All three of these investigators were critical of Kōra's thesis[29] on Morita therapy. Although these

23 Reynolds, D. K.: Morita therapy in America. In *Gendai no Morita Ryōhō* (Present-day Morita Therapy), edited by K. Ōhara. Hakuyōsha, Tokyo (1977). (Printed in Japanese)

24 Elzinger, R. H.: Quote from H. Iwai's Gaikoku bunken wo tōshite mita Morita ryōhō (Morita therapy taking a general survey of the foreign literature on this subject); op. cit.

25 Kim, S.: Morita ryōhō e no rikai to sonkei (Toward understanding of and respect for Morita therapy); op. cit.

26 Kumasaka, Y.: Discussion on Morita therapy. *International Journal of Psychiatry* 1(4) (1965).

27 Levy, N. J.: Discussion on Morita therapy; op. cit.

28 DeVos, G. A.: Discussion on Morita therapy; op. cit.

29 Kōra, T.: Morita therapy. *International Journal of Psychiatry* 1(4):611–640 (1965).

investigators base their criticisms on differing academic criteria, their criticisms all stem from a psychodynamic standpoint.

Kumasaka, who takes a psychoanalytical position, considers the therapist-patient relationship as being one in which a therapist stands for Nature. A therapist's discernment of a patient is neither emotional nor intellectual, instead being directed toward giving the patient a realization of his or her position in Nature. To a Japanese patient, Nature is something that has a character beyond control. A Japanese patient who attains discernment of Nature displays an attitude of living while harmonizing with universal Nature.

Differences in culture between the Occident and Orient pose a large obstacle to an understanding of Morita therapy. Kumasaka comments that Nature, in the Occident, is something to challenge rather than accept, particularly in the United States. Consequently, *arugamama* is not accepted in the West as it is in the Orient. However, because Morita therapy is a type of self-training therapy, it is considered to be effective even in the West for the management of certain forms of neurosis, for example, obsessive neurosis. Kumasaka concludes, however, that in the United States, Morita therapy must be reconstructed in terms of a psychoanalytical concept in alignment with the culture of that country.

The author is of the opinion that the interpretation of *arugamama* in Kumasaka's paper is a common misinterpretation, similar to that found in other theses. Kumasaka remarks that Nature is something that must be conquered, not accepted in the sense of peaceful coexistence with it; if a mountain stands in the way, it must be moved. The process of aging in human beings is deteriorative, he says, and its marks need to be covered by beautifying substances or clothing; consequently, it is not possible to accept *arugamama.*

In Morita therapy, however, the desire for beautification or clothing arises because it is recognized that human beings do deteriorate as a result of the aging process. Ideas and inventions are created not because deterioration is thereby negated but precisely because deterioration is recognized as such. This recognition is a fact of Nature that cannot be negated in the least. The desire to negate it is not necessarily the same as the possibility of negating it.

Neurotic *toraware* appears as an obsession from the standpoint that one can negate whatever one anticipates. The *arugamama* in Morita theory is not passive resignation or negation, as Kumasaka sees it but, rather, only a frank acceptance of fact as fact. Various real changes in the human condition can be dealt with efficiently only because of this genuine recognition of reality.

The author's viewpoint on proper interpretation of *arugamama* has been explained in reference to Leonhard's thesis.

Norman Levy of the Horney Clinic says that the principal feature of the therapist-patient relationship in Morita therapy is that Japanese patients are obedient to their therapists, and this obedience leads one to presuppose a compulsory, authoritative situation. He also points out, as does Kelman, that any such authoritative therapist will not win acceptance in the United States, where emphasis is placed on horizontal relational and situational values. However, Levy perceives the position of a therapist in Morita therapy as being one that is rational and also says that the therapist uses a suitable distribution of the word "should" as a direct method to bring a patient to think about the value of constructive efforts and to improve and develop concretely the daily life of the patient. Levy concludes that specialists in Morita therapy or psychoanalysis should define, together with their patients, the ultimate goal of therapy and the gains to be made if the long period required for treatment with psychoanalysis is taken into consideration. It is the obligation of both Morita therapists and psychoanalysts to effect an interchange that enables a correct mutual evaluation of theory and technique.

DeVos,[17, 28] together with Caudill, wrote a large number of papers couched in cultural and anthropological terms on the imminent evolution of ethical regulations in Japan, correlated with the actions of Japanese adults. On that basis, he says that the Japanese differ from Americans when engaged in activities that family members or social superiors anticipate. Emphasis is placed on incompleteness or incompetence for attainment, rather than on insufficiency or reluctance to request it. Incompleteness is suppressed in Americans, but in the Japanese, it is reluctance that is suppressed. Japanese adolescents consciously avoid the self-sacrifice required of students or professional workers, and Japanese women avoid absolute mother-role devotion to their children or husbands.

DeVos believes that the resistance to this "should," which is unconsciously motivated, can be observed in the hypochondriacal type correlated with the physical incompletion that is characteristic of patients with *shinkeishitsu*. According to him, Morita therapy is descriptive psychiatry mixed with the traditions of an indigenous *samurai* culture. The therapeutic system is intended to liberate a patient from interference by a resistive, suspicious and observant self, in a manner similar to liberation through the practice of Zen discipline.

DeVos considers this liberation to occur by means of self-acceptance of one's incompleteness. It is this liberation, he says, that is *arugamama* and that constitutes freedom from authority, specifically freedom from the familial superego that has been made imminent.

DeVos perceives the Japanese as striving constantly to liberate the self from the role of doing what is anticipated socioculturally. In this regard, the Japanese are similar to the Calvinists of Northern Europe, who consider the contemporary solution to the problem to lie in diligence.

It is true that elements of old, traditional culture persist, as DeVos mentions, and it is recognized that Oriental philosophy or Buddhist humanism lies in the ideological background of Morita therapy. Further, it is undeniable that great importance is placed on human relationships in Japanese society within a framework of a vertical superiority. What is not understandable is DeVos's interpretation that an attitude of self-sacrifice or an ethic rooted in the diligence of accomplishing one's duties under the authority of a monarchical or family system constitutes the roots of Morita therapy.

The overall evaluation of Morita therapy within the field of general psychotherapy is summarized in the paragraphs that follow.

During the barren age of Morita therapy, it was criticized strongly by mainstream German psychiatrists, even by those from the psychoanalytical subsector, and could win no acceptance. What could be called general psychotherapy at that time consisted of therapies that revolved around rest cure, persuasion, suggestion or hypnotic methods of a disordered nature. Morita theory, with its background of Oriental ideology, could not win favorable attention, even if clarification of the pathological basis of neuroses and management directed toward the underlying cause were given emphasis, but it was also disregarded as being too difficult to understand.

In the next period, attention was directed toward Japanese psychotherapy as one aspect of the upwelling of interest of the Western world in Japan's traditional culture, but much of this interest was simple curiosity.

The seeds of self-criticism that germinated in the field of mental science in the West, however, aroused further interest in the real progress of Western psychotherapy, with the goal of achieving true cures. A number of foreign investigators, particularly in the United States and Europe, began to direct serious attention to the cure experience indicated by Morita therapy, which is based on Oriental culture.

In the most recent period, dating from the first half of the 1960s, in which the aim has been development, Morita therapy has been increasingly examined as demonstrating considerable possibilities for illuminating general psychotherapy, even though it is applicable to a small group of neuroses, and in spite of the fact that it differs in objective from the scope of illumination provided by psychoanalysis. It is simply not possible for Morita therapy to replace psychoanalysis in the future, as Wendt points out, but the older attitude of considering it as being foreign matter that has no understandable substance will tend to diminish.

The self-complacent notion that only psychoanalysis can enable human beings to attain understanding of life and to live in independent freedom, with no true liberation from the immature, self-centered concepts of human life common throughout the world at present, will, as Boss[30] points out, no longer be permissible.

The author has attempted to position Morita therapy in the niche where it should be, but there remains the possibility that certain critics will dismiss this attempt as overly optimistic. With the exception of a few investigators who belong to the behavior therapy or neo-Freudian school, most authors who were critical of Morita therapy in the past now believe that it differs entirely from European and American psychotherapies, particularly orthodox psychoanalysis.

Morita therapy is, however, a treatment modality that operates only on the surface layer of consciousness, with no deep probing of the psychodynamics beneath that level that act to induce symptoms. For this reason, it is distinctly possible for the attitude of a Morita therapist, and the therapy, to become authoritative and directive and for a patient to acquire an attitude of submission to authority. The vertical therapist-patient relationship that is characteristic of Morita therapy suggests, to DeVos, that it is difficult to anticipate application of this therapy in Europe and the United States, where horizontal situation values are given priority.

Taking into account this general opinion, what can be done in the future to improve the Western world's understanding of Morita therapy?

At the beginning of this chapter, the author said that it is necessary to define a methodological criterion within which productive discussion can take place, while striving to surmount sociocultural differences, but definition of such a criterion is, of course, difficult. However, some past investigators have shown a deeper understanding of Morita therapy. With regard to its future, there are also a few contemporary critics who have suggested harmonizing Morita therapy with Western psychotherapy.

One way to attain this harmonization may be to discuss in detail what these critics anticipate from Morita therapy. If certain points of criticism lie in misunderstandings that arise chiefly from a lack of mutual proficiency of expression to explain certain phenomena, the removal of this barrier will not be too difficult, if more suitable expressions can be developed. (One such attempt, for example, is the author's commentary on Leonhard's and Kumasaka's interpretations of *arugamama.*)

The cumulative understanding that can come from individual efforts is hardly insignificant to the future of Morita therapy.

30 Boss, M.: *Indienfahrt eines Psychiaters.* Grunther Neske, Pfullingen (1959). Translated by T. Shimoyama and M. Ohno. Misuzu Shobō, Tokyo (1972).

25

Expectations of Morita Therapy and Self-Examination of the Morita Therapist for Future Development

It is not possible to cover all the issues involved in critical evaluations of Morita therapy, so the author will discuss a few issues that can be considered as having special relevance for general psychotherapy with respect to the future development of Morita therapy.

For example, Horney[1] mentions that there is a need for mutual exchange of knowledge between Japan and the West concerning therapy for neurosis within the context of the future development of psychotherapy and stresses that exchanges should be based on a thorough understanding of social and cultural differences between Japan and the West. In seeming compliance with this view, Kelman[2, 3] states that it would be meaningful to future psychotherapy if a genuine interchange between psychoanalytical thought and Oriental thought could be achieved.

These opinions are appropriate for fields of study that overlap different sociocultural spheres, as does psychotherapy, but, such an interchange is difficult to put into practice. The proposal by Kelman, in particular, requires discussion of the subject by transcultural methodology, but it is probably difficult for the nuclei of Morita therapy and psychoanalysis to truly intersect.

For example, the condition of *arugamama* in Morita therapy is that of an aggressive self-acceptance that includes no mental discretion, and it is the point at which the process of self-illumination begins. This condition of self-acceptance is one that can be construed as signifying self-surrender or aggressive self-submission. When this condition is evaluated by American thought, its content is one of a parallel that will not intersect, and thus cannot win acceptance.

The reason is that the suffering of a patient, caused by instinctive, aggressive or destructive impulses, not to mention all kinds of everyday uneasiness, is a condition that should not be accepted. Rather, the suffering can and should be controlled intellectually. However, the self-surrender that is accelerated in the process that moves a patient toward self-illumination in Morita therapy is neither resignation nor simple, passive submission, much less the abandonment of self-consciousness. A strong mentality with a concealed core of maturation is achieved. Consequently, from the standpoint of Morita therapy, the question of whether or not a life in which there is no self-surrender is worth living needs to be reconsidered.

The one person who thoroughly understands the differences that make the intersection of Morita therapy and psychoanalysis both difficult and still hoped for, so that Morita therapy can have a role in universal psychotherapy, is Wendt. Her understanding is that, in Morita therapy,

[1] Kōra, T.: Kōra's Introduction to K. Horney's "A lecture on developments of new psychoanalysis" (in Japanese). *Nihon Iji Shimpō* 1491 (1952).
[2] Kelman, H.: Eastern influences on psychoanalytic thinking. *Psychologia* 2:2 (1959).
[3] Kelman, H.: Psychotherapy in the Far East. *Progress in Psychotherapy* 4 (1959).

a patient rediscovers the creative, vital energies hidden in the self only by enduring his or her suffering.

The insights of such therapists have important implications. The proposal to the effect that theory and technique in Morita therapy and psychoanalysis can be reevaluated and an interchange addressed to the problem of precisely defining the final goal of psychotherapy and what is truly beneficial to the patient, as stated by Levy, will be worthwhile to pursue on that basis.

In the author's view, if the true goal of psychotherapy is self-discovery by a patient for subsequent self-treatment, it can be said that Morita therapy is undoubtedly suitable for achieving this goal. The objective in Morita therapy is for a patient first to discover his or her authentic nature as a human being and then to develop and improve himself or herself accordingly. This life process derives from the same mode of thought as the process for curing a patient's neurosis as such, and the patient moves forward toward natural activities that make use of creative, vital energies (*sei no yokubō*) in a state of liberation. The true effectiveness of this therapy is not the result of knowledge imposed on a patient by a therapist or an authoritative attitude but, rather, the experience of the patient.

Reynolds[4] is one investigator who comprehends the true importance of Morita therapy for a patient. He firmly believes that Morita therapy has, hidden within it, the power for effective application in both the Occident and the Orient, pointing out that human beings are originally matter-of-fact animals and therefore normally evaluate the extent or method of examining things or modes of thought in terms of practicality. Reynolds evinces strong practical support and expectations for Morita therapy, but his comments alone are insufficient for promoting the further development and popularization of Morita therapy.

Basic psychology has, of course, an immense influence on popularization of any form of psychotherapy, not only Morita therapy. Further, differences arise in accord with the degree of affinity that people have for the philosophy and culture that underlie Morita therapy. With few exceptions, there have been wide differences between the Japanese and foreign peoples in the degree of affinity and support demonstrated for Morita therapy. This contrast has been evident irrespective of whether the person has been a therapist or a patient. How to surmount this massive obstacle is a major problem that must be faced and solved in the future.

As a first step, we need to develop more suitable, concrete descriptions that incorporate psychopathology, which is the theoretical and rational side, and therapeutics, which is the experiential and practical side of Morita therapy. We need to explain these descriptions with great patience, and we then must exert the utmost effort to implant an accurate understanding of the social and cultural conditions in Japan, past and present, that form the underlying basis of Morita therapy.

As one example, we would like to reach a final understanding on the issue of the authoritative character of Morita therapy, which has been the subject of so much dispute, and to reeducate therapists on that issue so that we may be better able to respond to future criticism and so that they may be able to reconsider Morita therapy in a more positive light in the future.

4 Reynolds, D. K.: Morita therapy in America. In *Gendai no Morita Ryōhō* (Present-day Morita Therapy), edited by K. Ōhara. Hakuyōsha, Tokyo (1977). (Printed in Japanese)

26

Criticisms of the Authoritative Nature of Morita Therapy

The authoritative stance taken by Morita therapists toward their patients has been sharply questioned and frequently criticized. Therapists and investigators of Morita therapy have not thoroughly studied these criticisms in the past and have not responded to them.

Critiques of this kind began to appear in Japan in the 1950s but aroused no evident refutation. The reason is not clear but is probably not simple. However, it is believed that psychotherapy at the time tended to focus on Rogers's client-centered therapy rather than on psychoanalytical thought. Therapy based on nondirective methods was favorably accepted in general by therapists in a field that had become rapidly influential after the Second World War.

Another background factor was the postwar political and social democratization of Japan, as a turning point that gave rise to various collisions between the so-called old and new cultures regarding those reforms. The Japanese mentality had gradually become accustomed to a democratic, horizontal type of social thought.

It is probably not unexpected that the technique of Morita therapy and the attitude of Morita therapists appeared to be directive and authoritative to investigators who were particularly vulnerable to the effects of such cultural reforms. Further, it is believed that the advocates of Morita therapy made almost no rebuttal to such criticisms, which were based on a novel methodology stemming from an entirely different viewpoint in line with the general trend of the time.

However, apart from that trend, it is believed that Morita therapy attracted considerable attention because of its originality. It was a reevaluation of a traditional culture within the context of a new postwar culture. In that light, there was little meaningful basis for criticizing the authoritative nature[1] of Morita therapy from so disparate a viewpoint.

Nonetheless, the author believes that the time is ripe for an inquiry regarding the authoritative aspects of psychotherapy in general. Moreover, the specific issue of the authoritative nature of Morita therapy must be addressed assertively.

Authoritativeness of Therapy and Resistance of Patients

The authoritative stance taken by Morita therapists has often been criticized by nondirective therapists in Japan, as has been mentioned, but numerous discussions were carried out actively in the latter half of the 1940s in the United States. The criticism of authoritativeness is based partly on unpleasant semantic confusion that equates expression of authority or authoritativeness with fascism or Stalinism.

---

[1] It should be made clear at this point that this authoritative stance does not imply authoritarianism.

Further, criticism of authoritarianism by comparison with liberalism is deep-rooted in the United States and forms the basis for the refutation of any authoritative attitude adopted by a therapist.

Human beings do, in general, resist interference or advice from other persons, and the fact that human beings have customarily lived in social settings means that they have lived under the influence of some sort of authority or authoritativeness, in both sociocultural or ideological history and tradition, and that they have had to struggle to achieve true liberty by contending with those historical forces.

The situation is much the same in psychotherapy. It is true that an authoritative atmosphere is absent in the setting of nondirective therapy, but such therapy cannot be said to be completely nonauthoritative as long as a consultative relationship exists. Saying that silence is equivalent to not speaking is, in itself, a breach of silence. Similarly, it is doubtful whether not being authoritative is equivalent to being nonauthoritative. Further, the therapeutic efficacy of being nonauthoritative cannot be determined simplistically.

If there is an instance in which a nonauthoritative method has been effective, it is because the patient was capable of taking complete responsibility. To assume that a patient can do so would be a waste of time in the vast majority of cases. The discernment of this fact is part of the authority that a therapist must exercise.

The notion that there is no effective type of psychotherapy other than nondirective therapy is, in itself, an authoritative declaration. It seems reasonable to point out that, in all senses, life without some form of authority is not possible in the real world.

In general, the term "authority" is defined as[2] the power of coercing an inferior and making him or her obedient. This power includes the mental, moral, social and legal powers to command approval, obedience and obligation from other persons. These powers are based on beliefs or reflections of values invested in a superior dignity or on awe for the sanctity of tradition and a fear of intransigent opposition. Authority also has a second definition: a distinguished specialist or other person conversant in a specific field.

There are considerable differences in the attitudes that people take toward authority of either definition. The differences relate to whether a person is active or passive, or compliant or rebellious. It is also true that there have been considerable historical differences in this regard. Similarities existed in forms of obedience to authority in Japan and the Western world until medieval times, but thereafter a great divergence occurred.

In the Western world (from the emergence of Protestantism until the era of Emmanuel Kant), emphasis was increasingly placed on assertion of one's individuality and on acquisition of the will to achieve personal freedom. The modalities of personality formed by historical differences of this kind are obvious. The Japanese have a tendency to approve, as it is, the environment or the objective conditions in which they live.[3] They actively show approval for and respect, without much doubt, traditional values, existing concepts and superior personalities. This attitude has served as a basis for criticism by champions of nondirective therapy, who insist that the Japanese have a strong sense of dependence on authority and are inclined to accept external authority voluntarily. This temperament is equated with the attitude of reliance and dependence that a patient shows toward a physician and therapist in medical treatment.

These Japanese attitudes do not, however, fit the definition of authoritarian character expounded by T.W. Adorno et al. (*The Authoritarian Personality*, 1950). The principal mean-

[2] Edited by Shinmura, I.: *Kōjien*, Iwanami Shoten, Tokyo (1955).

[3] Nakamura, H.: *Tōyōjin no Shii Hōhō* (Ways of Thinking of Eastern Peoples) (3). In *Nakamura Hajime Senshū*, Vol. 3. Shunjūsha, Tokyo (1962).

ing of authority in psychotherapy is the capability that any such professional specialty provides. However, it is first of all necessary to grasp dynamically the character of the therapy and the therapist-patient relationship that exists and develops when considering its authoritative nature.

The character of any system of psychotherapy is generally classified on the basis of several criteria. One method is classification as directive or nondirective, in accordance with the method used by a therapist or the attitude that he or she takes in associating with a patient.

Morita therapy belongs to the directive type in this classification, and psychoanalysis, or client-centered therapy, to the nondirective type. A directive therapist deals with a patient actively, using persuasion, guidance, advice, reassurance, reeducation or training techniques, and leads the patient in the direction that he or she sets. There is no doubt that, in a broad sense, Morita therapy is directive. In a narrow sense, however, Morita therapy does not belong to either category because it is an overall self-training method that patients learn so they may acquire an integrated mind-body unity.

If an authoritative condition similar to a teacher-student relationship in ordinary education exists in the therapist-patient relationship in directive therapy, such therapy is generally said to be authoritative. This authoritative nature comes into question chiefly in terms of instruction based on a specialized knowledge that a therapist possesses but is not restricted to a deductive function in the therapist-patient relationship.

However, this relationship is not a simplistic one. For example, even if a therapist meets with a patient as a specialist, there still exists a friendly, comforting relationship on the same level. Communication aimed at self-illumination is mutual. A patient does not communicate with a therapist only by means of the intellect but begins to comply with therapy as a whole being. What a patient desires from therapy is liberation from anxiety and fear, and to that extent a therapist directs the goal of therapy in line with his or her response to the patient's request (in the patient's awareness, setting aside the full intention of the therapist).

Guidance by a therapist in his or her superior role as a specialist is strongly anticipated by a patient. The reason is that the effort made by a patient to expose his or her human suffering to another person, even if that other person is a therapist, is a serious determination in itself.

The acceptance of the superiority of both the personality and the specialized knowledge of a therapist is an absolute to a patient. A quasiauthoritative relationship can easily spring up in any such therapeutic situation. The author will define such a relationship as "therapeutic authoritativeness." This type of authority is most conspicuous in directive therapy, but in general it is true that therapeutic authoritativeness is granted to a therapist as a professional responsibility in his or her association with a patient, irrespective of whether the therapy is directive or nondirective, and this granting of responsibility does have an active therapeutic effect. There is no exception, not even nondirective therapy, which claims to have no authoritative atmosphere. The only difference is whether the authoritative aspect appears readily or is kept well-concealed.

Even in therapy of the same school, the attitude of a therapist includes concern with this authoritative situation during association with a patient. Whether or not the patient becomes strongly conscious of the authoritative aspect depends on his or her mental condition and motivation for going into therapy. What is important is that the form of therapeutic authoritativeness is determined by the mode of association between a therapist and a patient. Even if the therapist tries his or her utmost to conceal authoritativeness, there are still cases in which resistance to therapy crops up.

The relationship between a patient's resistance and therapeutic authoritativeness is worthy of further examination. Therapeutic authoritativeness can readily appear in directive therapy when persuasion and guidance are conducted directly, but even in that case, the resistance of a patient to directive therapy will tend to be suppressed or eliminated if the patient's suffering is relieved or disappears. The patient will then tend to feel gratitude or praise for the therapist. The opposite situation will probably increase the patient's resistance. Even in the same type of directive therapy, there are approaches in which the authoritative role of a therapist is not shown conspicuously, by guidance that develops self-acceptance by a patient independently. Even in that instance, however, there are patients who resist cooperating with their therapists, although the resistance may not be intentional, and will not open their minds to them.

One reason is that patients resist being directed by therapists, even while being helped, because of the wish to help oneself by oneself, by one's own power. Psychotherapy is, however, carried out on the basis of that human disposition. Consequently, depending on the technique of a therapist, the independent attitude of attempting to formulate one's plans and to educate oneself will eventually appear, if a patient lives his or her life by cooperating with the directives of therapy.

This situation does not end simply in obedience because the feeling of unity with a therapist begins at the point when a patient feels that the internal discipline, which soon becomes integrated by means of internal discussion carried out repetitively within oneself, is his or her self-discipline. The awareness of an individuality characterized by the resistance that indicates the patient's sense of self-subsistence is suppressed at its base.

In other words, psychotherapy leads a patient in the direction that the patient desires, with use of basic human resistance as a functional premise. The task of a therapist is to determine the best method for obtaining the cooperation of a patient so that he or she can discover the internal form of living that is most acceptable to the patient. Therapeutic authoritativeness is merely the key for solving this problem, and it is probable that the structure of the internal discipline that is formed in a patient is determined by the turning of that key.

Fromm[4,5] has frequently remarked on the authority that comprises this so-called key; his viewpoint can be summarized as follows.

Authority is not limited to persons or systems that order one to do this or not to do that. Such authority can be called external authority. Apart from this authority, there is internal authority, called duty, conscience or superego. The development of modern ideology from Protestantism to Kant's philosophy can be characterized as a process in which internal authority replaced external authority. The privileges of external authority were lost in the political victory achieved by the sudden increase of power of the middle classes, and the prior position of external authority was replaced by the internal conscience of the individual human being. The factor that resists submission to discipline imposed from outside and that controls the natural requirements of human beings is internal discipline, which is characterized by reasoning, will and conscience, and it is believed that internal discipline is the substance of human freedom.

Recently, however, the importance of conscience has been diminished. What has power in an individual life is neither external nor internal authority at present. Nonetheless, authority has not died out; it has only become invisible. This invisible authority could be called "anonymous authority." Its characteristics are common sense, science, mental health and normalcy, or public opinion. Anonymous authority penetrates one gently, without compulsion.

Ultimately, what governs the entire lives of contemporary human beings is an anonymous authority that has this delicate, suggestible character, and it is more effective for self-realization than is visible authority.

---

[4] Fromm, E.: *Man for Himself.* Holt, Rinehart, New York (1947).

[5] Fromm, E.: *Authority and Family.* Translated by I. Yasuda. Seidosha, Tokyo (1977).

When the relationship between authority and human resistance in light of Fromm's opinion is replaced by the condition called therapeutic authoritativeness, there is a problem correlated with psychotherapy.

According to Jaspers,[6] there are three types of human resistance. The first type is similar to that which is encountered in animal training. It is an absolute resistance, with no meaningful change, but it is formed only by external force. The second type is the resistance that is formed internally, by such means as education and self-discipline. The third type is basic self-subsistence resistance. This resistance is one in which the self struggles to attain true self-subsistence, that is, genuine human existence.

In general, an authoritative factor will appear when a patient and therapist come into association in a therapeutic situation. If the therapist confronts the patient in a manner that arouses the first type of resistance, the patient is dealt with as a mere object in a confrontation that disregards the patient's mind. The outward training form does not pursue value in relation to content to exert therapeutic authoritativeness. Authority is imposed automatically by its own power.

The second method is that of educational communication. When this situation is considered in a broad sense, including counseling, it corresponds to directive or nondirective methods, and a patient's mind becomes relatively open. However, the communication includes a certain psychological distance. The patient encounters his or her internal resistance, and an attitude of self-planning and self-education takes place by means of conversation, which is developed by therapeutic authority (from external and internal authority to anonymous authority).

The third method is one of existential communication. A patient tries to restore the true self, which has been lost and subordinated by communicating with a therapist on the same level. Only in this existential communication can both the therapist and the patient start the struggle for self-existence. Both persons try to attain true freedom and subjective self-illumination by refusing acceptance of all authority and superiority. However, the more that existential communication is activated, the farther it moves from universally applicable therapy.

What a therapist must consider is the problem of the limitations of therapeutic authoritativeness. One such limitation relates to a patient's resistance. When a person decides to receive psychotherapy, it means that he or she is obliged to open up the depths of his or her mentality to the therapist. This decision is a critical one. Receiving treatment by overcoming resistance to it leads to consciousness of human weakness, or consciousness of a specific illness, as Jaspers has said.[7]

Nevertheless, some patients do not wish to be treated as mere objects. Such patients accept therapy in a state of mind in which what they wish to become or what they desire from therapy is still unclear. Conversely, other patients simply entrust themselves, as having both physical and mental illness, to their therapists as mere objects.

These opposite types of patient set limitations to therapy or to the effectiveness of therapeutic authoritativeness, although their respective implications in these regards differ markedly. Another limitation is inherent to therapists. Whether a patient accepts or refuses the direction set by a therapist, he or she does become an object to the therapist the instant the therapist entertains any sense of superiority. As a result, the therapist may try to protect his or her scientific authority by utilizing to the utmost the empirical skills of acting like a scientist, as mentioned by Jaspers,[8] or by demonstrating the value with which only he or she is imbued.

---

[6] Jaspers, K.: *Allgemeine Psychopathologie* (1948). Translated by Y. Uchimura et al. Iwanami Shoten, Tokyo (1958).
[7] Jaspers, K.; ibid.
[8] Jaspers, K.; ibid.

Absolute authority, based on a therapist's belief that his or her theory is truth, exists in such a situation. A patient can be treated to some extent as an object given over to the techniques and skills of a therapist, but clarification of the patient's sense of self-existence cannot be anticipated. However, if the therapist completely discards all specialized superiority, that it, therapeutic authoritativeness, and places himself or herself together with the patient in a predetermined community setting as another human being seeking self-existence, this approach exceeds the general framework of psychotherapy.

How, then, should a therapist behave? What part should he play to make therapy most useful to patients who are in a median position, halfway between the condition of being shackled by fear and anxiety and the condition of aiming for true freedom by self-control of the resistance that springs from the factor of self-subsistence?

Perhaps the question should be: What is the true goal of therapy? The goal of a patient in seeking therapy is the elimination of anxiety and pain, and for this purpose the patient makes a decision to permit the therapist to penetrate deeply into his or her mind, albeit reluctantly, but the therapist must have something that is helpful to respond to the patient effectively.

This condition is true therapeutic authoritativeness. It is not pretended dignity or pressure, nor is it a miraculous power. It is a superior form of intelligence and abundant human nature. This condition is what Fromm means by the authoritativeness of anonymity. Deep thinking and correct discrimination by a therapist are possible in this condition, and both the limits of therapy and the true goal can be discerned. In this sense, therapeutic authoritativeness can truly respond to the request of a patient; in other words, capability as a specialist is a necessity. It is not authoritarian in being authoritative.

Even for patients who criticize and resist their therapists' instructions, such resistance is a hidden subjectiveness based on *sei no yokubō* (in Morita therapy). A therapist can exert efforts to carry out treatment in a manner that becomes a motive for drawing out "the desire to live" into the open, but only because the therapist has the capability for responding to this desire. This authoritative character is something that can be called rational authority (Fromm).

By contrast, if there is no resistance, and a patient desires to integrate himself or herself completely with the authoritativeness of a therapist, a kind of faithful adoration results and therapy is interrupted. Faithful adoration is a response to the absolute authority adopted by the founder of a religious sect, but this attitude is utterly unnecessary in psychotherapy. It is similar to irrational authority (Fromm).

Some criticisms of directive methods that are still heard on frequent occasions will be examined. For example: "It is generally difficult for most patients to resist attempts to impose direction at a place of authority, and this is due to the fact that, from the patient's point of view, the psychotherapist appears to be a symbol of authority." Also: "Once the psychotherapist takes an authoritative attitude, the patient cannot be expected to comply with it, even if the attitude is later changed." And: "Most people generally feel unpleasant in the face of direction backed by authority."

What is the actual status of the therapist-patient relationship in Morita therapy? As has been mentioned, Kelman[9, 10] says that the Japanese readily accept directives from Morita therapists because they have a tendency to demonstrate obedience to authority willingly; however, it is difficult to conduct Morita therapy in the United States because the attitude of American patients toward authority is different. It may be true that this tendency is inherent in the Japanese but, as has been mentioned, patients indicate an attitude of accepting assistance from therapists, on the one hand, but, on the other hand, desire to recover with their own strength

---

[9] Kelman, H.: Eastern influences on psychoanalytic thinking. *Psychologia* 2:2 (1959).

[10] Kelman, H.: Psychotherapy in the Far East. *Progress in Psychotherapy* 4:296 (1959).

while opposing therapy. Although the expression of this resistance by patients differs in various ways, Morita therapists frequently encounter this resistance.

This phenomenon is no recent discovery, being readily apparent during Morita's lifetime. The Japanese are not completely obedient and do not depend on authority in all instances. Also, it is not the characteristic phenomenon of indicating resistance toward authority, particularly in the instance of contemporary young people, who have become accustomed to a horizontal sense of ideological values in human relationships.

Human beings have individuality by nature, and they indicate resistance with anxiety and with unpleasantness to heteronomous control directed toward something that they do not desire or cannot foresee. Morita therapists mollify such resistance and assist in the adjustment of a patient's internal order by exercising therapeutic authoritativeness in a rational manner. This assistance cannot be provided by direction and persuasion alone.

In response to such resistance by patients toward therapy, Morita explained to them that the determination of a patient who receives therapy is similar to the mental attitude of a researcher starting an unknown experiment. The patient has made an important decision to undergo therapy, although he or she initially feels anxiety and has misgivings in facing the therapist and following instructions. Consequently, the only thing the patient can do is to undergo therapy obediently with an attitude of obedience. The patient needs only to accept realistically the subsequent progress and make his or her own judgment.

The feeling of starting an experiment is complex, with anxiety and anticipation intermixed, and therapy is similar in this regard. If a patient has to obey what a therapist says without anxiety or distrust, this condition is simply blind obedience. It must therefore be understood that the submissiveness (in appearance) of a patient receiving Morita therapy differs from a desire for self-prostration, as claimed by the psychoanalytical school of thought.

However, the rational advice given in Morita therapy can appear to be authoritative from a standpoint in which the horizon of thinking differs. For example, Levy[11] mentions that patients receiving Morita therapy are brought to consider the value of constructive efforts for recovery of human nature. The position of the therapist, who advises and guides efforts for improving the patients' daily lives, is rational. Even then, there is something that makes a patient consider Morita therapy as being a compulsory, authoritative method of treatment.

From the author's point of view, however, most such deep-rooted, disapproving criticisms of therapeutic authoritativeness are due to the coercive, negative image that the word "authority" suggests, as the symbol of a continuing human struggle to resist all forms of authority. The criticisms advanced by investigators who strongly reject all directive methods of therapy, based on a premise that seeks to connect nondirective methods with democratic ideology, consist of an emotional prejudice and are not rationally supportable. The notion that therapeutic authoritativeness is nondemocratic is substantially different from the criticism of the therapy. There are cases in which a directive method is also used in psychoanalytical technique, and even if such a method is not used, the interpretations and explanations made by the therapist are still based on therapeutic authoritativeness, in other words, anonymous authority.

By participating in the absolute, isolated bed rest and work periods with the guidance of a Morita therapist, a patient confronts the basic problems of his or her condition independently, even if this situation seems experimental, and eventually the experience of accepting the condition causes a process of comprehension and insight to take place, which is not due simply to direction and persuasion by the authoritative pressure of the therapist but which the patient understands. Consequently, the basis of therapy is the ability to judge correctly the therapeutic condition, which a therapist changes in various ways throughout the therapist-patient relation-

---

[11] Levy, N. J.: Discussion on Morita therapy. *International Journal of Psychiatry* 1(4) (1965).

ship, irrespective of whether it is by a directive or nondirective method. The real problem here is the professional qualifications of the therapist.

27

Professional Qualifications of Morita Therapists

At first, education and training of therapists to carry out Morita therapy were provided directly by Shōma Morita. The students of Morita, through their practice, trained subsequent therapists. There has been no basic change in this system to date.[1,2] This so-called handed-down approach is a personal one. Therapists are placed in situations that are readily subject to such factors as depth of experience and character, even therapists who are involved in clinical psychiatry. Psychotherapy is based on clinical psychiatry. Its direct objective is training and strengthening of the ego, but the final result of this process is the liberation of patients who are captivated by mental suffering and weakness of character.

This liberation, in turn, leads the patients to self-discovery and self-realization, which are the roots of human existence.

In other words, clinical psychiatry delves, at length, into the fundamental elements of human nature. Psychotherapy reaches the ramparts of philosophy, buttressed by the clinical supports of psychiatry and psychology. Jaspers[3] remarks that psychotherapy confronts the facts of situations that extend to the outer limits of therapeutic efforts and incorporates the datum of the individual as-is (*Sosein*), and such therapy inevitably touches on the problem of a world view. This problem is neither psychological nor medical, but a subject that can be dealt with only through the faith and fundamental philosophical attitude that envelopes therapist and patient alike.

Two attitudes that are important to therapists can be considered within this context. One is the attitude of observing patients from the standpoint of psychiatric experience and exercising judgment that is adaptable. This attitude is put into practice by accurately grasping the situation within the range that therapy can attain. The other attitude is that of close association with a patient as two persons bound up in a fateful, cooperative unit, encouraging the patient to achieve the freedom in which one seeks to form one's life as a genuine human being. A therapist placed in that position is engaged in existential communication on the same level as the patient and does not function as a therapeutic technician.

Because psychotherapy is carried out by such intimate communication, therapists must take into thorough consideration the prospect that some sort of mental effect will be engendered, irrespective of whether or not patients desire it.

The personality of a therapist becomes the motive power for the curative process in psychotherapy. In general, affection, sensibility and apperception are the common prerequi-

---

[1] Nomura, A.: Morita ryōhō ka ikusei no jōken (Conditions of training of psychotherapists in Morita therapy) (in Japanese). *Japanese Journal of Psychiatry* 3(2) (1977).

[2] Ōhara, K.: Morita ryōhō ka no shikaku (Qualifications of the psychotherapist in Morita therapy) (in Japanese). *Ima ni Ikiru* 32 (1969).

[3] Jaspers, K.: *Allgemeine Psychopathologie* (1948). Translated by Y. Uchimura et al. Iwanami Shoten, Tokyo (1958).

sites of the temperament of therapists, especially Morita therapists. In addition, therapists must be thoroughly trained to have a personality rich in useful content.

Present Training and Considerations for the Future Training of Morita Therapists

Systematic education and training have not been provided to Morita therapists. Rather, training has been accomplished by a handed-down approach on a one-to-one basis and within a limited scope. This condition will be described more concretely to furnish information for a discussion of the future training of Morita therapists.

The need for systematic education and training of Morita therapists became a subject for discussion during the latter half of the 1960s. The reasons that this need has not been addressed are not clear, although the following possibilities can be surmised.

A relatively large number of the students who later became Morita therapists were strongly influenced by Shōma Morita or had received instruction in the psychiatric department of the university in which Morita was a professor. They had received treatment from Morita or his immediate successors. A program for the systematic training of therapists to replace the handed-down approach has been discussed as the number of potential students has continued to increase. Nonetheless, contemporary education and training are still supervised in much the same way by Morita's successors.

Education and training of other therapists in Japan has been for the most part almost identical to the education and training of Morita therapists, in that they have not been carried out systematically. However, education and training of psychoanalytical therapists have been more systematic in regard to instruction in theory. Educational analysis and supervision have often been more systematic. These systems have become important as special processes required to establish a professional identity, in training of nonphysician therapists.

The legal system in Japan specifies that medical therapy must be carried out by a physician. In truth, however, the situation is that similar functions are carried out by nonphysicians in the form of consultation with patients by nondirective methods. This situation leads to difficulties, however, because licensing for practice of nonphysicians is not legally granted, even to those who are the most specialized therapists.

With respect to the qualifications and training of Morita therapists, students who have received training in general medicine go on to specialize in psychiatry and receive training on the premise that a therapist must be a physician. They acquire an elementary knowledge of psychopathology and of general psychotherapy, in addition to practical training at a psychiatric clinic from a resident instructor.

Instruction in the theory and technique of Morita therapy is carried out within the scope of transmission that is possible in any such progression of study and training. However, to acquire competence as a genuine therapist, teaching by the instructor must be supplemented by therapeutic experience encountered in one-to-one relationships with patients. Such experience, of course, has an important role in training, and together with acceptance of the specialized authoritative stance of an instructor and his or her temperament, the characteristics of a student therapist, which differ from those of Morita and his successors, will tend to emerge.

It is not possible to eliminate a person as being unqualified as a therapist because there is no system in Morita training to control the qualifications of therapists. There have been problems regarding the suitability of the technique, ability or temperament of student therapists. For example, there have been students who identified excessively with Morita or his successors, indicating an overly sympathetic attitude toward their patients' complaints, strongly manifesting, albeit unconsciously, their temperament or transmitting to patients a wastefully authoritative impression by acting like the head of a religious sect.

If any such attitude appears during the therapeutic process, it is not a desirable phenomenon, at least from the perspective of patients, and the suitability of therapists who have such attitudes must be questioned. However, this problem is overlooked as long as a therapist does not become aware of it. When a therapist is aware of having such an attitude, it becomes a problem for him or her as well as a matter of concern to all Morita therapists. For such therapists to continue to have suitable relationships with their patients, they need to exercise self-illumination (including therapeutic retrospection).

This process is, of course, one that is inherent in psychotherapy, and it is continued by the desirable situation of a therapist and patient exercising mutual influence. In this respect, therapists must always be aware of that human being called oneself and the actions of that self, always casting illumination on oneself.

Therapists who cannot help themselves cannot give genuine assistance to their patients. The therapeutic goal of a patient is one that should not be avoided by a therapist.

The self-realization of *arugamama* is the objective of Morita therapy, but this *arugamama* is a natural condition of the mind, and its acceptance is true human freedom, closely related to self-realization. Therapists are no exception. Human beings are imperfect, subject to uncertainty and instability. No human being can negate his or her ontological anxiety. A condition of complete emotional stability is not possible.

Patients tend to suppose erroneously that even reactions of authentic human nature, which crop up in life, are something undesirable and abnormal (contradictoriness in thinking). It is this emotional instability that leads patients to demand that therapy must produce stability. This demand arises from nonacceptance of *arugamama*, that is, the facts of human nature, but therapists not only need to have intellectual acceptance of *arugamama* but also must have experienced this state of mind. If therapists have not had such an experience, they will attempt to provide instruction to their patients simply from their own store of abstract knowledge. Only the impression of an authoritative compulsion will remain, and an attitude of true acceptance on the part of a patient will not appear.

The human mind is ever-changing, or fluid; it does not follow a fixed path according to a fixed form. Because human beings do have options, one can feel cast out into an unknown future and thus be anxious. Consequently, therapists also must seek emotional stability in the development of their lives and, likewise, must look forward to self-realization. The acceptance of *arugamama* means that the attitude of an anxious mind is characteristic of the mind itself. This characteristic applies to patients and therapists alike, and this is why therapeutic assistance to relieve a patient's suffering is possible.

Acceptance of *arugamama* in terms of the human, emotional anxiety that therapists and patients alike suffer is the basis of constructive power in the therapeutic process, as mentioned by Fromm-Reichmann.[4]

---

[4] Fromm-Reichmann, F.: Personality of psychotherapist and the doctor-patient relationship (1952). In *Seishin Ryōhō no Riron to Jissai* (Theory and Practice of Psychotherapy), edited by K. Okonogi. Igaku-Shoin, Tokyo (1964). (Printed in Japanese)

Is Therapy in Training a Necessity for Morita Therapists?

The proposition that a therapist who has not achieved self-illumination cannot properly illuminate a patient[5] is unquestionably a governing principle of Morita therapy. Is therapy in training, as is customary for psychoanalytical therapists, necessary for Morita therapists?

A correct reply to this question is possible only when a therapist places himself or herself in the position of a patient who is about to receive therapy. The therapist will then grasp the patient's distrust and dissatisfaction toward the *fumon* (disregard of symptoms; see Chapter 17) that he or she exercises or the skepticism and sense of resistance experienced by the patient, who is expected to obey his or her instructions for absolute bed rest and work therapy.

Why is it, then, that systematic training of therapists to understand the position of their patients or to know themselves thoroughly through continual self-illumination has not been carried out for Morita therapists?

It is believed that the reasons lie in the method by which Morita therapy is practiced and in the mode of training to date.

Morita therapy differs from psychoanalysis in being a therapy that is almost always conducted in a hospital setting. Moreover, Morita therapists live with their patients in most cases. As a result, Morita student therapists do receive characteristic training.

One pertinent episode is related to Morita's creation of the therapy that bears his name. Morita took into his home a patient with an obsession who had symptoms of anxiety that had been difficult to cure, made her rest in bed without direction, left her in that tedious condition and observed the course of the disorder. He directed his attention during this time to changes in the patient's attitude of practical orientation, changes that were unintentional. He later incorporated the process of change into his therapy as an inevitable phenomenon.

Morita then continued to deduce therapeutic principles by accumulating therapeutic experience from living with his patients. That clinical experience gave rise to his recognition that patients suffering from *shinkeishitsu* are not sick persons but, rather, human beings in a condition of normality stretched to the limit, and thereby increased his understanding and observation of patients. Morita's successors began to accumulate experience basically similar to Morita's, and followed Morita's policy of giving instruction that has genuine meaning for the patient and therapist alike.[6]

This practical and strict training method was handed down for training of therapists after Morita's death, but this approach to education and training does have advantages and disadvantages, which will now be addressed.

• Student therapists have numerous opportunities for self-study by means of human contact; self-study should lead to self-discovery and a concomitant discovery of the most important characteristics of human beings in general. The basic attitude in psychotherapy of extending a helping hand from one human being to another is induced in that training context and is bereft

---

[5] Jaspers, K.; ibid.

[6] Morita gathered together patients who had been discharged from clinical treatment and patients who were still receiving treatment (in the work therapy stage) to carry out periodic group counseling. Morita Keigai-kai physicians who wished to become therapists attended the sessions. Morita provided this counseling not only for the patients but also for the therapists as a form of practical training in their education. He also provided guidance by responding to the entries in patients' diaries and by giving concrete instruction in practical work so that his patients could concentrate on constructive living. This guidance, again, was beneficial not only for the treatment of his patients but for the training of student therapists as well.

of human contempt. Each human being has a "root anxiety" of some sort about human life and, at the same time, questions the meaning of life and takes on the true character of aiming for constructive living to fulfill his or her potential.

• A desirable situation is developed through personal communication between the instructor and the student, centered around patients, in the practice of Morita therapy. Nonetheless, there have been cases in which student therapists have identified with the instructor (Morita and his successors) and have acquired an image of a therapist that is confined to a specific form. If that happens, the subjecthood of a student is not manifested as a therapist. Also, with Morita therapy codified and regulated by Morita and his successors, and with instruction undertaken with this as the nucleus forming an orientation of a world view, it is possible that group activity will resemble the birth of a religious sect of some sort. Group activities can obstruct the true development of Morita therapy. There is a clear need for Morita therapists to monitor closely any such activity, to maintain a distinct line between therapy and sectarian religious activities.

The human relationship that exists between Morita therapists and their patients is undoubtedly one of personal communication, but it is not a form of communication of "total personality," as in the case of the "absolute" factor in a religious sect. A nonpersonal character of personality, which is the requisite technique in Morita therapy, must always be active.

When the need for training of Morita therapists is considered, the temperament of a therapist remains as a factor that is not closely related to the rules of systematic criteria, even if acquisition of technique is carried out rationally within certain limits or even if qualification by technical proficiency can be considered objectively in systematic training. This personality factor is not negative, as long as training is not carried out on a one-to-one basis, as was customary in the past.

The mode of thought acquired by therapists who receive one-to-one training is generally rationalistic and intellectual. Although such therapists are easy to approach, as a rule, they are readily inclined toward technical conduct in the practice of therapy. What is most important in the practice of Morita therapy is the personality of a therapist. Therapists who must deal with problems of human life, as is true of Morita therapists, must have the true mental health of constantly striving for self-illumination, volitionally rather than intellectually, to truly act out their role as therapists by working to relieve the suffering of human life together with their patients.

If systematic training of therapists would harm the true personal value factor of therapists, which can be said to be the decisive factor in practice, the author believes that continuation of a nonsystematic training method is unavoidable.

In the author's attempt to respond to numerous criticisms and unrealized expectations of Morita therapy in the Western world, he has perhaps been more self-justifying than self-critical. The reason is that many criticisms are based on misunderstanding rather than on insufficient understanding, if the author understands these criticisms correctly. In the end, the author has tried to impart an accurate understanding of Morita therapy and sincerely hopes that this effort will be beneficial to general psychotherapy in the future.

Reynolds's *Morita Psychotherapy* (1976) was published about 50 years after Morita therapy was developed, and that book was a milestone for communicating Morita therapy to countries outside Japan. The author hopes his effort will be considered in the same light.

The current popularization of Morita therapy confers the feeling of a new world by comparison with the situation that existed while Morita was alive. However, the author is keenly aware, nevertheless, that the future will present many more challenges of communication that must be faced squarely and, with a proper amount of determination, dealt with and resolved to the satisfaction of all concerned.

Postscript

It has been a rather reckless venture for this author to attempt to produce a book on Morita therapy in the English language. Nevertheless, the book, at long last, has been finished. This is due to several significant persons who stepped in to help me step past the "language barrier"; in particular, Mr. William E. Dyne, who assisted with rewriting of the original manuscript, and Mr. N. Maya and Mr. M. Fujino for their invaluable editorial expertise.

If it had not been for their help, it is doubtful that this book could have reached the publication stage. Behind that, however, was my personal determination to fulfill Shōma Morita's original ambition to publish his complete system of Morita therapy in book form for international dissemination. Only in that way, he was sure, could Morita therapy be further developed for clinical development and application outside the national borders of Japan.

The plan for publication of this book was first proposed to me by the publisher in 1969. Quite frankly, I felt it was a rather precipitate idea at that time, but later noted strong interest in Morita therapy emerging rapidly in various fields, both at home and abroad.

The late Professor Morita did intend to introduce his system of therapy worldwide, for critical evaluation. Unfortunately, he died before he had a chance to do so. In that light, I decided to accept the publisher's proposal, because I did wish to present Morita therapy correctly and to have it put into practice by therapists in other parts of the world.

The greatest obstacle I faced, of course, was the language barrier–in terms of precise definition and elucidation of Morita therapy concepts and practices, native to Japan, in a foreign (English) language.

This struggle with linguistic precision and expression is one of the reasons why the complete preparation and publication of this book have taken more than a decade. I thought of giving it up any number of times, but rallied again and again to the challenge, thanks to the full understanding and constant encouragement of those most concerned.

I wish to state clearly that *Shinkeishitsu no Hontai oyobi Ryōhō* (The Substance of *Shinkeishitsu* and Its Therapy) is the original book on Morita therapy and the nucleus of my own exposition, but expanded by my own comprehension of Morita therapy and my clinical experience over the years.

I regret that the case histories and literature (both in reference and quoted) which I cite are dated mostly prior to 1980, because of the decade or so that has passed while this book was in preparation. I have, however, endeavored to include more up-to-date data in footnotes to each page.

The true value of this book rests wholly on its basic presentation of Morita therapy, which remains valid in both principle and clinical practice to the present day. I am fully responsible, of course, for any flaws, omissions, distortions or oversights that my own exposition may contain, in the difficult transition from the original Japanese to this foreign-language edition.

I do hope, however, that the book will serve its principal purpose: to bring Morita therapy, in principle and clinical application, into universal use for treatment of *shinkeishitsu* patients.

During the long period of time that this book was still in preparation stages, a number of notable developments have taken place in popularizing and further disseminating Morita therapy.

One such development is broader clinical application by group studies devoted to the principles of Morita therapy. Another is the founding of the Association of Morita Therapy. The third meeting of this Association, under the auspices of the Jikei University School of Medicine, was held on November 8, 9, 1985, shortly before this book went to press.

The first of these two developments is most remarkable as the starting point of a new training concept embodied in the so-called *Seikatsu no Hakken Kai* (Society for Life Discovery) whose board chairman is Mr. Y. Hasegawa. The first session of this group's studies activity took place 15 years ago.

Even before that, some 28 years ago, the first issue of the *Hakken Kai* magazine was published. The month of April,1985, marked publication of the 300th issue. This headquarters group now has affiliate branch groups in about 80 different locations throughout Japan. *Hakken Kai* training sessions are directed toward the goal of each member's achieving a full understanding of authentic human nature and a concomitant realization of personal growth.

In the United States, apart from Japan, Mr. David K. Reynolds has successfully applied Morita therapy in clinical treatment regimes.

He emphasizes, as a now characteristic feature of American-type Morita therapy, the broad use of principles which can be applied to most people, not only to those with the Morita *shinkei-shitsu* persona.

In all events, these life training movements that feature broad application of Morita therapy methods are emerging increasingly inside and outside Japan. This is a most gratifying development in the estimation of Morita therapists, provided that widespread applications of Morita therapy's principles are firmly based on a precise comprehension of the fundamentals of Morita therapy as such. It is hoped that this present book can make a certain contribution to that end.

November, 1985
Tokyo

Chihiro Fujita

Name Index

Subject Index